Closing the Gap

CLOSING THE GAP:
The Burden of Unnecessary Illness
Documentation and Intervention Strategies resulting from the
Health Policy Consultation of the Carter Center of Emory University,
November 26–28, 1984, Atlanta, Georgia

Co-Chairs
Former President Jimmy Carter
Edward N. Brandt, Jr., M.D., Ph.D.
Assistant Secretary for Health

Project Director
William H. Foege, M.D., M.P.H.
Editors: Robert W. Amler, M.D.
H. Bruce Dull, M.D.
Managing Editor: Daphna W. Gregg

Planning Committee:
Robert W. Amler, M.D.
Andree Carriere
Donald L. Eddins
Annemarie Kasper
Craig C. White, M.D.

Project Officers:
Nancy N. Fajman, M.P.H.
Erica Franks, M.P.H.
William H. Herman, M.D.
Daniel Horth, M.P.H.
Thomas K. Welty, M.D., M.P.H.
Craig C. White, M.D.

Health Policy Task Force:
Donald O. Nutter, M.D., Chair
Paul B. Hoffman
Richard M. Levinson, Ph.D.
James W. Phillips
Douglas C. Rundle, D.D.S.
Thomas F. Sellers, M.D.
W. Douglas Skelton, M.D.

Editorial Staff:
E. W. Barringer
Martha E. Hagan
Jerelyn H. Jordan
Anne D. Mather
Marie S. Morgan
Barbara B. Reitt

Conference Support:
Mary Ellen Cates
Shirley Gambrell
Julia Fuller
Betsy R. Morgan
Freida R. Quarles
Angela Tucker
Pamela Willoughby

EMORY UNIVERSITY
James T. Laney, President

THE CARTER CENTER OF EMORY UNIVERSITY
Jimmy Carter

Executive Director
William H. Foege

Deputy Executive Director
William C. Watson, Jr.

Fellows:
Harold Berman (Soviet Studies, Human Rights)
Linda Brady (Arms Control)
Thomas Buergenthal (International Law)
Karl Deutsch (International Relations)
William H. Foege (International Health)
Ellen Mickiewicz (Arms Control)
Robert Pastor (Latin America)
Dayle E. Powell (Conflict Resolution)
Kenneth W. Stein (Middle East)

Past Executive Directors:
James L. Waits, 1982–1984
Kenneth W. Stein, 1984–1986
Dayle E. Powell, 1986 Acting

ME: Healthy Policy Consultation (1984 : Atlanta, Ga.)

Closing the Gap):
The Burden of Unnecessary Illness

Edited by
Robert W. Amler
H. Bruce Dull

Oxford University Press   New York, Oxford 1987

Library of Congress Cataloging-in-Publication Data

Health Policy Consultation (1984: Atlanta, Ga.)
    Closing the gap.

    "Documentation and intervention strategies resulting from the Health
Policy Consultation of the Carter Center of Emory University, November
26–28, 1984, Atlanta, Georgia"—P. facing t.p.
    Includes index.
    1. Medicine, Preventive—United States—Congresses. 2. Public
health—United States—Congresses. 3. Health behavior—United States
—Congresses. I. Amler, Robert W. (Robert William) II. Dull, H. Bruce.
III. Emory University. Carter Center. IV. Title. [DNLM: 1. Health
Promotion—congresses. 2. Preventive
Medicine—congresses. WA 108 H434c 1984]
    RA445.H343   1984   362.1'0973   87-24829
    ISBN 0-19-505483-0

THE
CARTER CENTER
OF EMORY UNIVERSITY

April 1987

Greetings,

I am delighted to introduce to you one of the fine products of The Carter Center's early years -- the final report of a consultation entitled "Closing the Gap", held here in November 1984. This consultation focused on what Americans can do as individuals and as a nation to improve their health.

When The Carter Center was established in 1981, I hoped that through it I could use my experience to further the search for solutions to problems on the national and international agenda. I believe that a first step towards solving most problems is to inform Americans more thoroughly. We want to make informed choices, yet can do so only when all the facts are presented to us clearly and without bias.

This is particularly true for an issue as complex as health. Too often, Americans are confronted by messages about health that leave us with little or no hope. If smoking doesn't kill us, then alcohol, cancer and cholesterol lie in wait. Frequently, there is no mention made of what I as an individual, or what we as a society, can do to arrest this relentless onslaught on our health.

The purpose of the consultation, and of this final report, is to clear up some of the confusion that abounds, and to highlight the steps we can take. By gathering together the nation's foremost experts on public health in a single meeting, we have tried to look at the major risks to good health in the U.S. today, to place them in their proper perspective, and then outline the preventive actions that could result in fewer deaths, saved dollars, improved health and quality of life, and greater productivity. The results were heartening. Approximately two-thirds of all reported deaths can be delayed, which means that 1.2 million lives and 8.4 million years of life can be preserved each year.

I am committed to helping search for solutions to the problems faced by Americans. The publication of "Closing the Gap" is a promising step in that direction. I hope you think so too.

Jimmy Carter

THE CARTER PRESIDENTIAL CENTER, INC. · ONE COPENHILL · ATLANTA, GEORGIA 30307
(404) 522·8900 · TELEX ITT 493·0231 CARTR

Foreword

Closing the Gap. What a marvelous expression, especially when that can be translated into decreased suffering, decreased disability, and a markedly improved quality of life. The gap is clearly documented in this volume. Far too many people suffer pain, loss of function, or premature loss of life from preventable causes. The gap can be closed. Sometimes, relatively simple steps are required such as getting people to wear seatbelts, not drink while driving, and continue to take their prescribed medication. In other instances, more complex steps are required as is true when we consider homicide and suicide.

This book includes the proceedings of a conference held in November 1984, at the Carter Center in Atlanta, Georgia. The material included details clearly the nature of the problems *and* steps to solve them. All of this material tells one major story: the gap is real, but it can be narrowed and, in many instances, closed *if* each of us adopts a prevention ethic. If we are willing to change our behavior and to assist others in changing theirs, it is possible to decrease unnecessary suffering, disability, and premature death as well as decrease both the direct and indirect costs of poor health. Clearly, the most important benefit is an improved quality of life, with all of the joy that such brings.

The contents of this book are important. It is critical that each of us as individuals and all of us as a society learn this information and, more importantly, implement those steps necessary for closing the gap.

Edward N. Brandt, Jr., M.D., Ph.D.
Assistant Secretary for Health
April 1987

Preface

The Health Policy initiatives of The Carter Center of Emory University are becoming increasingly well-known. Those who practice and teach Preventive Medicine have taken particular note of the Center's emphasis on prevention and have been especially supportive of its pragmatic, practical approaches. Asking questions like, "What can we already do to prevent unnecessary deaths and disability, and how can we get on with it?" is important both for domestic and international health policy-making.

All of us associated with the American Journal of Preventive Medicine are pleased to publish, as the initial supplement to the Journal, the full documentation of a Health Policy Consultation of the Carter Center, Closing the Gap: The Burden of Unnecessary Illness. The consultation in November 1984 was, in fact, only one part of an ambitious five-year health project. The objective of the research, planning, and implementation phases of the project is to highlight missed opportunities for preventing premature deaths and unnecessary disability in the United States using prevention strategies already in hand.

About a decade ago, in the mid-1970s, a somewhat analogous survey was made of the scientific knowledge and skills available to preventive medicine. Eight separate task forces were appointed, sponsored by the Fogarty International Center, National Institutes of Health, and the American College of Preventive Medicine. After more than a year of comprehensive analysis of the field, a National Conference on Preventive Medicine was held in Washington, in June 1975. The Task Force reports represented the efforts of more than 300 specialists and had the endorsement of national health organizations and professional societies. The reports became the basis for the prevention theme of The Forward Plan for Health, 1976–1980, prepared by the Department of Health, Education, and Welfare. They were also published separately in 1976 with the title, *Preventive Medicine USA* (Prodist, New York, 1976).

Like its 1975 predecessor, *Closing the Gap* is an exceedingly valuable statement of contemporary knowledge, skills, and concepts with which to prevent premature death and unnecessary disability.

In choosing to publish documentation of *Closing the Gap* in 1987, nearly three years after the investigative reports and recommendations were prepared, questions of timeliness arise. However, they seem relatively unimportant in contrast to the considerable scope, depth, and inherant professional value of the material. Because the scientific reports are collaborations of experts and were reviewed in detail by specialists in each field represented, additional scientific review has not been done. Undoubtedly some facts and perceptions will have changed, but to have tried to update or re-verify such a comprehensive series of interrelated documents would have jeopardized the integrity of the project and risked producing a far less coherant result.

The reader will find in this publication a vivid summary of the current status of preventability, preventive medicine, public health, and proposed prevention strategies for the United States. It is sure to be relevant for some time to come. We can justifiably express our appreciation to the many persons who organized and managed *Closing the Gap* and to those who prepared and edited its extensive documentation.

H. Bruce Dull, M.D.
Associate Editor, AJPM
April 1987

Contents

Contributors

Deborah C. Abels, M.B.A.
Emory University School of Medicine
Atlanta

M. J. Adams, Jr., M.D.
Center for Environmental Health
Centers for Disease Control, Atlanta

Susan S. Addiss, M.P.H.
President, American Public Health Association
Chief, Bureau of Health Planning and Resource Allocation
Connecticut State Department of Health, Hartford

James Alley, M.D.
Georgia Department of Human Resource
Division of Public Health, Atlanta

Robert W. Amler, M.D., M.M.S.
Medical Epidemiologist
Office of the Director
Centers for Disease Control, Atlanta

Susan P. Baker, M.P.H.
Professor
Department of Health Policy and Management
Johns Hopkins School of Hygiene and Public Health, Baltimore

John V. Bennett, M.D.
Assistant Director for Medical Science
Office of the Director
Center for Infectious Diseases
Centers for Disease Control, Atlanta

Donald A. Berreth
Centers for Disease Control
Director
Office of Public Affairs
Centers for Disease Control, Atlanta

Edward N. Brandt, Jr., M.D., Ph.D.
Assistant Secretary for Health, Washington

Alfred W. Brann, Jr., M.D.
Director
World Health Organization Collaborating Center for Perinatal
Care and Health Services Research in Maternal and Child
Health, Atlanta

Lester Breslow, M.D., M.P.H.
Co-director
Division of Cancer Control
Jonnson Comprehensive Cancer Center
University of California, Los Angeles

William F. Bridgers, M.D.
President, Association of Schools of Public Health
Dean

School of Public Health
University of Alabama, Birmingham

Arnold Brown, M.D.
President, Association of American Medical Colleges
Dean
University of Wisconsin Medical School, Madison

Thomas E. Bryant, M.D., J.D.
Public Committee for Mental Health, Washington

James W. Buehler, M.D.
Division of Reproductive Health
Centers for Disease Control, Atlanta

William Burnett, M.D.
Bureau of Chronic Diseases Prevention
New York State Department of Health, Albany

Judith M. Conn, M.S.
Statistician
Violence Epidemiology Branch
Center for Health Promotion and Education
Centers for Disease Control, Atlanta

Glenna M. Crooks, Ph.D.
Deputy Assistant Secretary for Health, Washington

Sherry Deren, Ph.D.
New York State Division of Substance Abuse,
Albany

Don C. Des Jarlais, Ph.D.
New York State Division of Substance Abuse,
Albany

Theodore C. Doege, M.D.
American Medical Association
Director
Department of Environmental, Public, and Occupational Health
American Medical Association, Chicago

Donald L. Eddins
Chief, Data Management Branch
Division of Immunization
Center for Prevention Services
Centers for Disease Control, Atlanta

Nancy N. Fajman, M.M.Sc., M.P.H.
Master of Public Health Program
Department of Community Health
Emory University School of Medicine, Atlanta

Henry Falk, M.D., M.P.H.
Director
Division of Environmental Health Hazards Evaluation
Centers for Disease Control, Atlanta

Laurence S. Farer, M.D., M.P.H.
Director
Division of Tuberculosis Control
Center for Prevention Services
Centers for Disease Control, Atlanta

William R. Felts, Jr., M.D.
Professor of Medicine
George Washington University
School of Medicine, Washington

William H. Foege, M.D., M.P.H.
Project Director: *Closing the Gap*
Assistant Surgeon General
Special Assistant for Policy Development
Centers for Disease Control, Atlanta

Erica Frank, M.P.H.
Master of Public Health Program
Department of Community Health
Emory University School of Medicine, Atlanta

Richard Frank, Ph.D.
Assistant Professor of Psychiatry and Economics
University of Pittsburgh, Pittsburgh

Michael E. Fritz, D.D.S., Ph.D.
Dean
Charles Howard Candler Professor of Peridontology
Emory University School of Dentistry, Atlanta

Eugene J. Gangarosa, M.D.
Professor and Director
Master of Public Health Program
Department of Community Health
Emory University School of Medicine, Atlanta

Kristine Gebbie, R.N.
President, Association of State and Territorial Health Officers
Administrator
Oregon Department of Human Resources, Portland

Linda S. Geiss, M.A.
Division of Diabetes Control
Center for Prevention Services
Centers for Disease Control, Atlanta

Richard J. Gelles, Ph.D.
Dean
Faculty of Arts and Sciences
University of Rhode Island, Providence

Paul J. Goldstein, Ph.D.
Principal Investigator
Narcotic and Drug Research, Inc., New York

Mary N. Haan
Human Population Laboratory
California Public Health Foundation, Berkeley

M. Alfred Haynes, M.D.
President, American College of Preventive Medicine
Dean
Charles R. Drew Postgraduate
School of Medicine, Los Angeles

Suzanne G. Haynes, Ph.D.
Research Associate Professor of Epidemiology
School of Public Health
University of North Carolina, Chapel Hill

Nancy A. Hedemark, M.P.H.
Graduate Research Assistant
Master of Public Health Program
Department of Community Health
Emory University School of Medicine, Atlanta

William H. Herman, M.D.
EIS Officer
Division of Diabetes Control
Center for Prevention Services
Centers for Disease Control, Atlanta

Marc C. Hochberg, M.D., M.P.H.
Director
Statistical Core Unit
Johns Hopkins Multipurpose Arthritis Center, Baltimore

Paul C. Holinger, M.D., M.P.H.
Department of Psychiatry
Michael Reese Hospital
Rush-Presbyterian-St. Luke Medical Center, Chicago

Scott D. Holmberg, M.D.
Medical Epidemiologist
Division of Bacterial Diseases
Center for Infectious Diseases
Centers for Disease Control, Atlanta

Cathy L. Holt, B.S.N.
Emory University School of Medicine
Atlanta

Dan Horth, M.P.H.
Master of Public Health Program
Department of Community Health
Emory University School of Medicine, Atlanta

Dana Hunt, Ph.D.
Principal Investigator
Narcotic and Drug Research, Inc., New York

Richard S. Johannes, M.D.
Assistant Professor of Medicine
Johns Hopkins University School of Medicine, Baltimore

Stephen N. Kahane, M.D.
Department of Medicine
Johns Hopkins University School of Medicine, Baltimore

Mark Kamlet, Ph.D.
Assistant Professor of Social Sciences
Carnegie-Mellon University

George A. Kaplan
Human Population Laboratory
State of California Department of Health Services, Berkeley

Trudy A. Karlson, Ph.D.
Center for Health Systems and Analysis
University of Wisconsin, Madison

Luella M. Klein, M.D.
President, American College of Obstetrics and Gynecology
Emory University School of Medicine, Atlanta

Jeffrey P. Koplan, M.D.
Assistant Director for Public Health Practice
Centers for Disease Control, Atlanta

John Kurata, M.D.
Assistant Professor of Medicine
Center for Ulcer Research
Veterans Administration Wadsworth

Reva C. Lawrence, M.P.H.
Arthritis Epidemiology & Data Systems Program Officer
National Institutes of Health, Bethesda

Michael R. Lavoie, M.A.
Georgia Department of Human Resources
Atlanta

Brian J. McCarthy, M.D.
Division of Reproductive Health
Centers for Disease Control, Atlanta

Frederic C. McDuffie, M.D.
Senior Vice President for Medical Affairs
Arthritis Foundation
Professor of Medicine
Emory University School of Medicine, Atlanta

Daniel P. McGee, Jr.
Programmer
Center for Health Promotion and Education
Centers for Disease Control, Atlanta

Albert I. Mendeloff, M.D.
Professor of Medicine
Senior Associate, Epidemiology
Johns Hopkins University School of Medicine, Baltimore

Meredith Minkler
Department of Social and Administrative Health Services
University of California, Berkeley

Jaromir Mikl, M.P.H.
Research Assistant
New York State Department of Health, Albany

Marilyn Miszcynski
Program in Epidemiology
University of California, Berkeley

Kenneth Mitchell, Ph.D.
Director
Rehabilitation Division
Ohio Industrial Commission
Ohio State University

Morey S. Moreland, M.D.
Head, Section of Pediatric Orthopedics
University of Vermont College of Medicine, Burlington

Philip C. Nasca, Ph.D.
Director

Cancer Control Section
New York State Department of Health, Albany

Donald O. Nutter, M.D.
Professor of Medicine
Emory University School of Medicine, Atlanta

Godfrey P. Oakley, M.D.
Center for Environmental Health
Centers for Disease Control, Atlanta

Barbara Reynolds, B.A.
Bureau of Chronic Diseases Prevention
New York State Department of Health, Albany

Frederick C. Robbins, M.D.
President, Institute of Medicine
National Academy of Sciences, Washington

Martha F. Rogers, M.D.
Medical Epidemiologist
AIDS Activity, Office of the Director
Center for Infectious Disease
Centers for Disease Control, Atlanta

Mark L. Rosenberg, M.D., M.P.P.
Chief, Violence Epidemiology Branch
Center for Health Promotion and Education
Centers for Disease Control, Atlanta

Harold P. Roth, M.D.
Director
Division of Digestive Diseases and Nutrition
National Institutes of Health, Bethesda

Richard Rothenberg, M.D., M.P.H.
Director
Bureau of Chronic Diseases Prevention
New York State Department of Health, Albany

Douglas C. Rundle, D.M.D., M.P.H., M.S.
Assistant Dean for Advanced Education
Emory University School of Dentistry, Atlanta

Carl W. Schieffelbein
Public Health Advisor
Division of Tuberculosis Control
Center for Prevention Services
Centers for Disease Control, Atlanta

Lawrence E. Shulman, M.D., Ph.D.
Director
Division of Arthritis, Musculoskeletal and Skin Diseases
National Institutes of Health, Bethesda

Gordon S. Smith, M.B., Ch.B., M.P.H.
Medical Epidemiologist
Injury Epidemiology and Control
Center for Environmental Health
Centers for Disease Control, Atlanta

Martin Smith, M.D.
President-elect, American Academy of Pediatrics
Gainesville, Georgia

Steven L. Solomon, M.D.
Medical Epidemiologist
Hospital Infections Program
Center for Infectious Diseases
Centers for Disease Control, Atlanta

Evan Stark, Ph.D.
Department of Public Administration
Rutgers University, New Brunswick

Jesse Steinfeld, M.D.
Former U.S. Surgeon General
President
Medical College of Georgia, Augusta

Alan Stoudemire, M.D.
Assistant Professor of Psychiatry
Emory University School of Medicine, Atlanta

S. Leonard Syme
Program in Epidemiology
University of California, Berkeley

Steven M. Teutsch, M.D., M.P.H.
Acting Chief
Technology and Operational Research Branch
Divison of Diabetes Control
Center for Prevention Services
Centers for Disease Control, Atlanta

Dennis D. Tolsma, M.P.H.
Director
Center for Health Promotion and Education
Centers for Disease Control, Atlanta

Lawrence Wallack, Dr. P.H.
Scientific Director
Prevention Research Center
University of California, Berkeley

Kenneth E. Warner, Ph.D.
Professor and Chairman
Department of Health Planning and Administration
University of Michigan, Ann Arbor

Thomas K. Welty, M.D., M.P.H.
Medical Epidemiologist
Chronic Diseases Division
Center for Environmental Health
Centers for Disease Control, Atlanta

Craig C. White, M.D.
EIS Officer
Behavioral Epidemiology and Evaluation Branch
Division of Health Education
Center for Health Promotion and Education
Centers for Disease Control, Atlanta

Lynn S. Wilcox, M.D.
Georgia Department of Human Resources
Atlanta

Margaret A. Zahn, Ph.D.
Professor of Sociology
Temple University, Philadelphia

Susan Zaro, M.P.H.
Georgia Department of Human Resources
Atlanta

Closing the Gap

Introduction and Methods

William H. Foege, M.D., and Robert W. Amler, M.D.

Closing the Gap seeks to focus national health policy on the burden of unnecessary illness, i.e., the "gap" between the current burden of health problems and the lesser burden that is achievable with knowledge already at hand.

To catalog such knowledge, consultants from various medical specialties were commissioned to investigate the burden imposed on the nation by cancer, heart disease, diabetes, and 12 other priority health problems. Each consultant convened an expert panel to oversee the investigation. Their findings were summarized and discussed at a national consultation on health policy held at Emory University, Atlanta, November 26–28, 1984. The consultation was attended by national leaders from private, public, voluntary, and academic institutions and was co-chaired by former President Jimmy Carter and Edward N. Brandt, Jr., M.D., then Assistant Secretary for Health, U.S. Department of Health and Human Services.

BACKGROUND

The Carter Center was founded in 1982 as an integral part of Emory University by former President Jimmy Carter and his wife, Rosalynn Carter. Their intent was to foster, in a strictly nonpartisan environment, scholarly and operational research on major global and domestic problems. The health field was identified as a priority from the beginning, along with arms control, conflict resolution, Middle East diplomacy, and Latin American studies. To ensure nonpartisanship, all substantive initiatives of the Carter Center have included, as key participants, officials from other administrations, both current and former.

Shortly after the Carter Center was established, a Health Policy Task Force was established to identify domestic problems in the health field. The principal problem identified was the gap between the observed burden to the nation of major diseases and conditions and the lesser burden that could be achieved, given full implementation of existing technical knowledge. Thus, the project was entitled *Closing the Gap*.

DESIGN CONSIDERATIONS

Usually, health policy studies focus on a specific health problem or a range of related problems and suggest interventions that address those specific problems. However, the purpose of *Closing the Gap* was to compare diverse precursors associated with health problems, using a standard set of measures for comparison for all the health problems. The project was intended to identify cross-sectional intervention strategies that addressed generic risk factors, or precursors, for several health problems, otherwise unrelated.

The project was also designed with a view toward sharing these methods with health officials in developing countries who wished to undertake a similar endeavor. In principle, any nation or community could benefit from a carefully designed analysis of major preventable precursors of health problems, whether long-standing and recognized (such as infection or malnutrition) or new and emerging (such as injuries caused by tobacco or motor vehicles). This desire for international comparisons influenced the choice of certain data classes. For example, the age of 65 was chosen as the end point for computing potential years of life lost. Although the growing life expectancy for North American adults might suggest that the age of 75 or even 85 be used for such computation, the use of the age 65 preserved the option for worldwide comparisons as well as the ability to underscore major killers of young people.

CHARGE TO CONSULTANTS

As the project began, each consultant convened an expert panel to investigate the assigned specialty area in terms of the health burden and potential interventions already known to be available:

Definition of the health problem(s). Each panel was asked to define the broad health problem (e.g.,

From the Carter Center of Emory University (Foege) and the Centers for Disease Control (Amler), Atlanta.

Address reprints requests to Dr. Amler, Centers for Disease Control, Atlanta, GA 30333.

cancer), to select the highest-priority specific problems (e.g., lung cancer, breast cancer), and to briefly describe the salient clinical manifestations of problems.

Documentation of health impact. Each panel was asked to use the suggested data classes to document the overall health impact and social burden of the problems selected, as described in Data Classes and Sources, below.

Description of risk factors and known interventions. Each panel was asked to describe primary, secondary, and tertiary preventive measures already known or available. Primary interventions aim to reduce or eliminate new cases and include such measures as immunization and smoking cessation. Secondary interventions are intended to diagnose and treat problems at their earliest manifestation, and include, for example, mammography and blood pressure screening. Tertiary interventions, when health problems cannot be prevented or promptly addressed, may limit disability or fatal complications, generally through optimal clinical management, such as for diabetes mellitus.

Potential benefit attributed to each intervention. Each panel was asked to quantify the potential benefit of each intervention in terms of attributable lives saved, hospitalizations averted, productivity preserved, and years of potential life gained.

DATA CLASSES AND SOURCES

Major data classes and definitions were established and reviewed by consultants at the beginning of the project (Table 1). These data classes were used to construct mock tables that were distributed to the consultants as they began to work. To enhance comparability, 1980 was used as a reference year. Consultants were encouraged either to report 1980 data or to adjust data from other years to 1980.

In the interest of time and efficiency, consultants also were encouraged to use existing data for the most recent years available, rather than to collect new data. The project staff offered consultants direct access to data sources maintained by federal agencies such as the National Center for Health Statistics (NCHS), the Centers for Disease Control (CDC), and the National Institutes of Health (NIH). Many consultants used these sources; several already had their own surveillance data or system.

In many cases, the most useful data sets were derived from the large national surveys conducted by the NCHS, especially the Health Interview Survey (HIS), the Hospital Discharge Survey (HDS), the National Ambulatory Medical Care Survey (NAMCS), and the Health and Nutrition Examina-

Table 1. Data classes requested of consultants

Health outcome	Requested data class
Mortality	Number of deaths
	Crude mortality rate
	Age-adjusted (to 1980) mortality rate
	Age-group-specific mortality rates
	Years of potential life lost before the age of 65
Morbidity	Incidence rate
	Annual period prevalence rate
	Days of hospital care
	Hospitalizations
	Physician visits
	Days lost from work or major activity
Complications	Blindness
	Paralysis
	Amputation
Direct costs	Hospital care (short-stay facilities)
	Physician and other professional care
	Pharmaceuticals
	Special equipment
	Long-term institutional care
Quality of life	Individual (disability, missed opportunity for education, training, employment)
	Family (transportation to health facility, financial and mental burden)
	Society (greater dependency, reduced productivity, financial burden)

tion Surveys (HANES-I, HANES-II). However, several large states contributed additional data from tumor registries and other sources. Population data from the 1980 United States Census and mortality data from coded death certificates (available from NCHS) also were used extensively.

SELECTION OF PRIORITY RISK FACTORS

A preliminary consultation for *Closing the Gap* was hosted by former President Jimmy Carter in Atlanta, August 27–29, 1984. Early findings from studies of the impact of selected major health problems in the U.S. were presented to a panel of health policy consultants (Table 2), along with the preliminary summary of a cross-sectional analysis of precursors. The purpose of this preliminary con-

Table 2. Members of preliminary consultation panel, August 27–29, 1984

Susan S. Addiss, American Public Health Association
Donald A. Berreth, Centers for Disease Control
William F. Bridgers, Association of Schools of Public Health
Arnold Brown, American Association of Medical Colleges
Glenna M. Crooks, U.S. Department of Health and Human Services
Theodore C. Doege, American Medical Association
Eugene J. Gangarosa, Emory University School of Medicine
Kristine Gebbie, Association of State & Territorial Health Officers
M. Alfred Haynes, American College of Preventive Medicine
Jeffrey P. Koplan, Centers for Disease Control
Donald O. Nutter, Emory University School of Medicine
Frederick C. Robbins, Institute of Medicine
Kenneth E. Warner, University of Michigan

Table 3. Eighteen generic precursors initially listed, August 1984

Tobacco
High blood pressure
Overnutrition
Gaps in screening
Alcohol
Injury
Gaps in clinical management
Gaps in primary prevention
Occupational hazards
Gaps in health education
Handguns
Unintended pregnancy
Substance abuse
Depression
Infant mortality
Dental problems
Chronic diseases
Violence

sultation was to assign priorities to generic precursors and interventions, to consider possible negative consequences of such interventions, and to select six intervention areas for further discussion at the principal consultation in November.

PANEL FINDINGS

Panel members listed all generic precursors suggested by the consultants' reports and by the cross-sectional analysis (see "Precursors of Premature Death in the United States"). Additional problems were identified that related to quality of life, such as sociodemographics and chronic illness, and they were added to the list by panel members. After lengthy discussion, a total of 18 generic precursors was listed (Table 3). These were ranked high, middle, and low priority by each member, considering the negative impact, the availability of interventions, and the likelihood of successful intervention.

The composite ranks were used to reduce the list to the nine highest-ranked precursors. Two, tobacco and alcohol, were unanimously ranked high (Table 4). The panel was asked to review the nine precursors and add any other important precursors that had been omitted or not ranked high enough. One such precursor was unintended pregnancy, including unwanted and mistimed pregnancy and accounting for 55 percent of all pregnancies. This precursor seemed especially important, considering its documented impact on infant mortality and its uncounted but probable contribution to social problems, suicide, domestic violence, and homicide.

The panel was then asked to consider specific intervention strategies that addressed the listed generic precursors and whether the Carter Center might be in an appropriate position to intervene. The precursors were ranked as high, middle, or low priority for the Carter Center. Four precursors were ranked high: alcohol, tobacco, injury, and unintended pregnancy (Table 5). Three additional precursors were ranked just below the top four: overnutrition (including obesity and high total serum cholesterol levels), handguns, and dental problems.

The panel recommended that the Carter Center use its unique orientation—part academic, part governmental, part voluntary—to encourage cooperation on a national scale to help close the gap. In addition, generic health problems, such as gaps in preventive care and mental health issues (violence, depression, and substance abuse), were later added to the final list.

ANALYSIS AND INTERVENTION STRATEGIES

The 15 chapters in this section contain the consultants' quantitative estimates of health risks presented in November 1984. These findings represent many months of intensive work and have been compiled with great care. In most cases, additional data, besides those published herein, have been compiled within the complete consultation report to the Carter Center. Persons wishing to examine these data should contact the consultants or write to: Presidential Materials Project, The Carter Presidential Center, One Copenhill, Atlanta, GA 30307.

Table 4. Nine priority precursors, August 1984

Tobacco
Alcohol
Overnutrition
Injury
Unintended pregnancy/infant mortality
Handguns
High blood pressure
Violence
Dental problems

Table 5. Highest-priority precursors, August 1984

Tobacco
Alcohol
Injury
Unintended pregnancy

Gaps in primary prevention[a]
Violence, depression, substance abuse[a]

[a] Added afterwards.

Following the general documentation is a cross-sectional analysis of the consultants' findings, ''Precursors of Premature Death in the United States.'' Considerable efforts were made in the course of that analysis to ensure comparability of data from different consultants. Nevertheless, it is important to note that the 15 consultants developed their estimates independently. Some of the consultants used different data sources and different assumptions. Thus, the cross-sectional findings drawn from these comparisons are imperfect but, we believe, numerically singular and valid for ranking precursors.

Following the reports on generic precursors are intervention strategies outlined by six working groups assigned to review the 15 consultants' reports and the cross-sectional analysis in November 1984. Each was chaired by a recognized leader in health policy. The working groups examined current intervention efforts at the national, local, community, and individual levels and, wherever possible, identified impediments to further progress and ways to surmount them.

Finally, each working group report contains a national agenda of opportunities for further intervention, as well as specific strategies that might be pursued at the Carter Center.

Documentation

Alcohol Dependence and Abuse

Alan Stoudemire, M.D., Lawrence Wallack, D.P.H.,
and Nancy Hedemark, B.S., M.P.H.

Alcohol abuse/dependence, defined strictly by diagnostic criteria, affects approximately 5 percent of the adult American population. According to less rigid criteria, 10 percent of the population are estimated to be problem drinkers. Almost 20,000 deaths a year are directly attributable to medically related alcohol problems, 24,000 deaths are caused by motor vehicle crashes in which alcohol played a role, and 30,000 deaths a year result from miscellaneous alcohol-related mishaps, such as falls, fires, and suicides. In addition, almost 300,000 disabilities result per year from alcohol use.

Alcohol abuse/dependence has emerged as a leading contributor to a plethora of health problems, including falls, burns, mental illness, injuries in motor vehicle crashes, gastrointestinal diseases, fetal alcohol syndrome, cardiomyopathy, suicide, and certain cancers. A comprehensive and concerted effort is obviously needed to decrease the far-reaching negative impact that alcohol-related disorders have on the American public.

Definition of terms. We refer to alcohol abuse/dependence as defined by the American Psychiatric Association.[1] *Alcohol abuse* refers to a pattern of pathological use of alcohol that results in impaired social or occupational functioning for at least one month. Symptoms of *alcohol dependence* include tolerance (the need for increased amounts of alcohol to achieve the desired effect or a diminished effect with regular use of the same amount) and withdrawal (the "shakes" or malaise, which are relieved by drinking after a period of cessation of or reduction in drinking).

Examples of pathological patterns include the need to use alcohol daily; the inability to cut down or stop drinking; repeated efforts to control or reduce excess drinking; binges (remaining intoxicated for a period of at least two days); drinking of nonbeverage alcohol; and amnesic periods (blackouts) while intoxicated. Impairments in social or occupational functioning because of alcohol use include violence while intoxicated, absence from work, loss of job, legal problems resulting from arrests for intoxicated behavior or traffic crashes while intoxicated, and unstable relationships with family and/or friends.

CAUSES OF ALCOHOL ABUSE/DEPENDENCE

The exact etiology of alcohol abuse/dependence is unknown but probably involves an interaction of multiple factors. Environmental and cultural factors influence how alcohol is made available and in what quantities and under what circumstances it is consumed. Cultural norms clearly influence social patterns of alcohol use. For example, epidemiologic studies have shown trends suggesting that the American, French, and Irish populations have relatively higher rates of alcoholism and alcohol-related morbidity and mortality than do Chinese, Japanese, and Jewish populations.[2] When drinking is absolutely forbidden, as in Islamic cultures, the chances of alcohol-related incidents are small. In other cultures, drinking may be practiced only in rituals (usually religious) or ceremonies, or on special occasions. Rates of alcoholism are highest in societies where people are allowed to drink for personal reasons, for example, to relax or to forget problems. Within the individual family setting, drinking habits are likely to be influenced by a child's exposure to the drinking behavior of parents and other role models.[3]

Even though most people in the United States are exposed to alcohol, only a relatively small percentage drink excessively or develop chemical de-

From the Emory University School of Medicine (Stoudemire) and School of Public Health (Hedemark), Atlanta, and the University of California, Berkeley (Wallack).

Address reprint requests to Dr. Stoudemire, Emory University Clinic, 1365 Clifton Road, Atlanta, GA 30322.

The prevention recommendations of the American Assembly for the Western Region on Public Policies Affecting Alcoholism and Alcohol-Related Problems, entitled "Bold New Initiatives in Alcohol Policy" held October 3–6, 1985, at the Mt. Alverno Center in Redwood City, California, were used as a resource for this paper. The final report of the American Bar Association's Advisory Commission on Alcohol and Drug Abuse was also used as a resource for prevention recommendations.

pendency. It has therefore long been accepted that alcoholism runs in families and that a strong genetic component influences vulnerability to the disorder. The lifetime risk for alcoholism in the sons of alcoholics exceeds the risk for males in the general population (20–30 percent versus 5–10 percent).[4-6] Genetic studies have shown that concordance rates for the development of alcoholism are as high as 54 percent in monozygotic twins and 28 percent in dizygotic twins.[5] In studies of children adopted away from alcoholic parents within the first several months of life, the risk for alcoholism developing in the children of alcoholics is four times that in adopted children of nonalcoholics.[7-9]

Enzymatic and neurotransmitter factors may play an underlying role at the biochemical level in the development of alcohol dependence. There are at least 15 isoenzyme fractions for alcohol dehydrogenase, which metabolizes alcohol to acetaldehyde, and four other forms of aldehyde dehydrogenase, which breaks down aldehyde to acetate.[5] Different ethnic groups show differential patterns in the activity of these enzymes. Enzymes involved in neurotransmitter metabolism, such as monoamine oxidase and dopamine beta hydroxylase, have also been shown to differ in activity in alcoholics as compared with nonalcoholics; no consistent trends, however, have been found.[10-12]

Taken together, both genetic and biochemical studies suggest that biogenetic factors may predispose certain individuals to alcoholism. As with other psychiatric disorders, underlying biological vulnerabilities may interact with family and environmental factors to cause the syndrome of alcoholism. Further refinements in genetic and biological markers for identifying susceptible individuals may provide methods for screening and case detection. The potential of genetic and biological markers for intervention at the present time remains speculative.

EPIDEMIOLOGY

Mortality. In 1980, 19,751 deaths were caused by illnesses directly attributed to alcohol use; 24,000 deaths (approximately 45 percent of total fatalities) occurred in motor vehicle crashes attributable to alcohol misuse;[13] and 31,914 deaths were indirectly attributable to alcoholism (falls, fires, homicide, suicide).[14] These figures represent a total of 75,665 deaths from alcohol abuse/dependence in 1980.

Morbidity. Only six-month prevalence rates for alcohol abuse/dependence are available; 7,521,338 cases among men and 1,439,627 cases among women (Table 1).[15] However, numerous studies using more liberal criteria have estimated that

Table 1. Alcohol dependence and abuse in men and women: Age-specific morbidity, United States, 1980

Age	6-month prevalence rates per 100,000 population	
	Men	Women
18–23	10.7	3.5
24–34	12.7	2.1
35–54	7.7	1.0
55–65+	3.4	0.1
Total rate	9.7	1.7
Total number of cases	7,521,338	1,439,627
Total number, both sexes	8,960,965	

Extrapolated from NIMH/ECA data by the Centers for Disease Control.[15]

"problem drinking" occurs in approximately 10 percent of the adult population. (Problem drinking includes acute and episodic difficulties associated with alcohol.) The facts indicating that approximately 5 percent of the population abuse alcohol or are dependent on it are conservative, as the survey misses many people characterized by occasional problem drinking.

A remarkable disparity exists between the number of men and the number of women who are categorized as alcohol abusers (Table 1). The reason for the disparity is still a matter of speculation. The postulation that female alcohol abusers are underreported because they are more likely than men to abuse alcohol in private has not been proved. The reason may be a cultural difference in drinking patterns, since alcohol use by men is often actively encouraged as an acceptable demonstration of "manhood."

Disability. Disability arises predominantly from injuries suffered in motor vehicle crashes. Disability cases may be categorized as follows: complete paralysis, approximately 5,100 cases/year; partial paralysis, 5,000 cases/year; complete loss of extremity, 900 cases/year; partial loss of extremity, 2,400 cases/year; complete disability, 70,000 cases/year; and partial disability, 201,600 cases/year. Disability from mental illness attributable to alcohol abuse affects approximately 2,420 per 100,000.[14]

COSTS

The Research Triangle Institute[14] estimated the total costs of alcoholism at $116.7 billion. The largest proportion (61 percent) is the indirect cost of reduced productivity and lost employment, which totaled 612 billion days in 1980. The next most costly

Table 2. Years of life and years of major activity lost as a result of alcohol abuse, United States, 1980

Specific problem[a]	Years of life lost[b]	Years of major activity lost[c]
Alcohol-induced illnesses	243,263	19,751
Related illnesses	137,907	11,120
Motor vehicle crashes	860,364	24,000
Other trauma	1,898,644	52,961
Total	3,140,178	107,832

From Research Triangle Institute.[14]
[a] Illnesses directly attributable to alcohol include: alcoholic cirrhosis, alcohol psychosis, alcohol polyneuropathy, alcoholic cardiomyopathy, alcoholic gastritis, alcohol dependence syndrome, and acute alcohol toxicity. Related illnesses include pneumonia, tuberculosis, and other disorders linked to generalized alcohol-related debilitation. "Other trauma" includes death from suicide, homicide, and unintentional injuries.
[b] Before age 65.
[c] Major activity is defined as primary occupation (work, housekeeping, school).

category (16 percent) is the imputed cost of alcohol-related mortality. In 1980, 75,665 deaths were *directly* attributable to alcohol, which accounted for 3,140,178 years lost prematurely (before age 65) (Table 2). Medical treatment costs, which are detailed in Table 3, make up 11 percent of the total. The remaining 12 percent of social costs are attributable to research support (1 percent), nonmedical costs of motor vehicle crashes (3 percent), crime related to alcohol abuse (3 percent), incarceration (2 percent), and other (3 percent).

MEDICAL COMPLICATIONS

The health problems resulting from alcohol use include a number of conditions that contribute to the morbidity and mortality more directly associated with illness than with alcoholism. In 1980 chronic liver disease and cirrhosis accounted for 12,938 deaths in the United States.[16] Nutritional deficiencies often result because alcohol disrupts the physiological and metabolic process of digestion.[17] Vitamin and trace element deficiencies among adults in the United States are most often linked to alcohol.[18] In addition, alcohol-induced debilitation often creates a susceptibility to other illnesses. Research has shown a high correlation (20–70 percent) between alcohol abuse/dependence and death from pneumonia or tuberculosis.[19]

Central nervous system impairments often appear in a person who has a history of abusive drinking, and nutritional deficiencies intensify or complicate the problem. One of the most serious impairments is the Wernicke–Korsakoff syndrome (alcohol amnestic disorder).[17] Few people recover completely from this illness, which is manifested by severe amnesia, confabulation, and personality alterations.[20] Structural changes and alterations in the central nervous system resulting from long-term abusive drinking behavior have also been demonstrated. Research on the extent to which alcoholism contributes to brain damage has found that central nervous system dysfunction is present in 50–70 percent of the alcoholic population entering treatment.[21]

An adverse relationship between alcohol consumption and the cardiovascular system has also been demonstrated. Long-term alcohol use is directly related to alcoholic cardiomyopathy, abnormalities in cardiac rhythm, and hypertension.

Included among the mental disorders associated with alcohol use is alcohol psychosis, which accounted for 454 deaths in 1980.[16] Delirium tremens is characterized by profound confusion; visual, auditory, tactile, and olfactory hallucinations; psychomotor overactivity; insomnia; fever; hyperhydrosis; and a coarse tremor. Acute alcoholic hallucinosis is characterized by auditory and visual hallucinations. Alcoholic hallucinosis also includes the mispercep-

Table 3. Direct costs of alcohol abuse, United States, 1980

Services	Costs (millions of dollars)			
	Specific illnesses	Related illnesses	Related trauma	Total
Hospitals	2,727	1,532	822	5,081
Community mental health centers	181	0	0	181
Halfway houses	54	0	0	54
Freestanding, correctional and other facilities	428	0	0	428
Physican visits	61	291	373	725
Assistance of other health professionals	144	104	39	287
Nursing homes	105	0	62	167
Pharmaceutical	327	249	173	749
Total	4,027	2,176	1,469	7,672

From Research Triangle Institute.[14]

tion or misinterpretation of environmental stimuli.[17]

Research is under way to determine the exact means by which alcohol exerts carcinogenic effects. Heavy drinkers are known to be at relatively higher risk than either moderate drinkers or nondrinkers for cancers of the tongue, mouth, oropharynx, hypopharynx, esophagus, larynx, and liver.[17] Combined, these sites represent 6.1–9.1 percent of the sites of all cancers in the white population and 11.3–12.5 percent in the black population in the United States.

Research has been undertaken in recent years to determine the effects of alcohol on pregnant women and fetal development. Studies have shown that pregnant women who drink, even moderately (four to five drinks per week), run a five times greater risk of having spontaneous abortions or low-birth-weight infants.[22] Fetal alcohol syndrome (FAS) is a problem that occurs in infants born to women who are alcohol abusers. The incidence is 1–2 per 1,000 live births, and a partial expression of FAS occurs in 3–5 per 1,000 live births. Signs of FAS include central nervous system dysfunction, including mental retardation, microcephaly, poor motor coordination, and hyperactivity in childhood; low birth weight and short body length; facial abnormalities; and malformation of organ systems, including cardiac, urogenital, and skeletal abnormalities.[23]

Mental depression may result from or be exacerbated by excessive drinking.[24] Although the exact role that alcohol plays in suicide is uncertain, it is known that persons who commit suicide are likely to have been dependent on or abusers of alcohol.[17] According to studies of autopsy reports, an estimated 25–37 percent of suicides involved alcohol use.[25] Kendall has delineated several variables that probably contribute to the suicide relationship. Alcohol use can result in the decline or breakup of a marriage and the loss of friends and job. The isolation resulting from the breakdown of social systems can predispose a person to suicide; the loss of self-esteem and resulting depression can predispose one to suicide; the interaction of alcohol with other drugs may be lethal; and alcohol may produce irresponsible behavior in a person who is not normally irresponsible.[25]

Mortality indirectly attributed to alcohol includes motor vehicle crashes, falls, and fires. Alcohol was implicated in approximately 45 percent (24,000) of all fatalities resulting from motor vehicle crashes in 1980.[13] Because of the effects that alcohol has on coordination and judgment, it also follows that drinkers are more likely than the general population to be involved in industrial accidents.

EFFECTS ON THE FAMILY

The potentially destructive effects of alcohol use on the family include violence, divorce, economic stress, and negative role models for the children.[26,27] In addition to the more dramatic and immediate effects the drinker has on the family, research has indicated that the longer-term effects on the family are subtle and obscure. Through their systematic research, Steinglass and his colleagues[28,29] found that a family attempts to adapt its behavior to the behavior of the drinking member so that the family structure will remain relatively stable.

Variables that might distinguish "binge" drinkers from "steady" drinkers in their relationships with their families have been studied. Jacob et al.[30] found that, as opposed to steady drinkers, binge drinkers generally drank away from home. Binge drinkers also exhibited greater levels of overall psychopathology than did steady drinkers. The binge drinkers experienced more adverse social consequences, such as involvement in fights, inability to keep a job, neglected family obligations, and more arrests for drunken behavior. Both groups had problems maintaining a marriage and friendships, and both groups experienced problems on the job.

POPULATIONS AT RISK

Some populations are at higher risk of becoming alcoholics or of having tendencies toward alcohol abuse or dependence. Individuals who have first-degree relatives with alcoholism are at greater risk, and genetic and possible biochemical factors were noted earlier.

Groups that commonly undergo periods of stress related to changes or shifts in lifestyle appear to be at higher risk for alcoholism. These groups include military personnel (whose drinking behavior is often rewarded by peers) and the unemployed (whose feelings of hopelessness and loss of self-esteem compound the problem). Drinking is often seen as a coping technique in stressful situations.

Certain work groups have also traditionally had high levels of alcohol consumption and problems related to alcohol use. Employees who have access to free or inexpensive alcohol, such as bartenders or brewery workers, are among this group,[31] as are members of certain trades, such as longshoremen and construction workers.

Teenagers and young adults are among the highest-risk populations. In 1977 the leading cause of mortality among persons aged 15–24 was motor vehicle crashes, accounting for 37 percent of all deaths.[31] Furthermore, this young population is approximately 2½ times as likely as the average driver to be involved in crashes in which alcohol is implicated.[13] In 1980, 43 percent of automobile crashes in which the driver was drinking alcohol occurred among drivers in the age range 16–24 years.[16]

PREVENTION EFFORTS

Efforts toward primary prevention of alcohol abuse/dependence have involved an array of programs aimed at specific segments of the population, but none of these programs has been proven to offer any conclusive long-term benefit. For example, the objectives of most alcohol education programs in the schools and through the media have been to develop a sense of responsibility toward alcohol consumption. It is assumed but not proven that increased knowledge about alcohol consumption and its consequences will result in responsible drinking behavior.[32]

Several assumptions underlie prevention messages about alcohol abuse, including the assumption that the media offer an effective mechanism for changing behavior and that the public's increased knowledge will lead to a change in attitudes and in behavior.[33] Television, radio, and print campaigns have been sponsored by agencies such as the National Council on Alcoholism, the National Safety Council, the National Highway Traffic Safety Administration, various insurance agencies, and private voluntary agencies. These campaigns emphasize the problems associated with drinking and driving and the other negative personal and social consequences of drinking.[33] The alcohol industry itself has been active in public information activities. Its messages tend to promote responsible drinking and knowing and respecting one's drinking limits.[34]

Primary prevention efforts undertaken through more specific segments of the population have also been studied. The role of bartenders, for example, has been examined for potential effectiveness in preventing alcohol abuse and related problems. Waring and Sperr[35] concluded that bartenders would be appropriate candidates for alcohol education aimed at reducing the harmful consequences of alcohol to customers. Through standardized interviews, they found that the majority of bartenders studied not only used discretion when dealing with customers who presented problems as a result of their drinking behavior but would be willing to take alcohol education courses.

Public information has been coupled with community outreach programs to address problems in specific high-risk populations. One such project sponsored by the National Institute on Alcohol Abuse and Alcoholism—the fetal alcohol syndrome

prevention project in California[36]—is geared toward women of childbearing age. It includes a combination of media campaigns, printed materials, and contacts (through presentations and seminars) with various groups throughout the target community. The effectiveness of the program has not yet been assessed. A similar program in Washington State takes a more integrated and comprehensive approach.[37] Components of the program include public education through the media and the training of professionals who provide prenatal care. The public health component encourages women of childbearing age to adopt health-enhancing behavior.

INTERVENTIONS

Most prevention efforts are geared to the individual or to specific high-risk populations. However, this strategy tends to ignore the cultural environment and social milieu that tolerate drinking and subsequent alcohol-related problems. Kinder et al.[38] reviewed alcohol education programs to determine their effectiveness on the target audiences. For the most part, they found that the programs, which were geared to both student and adult populations, made little or no impact. These findings are not surprising if we recognize that there is little support in our society for campaigns to prevent alcohol abuse.

A systems approach to prevention would view alcoholism as a problem that derives from many economic, social, and cultural factors and would intervene in all of these interacting systems—marketing and economics, cultural values, and social norms. No single intervention policy can solve society's problems with alcoholism, but all such initiatives, taken together, can help us move closer toward achieving the healthiest possible use of alcohol in our society. Such an ideal would be based on the following norms: (1) moderate consumption in low-risk situations is accepted, (2) any consumption in high-risk situations is actively discouraged, (3) abstinence is accepted, (4) heavy consumption in any situation is actively discouraged, and (5) safety and health protection mechanisms that apply to the entire population (e.g., drunk driving laws, seat belts, air bags) are a high priority.

The interventions we would recommend to facilitate these patterns of alcohol use are discussed below, along the lines of public policy initiatives.

Education. Comprehensive educational approaches that mobilize and coordinate multiple community resources including families, schools, churches, volunteer associations, sports clubs, industry, business management, social and professional organizations, and local media should be undertaken. Prevention programs should also focus on legislators, health care providers, school supervisors, principals, and teachers. While the general public may be the major target audience, specific groups should receive special attention.

For students, educational programs should begin by age 12, before children enter the teenage years when exposure to peer group pressure regarding alcohol use intensifies. Education on the potential risks of alcohol use and misuse is probably not sufficient in itself, since, as noted earlier, the long-term success of "educational" programs per se has not been proven. Particularly for the preteen and teenage population, interventions must focus on specific social skills that enable teenagers to resist peer pressure for the use of alcohol. The use of favorable role models for teenage alcohol prevention programs, such as popular musicians and television entertainers, may be an important component of intervention efforts at this level. Driver education should heavily emphasize the dangers and risks of drinking and driving.

Educational efforts should also be directed at the level of educators and professionals. Local and state Boards of Education should be encouraged to integrate formal, structured alcohol prevention programs into the curricula for students prior to the sixth grade, including social skills training to resist peer group pressure as noted above. With respect to professional groups, education, law, medical, and seminary schools should place a high priority on alcohol prevention education with implementation of formal curricula in this regard.

Specific educational warning programs for prospective and expectant mothers should be conducted both through the media and in the medical sector as well.

Warning labels. All alcoholic beverage containers and packaging should have mandatory labeling that: (1) discloses alcohol content, (2) discloses all other ingredients, including additives and preservatives, and (3) carries rotating health warnings on the potential dangers of alcohol (i.e., can be addicting, impairs driving ability, should not be used in conjunction with sedatives or tranquilizers, and is hazardous to unborn children). The primary regulatory authority over the content, labeling, and advertising should be vested with the Food and Drug Administration.

Increase price through tax policy. The real price of alcohol has declined significantly over the past quarter century. Since 1960 the real price of distilled spirits has declined 48 percent, beer 27 percent, and wine 20 percent. The federal excise tax on alcohol has not been increased since the Korean War. (Congress has recently approved a measure that slightly increases the excise tax on distilled spirits.)

Current tax policy has resulted in the decline in the real price of alcohol, which at least partially contributes to increased problems with alcohol. Furthermore, the low price suggests that by allowing alcoholic beverages to compete in price with soft drinks, alcohol is an acceptable alternative in any situation in which soft drinks are used.

Raising taxes on alcohol should be highly attractive to state governments. Enormous revenues have been lost because the excise tax on alcohol has not been indexed to inflation. The state of California, for example, has lost an estimated $189,000,000 since 1960 by not having the state alcohol tax indexed to inflation.

To reverse this trend, we recommend the following: (1) significantly increase the excise tax on beer, wine, and distilled spirits, (2) use alcohol content as a tax base, and (3) index the tax rate to the rate of inflation.

The expected effects of these revised tax policies would be a decline in overall consumption and a simultaneous decline in alcohol-related mortality and morbidity, particularly that resulting from cirrhosis and auto crashes. Tax revenue could remain constant with lower consumption at higher tax rates. Revision of the excise tax rate would reinforce the overall message that alcohol is a special product, one to be handled with care.

Remove income tax deductions. Existing policy allows personal income tax deductions for the cost of alcohol purchased for a broad range of loosely defined business purposes. Corporations and businesses are leading purchasers of alcoholic beverages. In 1979 corporate expenditures for alcohol were estimated at $5.6 billion, or 11.9 percent of the total market. All these expenditures are "discounted" by an estimated tax savings of 35 percent. These tax deductions are disproportionately distributed among persons whose incomes are high and those who benefit from corporate expense accounts.

The result of the existing arrangement is that alcohol problems are probably exacerbated by tax-supported incentives to drink. The total loss of tax revenue to the federal treasury is estimated at $3–$5 billion for each of the years 1979–1981. In addition, the federal government directly contributes to a business and corporate culture that supports higher levels of alcohol consumption.

The specific recommendation to reverse this trend is to prohibit tax deductions associated with the use of alcoholic beverages. The expected effects would be to increase the price of alcoholic beverages for businesspeople and to reduce consumption (and thus the associated problems). In addition, the change would generate additional tax revenue from drinking, which would no longer be subsidized through tax policy. Practically and symbolically, the removal of the tax deduction would signal that the public interest is not served by government incentives to drink, that alcohol is not an essential ingredient in business dealings, and that tax policy can be consistent with health policy.

Counteradvertising. Advertising has institutionalized inaccuracy by virtue of the regulatory acceptance of puffery. Although puffery may be acceptable for promoting more innocuous products, it can be dangerously misleading in advertising alcohol.

Alcohol advertising is noted for emotional appeals that are irrelevant to the product; the ads appeal to the viewer's wish to increase self-esteem, identify with wealth, gain greater peer acceptance, and increase sexual prowess. Warnings about the possible personal and public health consequences of alcohol use are never mentioned. A very partial and misleading picture is presented. Further, alcohol advertising has been found not only to increase consumption among adults but also to socialize youth to an alcohol-consuming system.

In 1982 more than $1.1 billion was spent on advertising alcoholic beverages, an increase of 9.2 percent over the previous year. In 1983, $550 million was spent to promote beer and wine on television. These figures do not include the extensive amounts spent to promote alcohol through sports and cultural events. Roughly 35 percent of the $1.1 billion spent on radio, television, newspaper, and magazine ads is tax deductible. The U.S. Treasury thus loses more than $350 million annually and is, in effect, subsidizing a misinformation campaign that runs counter to good public health policy.

Specific interventions to counter the alcohol industry's advertising include: (1) supporting existing legislation in the U.S. House of Representatives to mandate counteradvertising and to make an equivalent amount of broadcast time available for public health and safety messages regarding alcohol effects, (2) including health information in all alcohol advertisements, (3) prohibiting advertising that uses lifestyle themes such as glamour, sexually oriented messages, celebrities, and sports figures, (4) establishing a surcharge on all billings for alcoholic beverage advertising and using the surcharge to fund alcohol-related public education programs, and (5) banning any alcoholic beverage advertising that specifically targets adolescents.

The general effect of modifying and reducing alcohol advertising and changing its content would substantively alter social attitudes about alcohol. The changes would also be likely to increase the credibility of existing programs and public information programs.

Promote server intervention programs and dram shop laws. Most states now have third-party liability, or dram shop laws, which establishes the legal responsibility of those who serve alcohol commercially for the damage caused by an intoxicated patron. In recent years, suits based on dram shop laws have become common, and substantial damages have been awarded. In 1983 a California case was settled for $10.5 million.

The growing corporate and business concern about legal liability, coupled with extensive public attention to drinking and driving, has led to the development and increasing acceptance of server intervention programs. These programs seek to change the commercial setting in which alcohol is served in order to lessen the frequency of heavier drinking. Server intervention has two primary components: the education and training of managers and servers, and the establishment of clear guidelines for liability under state and local laws.

Under the current policy, dram shop liability laws vary from state to state, as does the legal responsibility of the server or the establishment. The lack of a clear policy results in a business-as-usual attitude, which can mean inappropriate serving practices that result in, for example, preventable traffic crashes.

We recommend: (1) implementing a model law that establishes uniform guidelines for responsible serving practices, (2) creating incentives for states to adopt the model law, and (3) creating incentives for all licensed establishments to provide continual training to servers.

Adopting these policies would also help establish a shared responsibility for alcohol problems and provide constructive role models for the drinker. Although overall consumption might not decrease, drinking in high-risk situations would. Perhaps most important, the changes would be a strong statement from the business and general community that excessive drinking is not acceptable.

Promote accurate portrayals of drinking on television. Television is not only a main source of health information, it may well be *the* single most pervasive source. In the past, much of the information presented about alcohol has been inaccurate and misleading. Research in this area has reported that drinking on television far exceeds the reality. Drinking is widespread and condoned; heavier drinking is the norm, often the source of comedy or amusement; and alcohol abuse is rarely disapproved of. Drinking is most often used in response to personal crises, as a social lubricant, or simply as something to do while standing around, a piece of stage business.

Recent observations have indicated that substantial changes in portrayals of alcohol use on television have occurred. Many of the problematic presentations found in previous work have greatly diminished. Nevertheless, despite some excellent television programs about alcohol, the alcohol story remains incomplete and inaccurately told.

Two recent initiatives in this area are notable. The first is the development of cooperative consultation. Developed by a team of social scientists, this process uses research, education, and consultation to work with writers, producers, and directors with the goal of producing more accurate portrayals of alcohol use. The second initiative grew from the first: The Hollywood-based Caucus of Writers, Producers and Directors issued a list of several ways in which members might be inadvertently contributing to alcohol problems. Members were urged to adhere to the suggested do's and don'ts, specifically: (1) promote voluntary compliance with the list of the Caucus of Writers, Producers and Directors, (2) create an independent agency to continue sponsoring cooperative consultation, (3) promote greater awareness of health issues to the National Association of Broadcasters, and (4) promote the development of local committees to work with media professionals on the presentation of alcohol-related issues.

Experience with cooperative consultation thus far indicates that people in the media will be responsive to concerns about alcohol portrayals. As these professionals respond, a greater understanding of the seriousness of alcohol-related problems is likely to spread through the population. This understanding will help form a supportive base for other policies and programs directed toward the prevention of alcohol-related problems.

Promote community involvement. State laws promulgated in the 1930s focused regulatory power at the state level. Although these laws vary considerably from state to state, they seem generally to minimize the role of communities in determining the availability of alcoholic beverages. Recent work suggests that the issue of availability can be at least partly addressed by controlling alcohol distribution outlets through local planning and zoning.

Current policy has resulted in communities that are, for the most part, powerless to control alcohol availability. Local availability has thus increased, with some areas having a high concentration of alcohol outlets. Greater numbers of outlets have been associated with higher levels of consumption and some alcohol-related problems. An excessive number of alcohol outlets in a neighborhood can effectively drive out other businesses.

Some communities are successfully controlling broad practices, for example, by eliminating "happy hours" and similar promotions that emphasize heavier drinking. Another local option is preventing the sale of alcohol in gas stations and convenience stores.

Our recommendations for promoting community involvement include establishing an incentive system that would encourage local authorities to regulate the distribution of alcohol, designing local reviews that involve community residents, and developing partnerships among state agencies that have authority over alcohol issues and the public and private organizations in communities. Specifically: (1) all new and renewed applications for alcohol retail outlets should be subject to environmental impact analysis, public hearings, and zoning regulations, (2) gasoline stations and convenience stores should *not* be licensed for the sale of alcohol, and (3) "happy hour" type promotions that encourage heavier drinking should be prohibited.

Prevention of alcohol-related automobile trauma. The primary focus of these recommendations has been the prevention of alcohol-related problems; however, there are other recommendations for preventing alcohol-related trauma, including (1) mandatory use of seat belts in all states, and (2) mandatory air bags in automobiles produced in 1989 and after.

Evidence also suggests that raising the drinking age to 21 will significantly reduce teenage driving fatalities. For example, although individuals between the ages of 16 and 24 constitute only about 20 percent of the total population and drive only 20 percent of the total vehicle miles in the United States, they are involved in 42 percent of all alcohol-related fatalities.[39] After Michigan raised its minimum drinking age from 18 to 21 in 1978, the figures of alcohol-related automobile deaths in the 18- to 20-year-old age group decreased 31 percent in one year. Similar dramatic reductions have been reported in other states after raising the legal drinking age.[40] Since contiguous states with different drinking ages create significant problems with crossing state lines to purchase alcohol, the age 21 limit should be uniform nationwide.

Other measures recommended to decrease alcohol-related automobile injuries and deaths include: (1) by state and local law, prohibit the consumption or possession of *any* alcoholic beverage in open or unsealed containers in the passenger compartments of motor vehicles, (2) lower the nation-wide blood alcohol content (BAC) for "per se" to .05 gm/dl, and require .00 BAC gm/dl for high-risk groups such as adolescents or those with previous convictions, and (3) provide for administrative revocation of licenses in all per se cases, with the license being surrendered at the scene of the arrest.

SUMMARY

We have put forth a series of policy recommendations that focus on some of the underlying, contributory causes to alcohol-related problems. Each of the areas targeted contributes to the "normalization" of widespread alcohol availability. Normalization means essentially that we accept certain problems as "normal and expected." In this way high levels of alcohol-related damage become institutionalized as given—the price we *must* pay for the pleasures of alcohol. Normalization thus makes it more difficult to raise questions about the appropriateness of existing policies.

Our recommendations have been selected from a range of possible alternatives. Increased attention to safety and consistent public information and education must take place. Our recommendations must serve as part of a comprehensive long-term effort that acknowledges the deeply rooted nature of drinking practices and problems in society. The sum of our proposals would significantly alter the social climate in which alcohol is used. Subsequent programs would benefit from the positive, supportive environment these policies would help establish—the potential result being more effective and efficient program outcomes.

It is important to emphasize that these policies cannot work in isolation. Policies to increase excise taxes or remove tax deductions for consumption and advertising of alcoholic beverages are dependent on the support of a population that is well informed about the health and social welfare benefits of such measures. Server intervention programs are dependent on the support of local communities and positive legal and regulatory guidelines.

For society to adequately address alcohol-related problems, it is necessary to shift attention away from the individual and focus on the system in which the individual acts. This does not suggest that traditional programs be abandoned. On the contrary, innovation in these programs is ongoing. It does suggest that the great imbalance that has characterized prevention efforts, leading to a lack of attention to the broader policy issues, needs to be redressed. Prevention means change, and change entails some sacrifice. If we are serious about re-ducing the enormous social and economic toll associated with alcohol, these policy initiatives will form a starting point for a more equitable distribution of the burden for prevention.

Special thanks to Dr. Alvin Cruze (Research Triangle Institute) for consultation and Mr. Don Eddins (Centers for Disease Control) for statistical assistance.

REFERENCES

1. Diagnostic and statistical manual of mental disorders. 3rd ed. Washington, D.C.: American Psychiatric Association, 1980.

2. Zucker R, Noll R. Precursors and developmental influences on drinking and alcoholism: Etiology from longitudinal perspective. In: Monograph 1: Alcohol consumption and related problems. Alcohol and Health Monograph Series. Rockville, Maryland: National Institute on Alcohol Abuse and Alcoholism, DHHS publication (ADM)82-1190, 1982:289–327.

3. Kinney J, Liton G. Loosening the grip: a handbook of alcohol information, 2nd ed. St. Louis: Mosby, 1983.

4. Schuckit MA. Alcoholic men with no alcoholic first-degree relatives. Am J Psychiatry 1983;140:439–43.

5. Schuckit MA. Trait (and state) markers of a predisposition to psychopathology. In: Cavenar JO, ed. Psychiatry, vol. 3. Philadelphia: Lippincott, 1985:9–11.

6. Cotton N. The familial incidence of alcoholism: A review. J Stud Alcohol 1979;40:89–116.

7. Schuckit MA, Goodwin DA, Winokur GA. A study of alcoholism in half siblings. Am J Psychiatry 1972;128:1132–6.

8. Goodwin DW, Schulsinger F, Møller N, et al. Drinking problems in adopted and nonadopted sons of alcoholics. Arch Gen Psychiatry 1974;31:164–9.

9. Bohman M, Sigvardsson S, Cloninger CR. Maternal inheritance of alcohol abuse. Arch Gen Psychiatry 1981;38:965–9.

10. Schuckit MA, O'Connor DT, Duby J, et al. Dopamine-B-hydroxylase activity levels in men at high risk for alcoholism and controls. Biol Psychiatry 1981;16:1067–75.

11. Schuckit MA, Shaskan E, Duby J, et al. Platelet monoamine oxidase activity in relatives of alcoholics: Preliminary study with matched control subjects. Arch Gen Psychiatry 1982;39:137–40.

12. Sullivan JL, Cavenar JO Jr, Maltbie AA, et al. Familial biochemical and clinical correlates of alcoholics with low platelet monoamine oxidase activity. Biol Psychiatry 1979;14:385–94.

13. National Highway Traffic Safety Administration. Facts of alcohol and highway safety. Washington, D.C.: US Dept of Transportation Office of Alcohol Countermeasures, 1984.

14. Harwood HJ, Napolitano DM, Kristiansen PL, et al. Economic costs to society of alcohol and drug abuse and mental illness—1980. Research Triangle Park, North Car-

olina: Research Triangle Institute, publication no. RTI2734/00-01FR, 1980.

15. Myers JK, Weissman MM, Tischler GL, et al. Six-month prevalence of psychiatric disorders in three communities: 1980–82. Arch Gen Psychiatry 1984;41:959–67.

16. Mortality Detail Data Tape. Hyattsville, Maryland: National Center for Health Statistics, 1980 (unpublished data).

17. Eckardt MJ, Harford TC, Kaelber CT, et al. Health hazards associated with alcohol consumption. JAMA 1981;246:648–66.

18. Leevy CM, Baker H. Vitamins and alcoholism: Introduction. Am J Clin Nutr 1968;21:1325–8.

19. Lyons HA, Saltzman A. Diseases of the respiratory tract in alcoholics. In: Kissin B, Begleiter H, eds. The biology of alcoholism: Clinical pathology, vol. 3. New York: Plenum, 1974;403–34.

20. Victor M, Adams R, Collins R. The Wernicke–Korsakoff syndrome. Philadelphia: Davis, 1971.

21. Lee K, Moller L, Hardt F, et al. Alcohol-induced brain damage and liver damage in young males. Lancet 1979;2:759–61.

22. Ouellette EM, Rosett HL, Rosman NP, et al. Adverse effects on offspring of maternal alcohol abuse during pregnancy. N Engl J Med 1977;297:528–30.

23. Clarren SK, Smith DW. The fetal alcohol syndrome. N Engl J Med 1978;298:1063–7.

24. Petty F, Nasrallah HA. Secondary depression in alcoholism: Implications for future research. Compr Psychiatry 1981;22:587–95.

25. Kendall RE. Alcohol and suicide. Subst Alcohol Actions/Misuse 1983;4:121–7.

26. Tinklenberg JR. Alcohol and violence. In: Fox R, Bourne P, eds. Alcoholism: Progress in research and treatment. New York: Academic Press, 1973.

27. Baily MB, Haberman PW, et al. Outcomes in alcoholic marriages: Endurance, termination or recovery. J Stud Alcohol 1962;23:610–23.

28. Steinglass P. The impact of alcoholism on the family: Relationship between degree of alcoholism and psychiatric symptomology. J Stud Alcohol 1981;42:288–303.

29. Steinglass P. The alcoholic family at home: Patterns of interaction in dry, wet and transitional stages of alcoholism. Arch Gen Psychiatry 1981;38:578–84.

30. Jacob T, Dunn NJ, Leonard K. Patterns of alcohol abuse and family stability. Alcoholism Clin Exp Res 1983;7:382–5.

31. Roman PM. Secondary prevention of alcoholism: The problem and prospects for occupational programming. J Drug Issues 1975;5:327–43.

32. Healthy people: The Surgeon General's report on health promotion and disease prevention. Washington, D.C.: US Government Printing Office, 1979; DHEW publication no. (PHS) 79-55071.

33. Staulcup H, Kenward K, Frigo DA. A review of federal primary alcoholism prevention projects. J Stud Alcohol 1979;40:943–68.

34. Wallack LM. Mass media campaigns: The odds against finding behavior change. Health Educ Q 1981;8:209–60.

35. Waring M, Sperr I. Bartenders: An untapped resource for the prevention of alcohol abuse? Int J Addict 1982;17:859–68.

36. Wittman F. Current status of research demonstration programs in the primary prevention of alcohol problems. In: Monograph 3: Prevention, intervention and treatment: Concerns and models, Alcohol and Health Monograph Series. Rockville, Maryland: National Institute on Alcohol Abuse and Alcoholism, DHHS publication (ADM)82-1192, 1982:3–57.

37. Little RE, Streissguth Pytkowicz A, Guzinski GM. Prevention of fetal alcohol syndrome: A model program. Alcoholism Clin Exp Res 1980;4:185–9.

38. Kinder BN, Pape NE, Walfish S. Drug and alcohol education programs: A review of outcome studies. Int J Addict 1980;15:1035–54.

39. Fell J. Alcohol involvement in traffic accidents, Washington, D.C.: Department of Transportation, DOT-HS-806-269, 1982.

40. Williams AF, Zador PL, Harris SF, et al. The effect of raising the legal minimum drinking age on involvement in fatal crashes. J Legal Stud 1983;12:169–79.

Arthritis and Musculoskeletal Diseases

Frederic C. McDuffie, M.D., William R. Felts, Jr., M.D.,
Marc C. Hochberg, M.D., M.P.H., Reva C. Lawrence, M.P.H.,
Kenneth Mitchell, Ph.D., Morey S. Moreland, M.D.,
and Lawrence E. Shulman, M.D., Ph.D.

Arthritis and heart disease are the two major causes of disability in the United States, each responsible for approximately 15 percent of the total.[1] Arthritis means inflammation of a joint, but in general usage the term has been extended to include any damage to a joint, particularly if it produces chronic pain. Certain chronic, painful conditions characterized by symptoms that appear in tissues in and around joints but that produce no demonstrable pathology (e.g., fibrositis, musculoskeletal pain syndromes, idiopathic back pain) are often included in the category of arthritis. Arthritis is thus not a single disease.

Research directed at uncovering the ultimate cause of arthritis must be strictly targeted to the individual forms of arthritis such as gout, ankylosing spondylitis, and psoriatic arthritis, each of which has its distinct etiology. But whatever their causes, all the chronic forms of arthritis produce similar problems for those affected. Patients have difficulty performing activities of daily living and working; they face high expenses for health care; and they must cope with the effects of arthritis on their emotional well-being and sexual relationships.

The causes of almost all the major forms of chronic arthritis remain unknown in spite of numerous advances in biomedical research that have pinpointed certain factors (such as heredity, infection, defects in regulation of the immune response, and the aggregation of proteoglycan molecules in cartilage) as playing important roles in these diseases. Therefore, we cannot yet identify the environmental hazards or lifestyles that lead to arthritis.

Arthritis is a prominent manifestation in more than a hundred diseases, but many are uncommon or produce most of their harmful effects by involving other organs. Therefore, we will focus our attention on the three most common and economically important forms of arthritis: osteoarthritis, rheumatoid arthritis, and back pain. Three other important health problems—gout, juvenile rheumatoid arthritis, and the inflammatory connective tissue diseases (systemic lupus erythematosus, scleroderma, polymyositis, and the vasculitides)—will be considered in less detail.

THE MORBIDITY OF ARTHRITIS

According to the 1980 National Health Interview Survey, approximately 37 million people (17 percent) in the United States consider themselves to have arthritis. Extrapolation from the Health and Nutrition Examination Survey (HANES) I data indicates that an estimated 32.6 percent of the adult population is affected by joint swelling, limitation of motion, or pain on motion.[2] However, obtaining complete and accurate data on incidence and prevalence is hampered by several factors, in particular the absence of standard case definitions and diagnostic criteria. Moreover, many rheumatic diseases have prevalence rates that are too low to be accurately measured by current national surveys.

Osteoarthritis

Osteoarthritis is the most common form of arthritis and probably represents the end result of a number of different pathologic processes. It involves primarily the fingers, feet, spine, hips, and knees. The process responsible for osteoarthritis begins in the cartilage overlying the ends of bones that form a joint and is initiated or accelerated by mechanical forces that disrupt the normal biomechanics of the joint. Meniscus tears, occupational stresses (e.g.,

From the Emory University School of Medicine and the Arthritis Foundation, Atlanta, Georgia (McDuffie), George Washington University, Washington, D.C. (Felts), Johns Hopkins Multipurpose Arthritis Center, Baltimore, Maryland (Hochberg), Department of Health and Public Health Service, Arthritis Epidemiology, Human Services (Lawrence) and the National Institute of Arthritis Musculoskeletal and Skin Diseases (Shulman), National Institutes of Health, Bethesda, Maryland, the National Industrial Rehabilitation Corp. (Mitchell), Dublin, Ohio, and the University of Vermont College of Medicine, Burlington (Moreland).

Address reprint requests to Dr. McDuffie, Arthritis Foundation, 1314 Spring Street, N.W., Atlanta, GA 30309.

on the spines of coal miners or the ankles of ballet dancers), disease affecting bony alignment (e.g., congenital dislocation of the hip, Legg-Calvé-Perthe's disease of the hip), obesity, and all other forms of arthritis have been implicated as causative factors in some persons. However, in most persons no predisposing factors have been identified. The symptoms are pain and limitation of motion of the affected joints.

People who have osteoarthritis are often in good health because the disease produces no systemic symptoms. Disability usually results from difficulty in walking because of disease in the knee or hip; hand involvement is not a great cause of disability.

Estimating the exact national prevalence of osteoarthritis is difficult for several reasons. The disease is measured by radiographic evidence, even though many persons whose X-ray findings are positive report no pain or disability. It remains unclear whether these persons should be counted as cases. Conversely, some individuals report pain but show no radiographic evidence of osteoarthritis. In addition, primary sources for data on osteoarthritis are based on the radiographs of only a few joints in each person. Therefore, most reports of prevalence are given only for specific joints because data are not available for all joints. Finally, prevalence rates vary, depending on whether mild and moderate cases are reported in addition to severe ones.[3]

The following estimates are based on radiographic evidence alone from the Health Examination Survey (HES) of 1960–1962[3,4] and the HANES I of 1971–1975.[3,5] The prevalence rate of mild, moderate, and severe osteoarthritis of the hands is approximately 32.5 percent for adults aged 25–74. It is 22.2 percent for the feet, 3.8 percent for the knees, and 1.3 percent for the hips. Osteoarthritis in all reported joints increases substantially with age. In the HES the frequency of osteoarthritis, based on radiographs of the hands and feet, increased from 4 percent among persons less than 24 years old to 85 percent among those aged 75–79. Overall, men and women are affected approximately equally when all ages are reported together, but prevalence is greater in men under age 45 and in women over age 55.

Rheumatoid Arthritis

Rheumatoid arthritis differs from osteoarthritis in that it involves multiple joints, usually commences at a younger age, is not caused by biomechanical factors, and begins as an inflammatory process in the joint lining or synovium rather than as a degeneration of the cartilage. The most commonly involved joints are the fingers, toes, wrists, knees, elbows, and ankles. Deformity and loss of muscle strength are common. Because rheumatoid arthritis is a systemic inflammatory disease, other structures may be affected. Subcutaneous nodules, pleuritis and pericarditis with effusion, splenomegaly, lymphadenopathy, episcleritis, and vasculitis involving skin and peripheral nerves are most common. Of the people who fit the diagnostic criteria for rheumatoid arthritis, 80 percent have autoantibodies to human IgG in their sera. These antibodies, or rheumatoid factors, are not specific for the disease, although high titers usually indicate a poor prognosis.

The etiology of rheumatoid arthritis is unknown. People who possess the HLA–DR4 gene are more likely to develop the disease because it is present in 60–70 percent of people who have the disease compared with 25 percent in a control population. All evidence points to the existence of an underlying infectious agent, probably a virus, but so far it has eluded identification.

The 1960–1962 HES is the only source of national rheumatoid arthritis data that are based on the American Rheumatism Association diagnostic criteria. Prevalence estimates from this survey were determined for cases defined as classical, definite, and probable.[6] Of the identified cases, 70 percent were in the probable category. According to the National Center for Health Statisitics (NCHS), it is likely that this subset includes cases of other arthritides or transient disease that could not be differentiated from rheumatoid arthritis in the survey. Only 15 percent of patients with probable rheumatoid arthritis develop chronic disease.[7]

The national prevalence of classical, definite, and probable rheumatoid arthritis, according to the HES data, is 3.2 percent of the adult population aged 18–79. Women have a rate of 4.6 percent, nearly three times the male rate of 1.7 percent. Prevalence rates increase with age in both sexes, as noted in Table 1.[6,8] If only classical and definite rheumatoid arthritis are considered, the overall prevalence rate becomes 1.0 percent, and the female–male ratio remains 3:1.

Back Pain

Back pain is a major cause of morbidity, disability, and economic loss.[8] It accounts for approximately one third of patients who have musculoskeletal complaints and who are seen by general practitioners. According to data from the NCHS,[9] in 1970 back pain was the most common cause of limitation of activity in workers younger than 45 and the third most common cause in those 45–64 years of age.

According to the HANES I survey,[5] 10.5 percent

Table 1. Prevalence of classical, definite, and probable rheumatoid arthritis, United States, 1960–1962

Age (years)	Classical, definite, and probable (% of population)			Classical and definite (% of population)	
	Male	Female	Both sexes	Male	Female
18–24	0.2	0.3	0.3	—	—
25–34	—	0.6	0.3	—	0.1
35–44	0.5	2.1	1.3	—	0.9
45–54	1.5	4.4	3.0	0.2	1.0
55–64	4.2	8.3	6.3	2.0	2.4
65–74	3.1	14.1	9.2	0.2	4.6
75–79	14.1	23.5	18.8	8.2	6.2
Total	1.7	4.6	3.2	0.5	1.4

Data from Engle et al.[6] and Kelsey.[8]

of respondents aged 25–74 have had pain in the lower back "on most days for at least a month." The frequency for women was 9.4 percent compared with 11.4 percent in men.

Prolapsed disc. Prolapsed, or "slipped," intervertebral disc is a major problem associated with back pain. According to the 1976 data, displacement of an intervertebral disc restricted the patient's activity in half of the cases and resulted in an average of 8.4 days in bed a year. The most recent prevalence data from the 1981 National Health Interview Survey (HIS) indicate that 3 million persons (14.1 per 1,000) are affected. A higher rate is reported in males than in females. The rate increases with age, peaking in the group 45–64 years of age (34.5 cases per 1,000).[10]

Scoliosis. One important and often preventable cause of chronic back pain is scoliosis, which is detectable in childhood before symptoms develop. If serious and not corrected at this stage, complications such as lung volume reduction, psychological effects resulting from hunchbacked appearance, and premature osteoarthritis may develop.

According to preliminary data from HANES II, scoliosis is found in 1.6 percent of children aged 12–17: 1.25 percent of boys and 2.1 percent of girls (personal communication, Jennifer Madans, Division of Analysis, National Center for Health Statistics, 1982). Only 10 percent of detected cases are progressive and require active treatment. Girls are more likely than boys to have progressive curves. Although some studies have found a prevalence rate as high as 5 percent among adolescents, the differences between estimates usually reflect the degree of curvature defined as the threshold for diagnosis. According to figures from the HANES I survey, approximately 3 percent of the adult civilian noninstitutionalized U.S. population aged 25–74 has scoliosis.[5]

Ankylosing spondylitis. Ankylosing spondylitis is a form of arthritis that produces chronic back pain and restricts motion in approximately 300,000 Americans.[11] In whites it is almost entirely limited to individuals who possess the HLA–B27 antigen, and it affects primarily young and middle-aged men. Because only a small proportion (fewer than 20 percent) of the persons who are B27-positive develop ankylosing spondylitis, it is believed that some environmental agent(s) triggers the disease in susceptible people.

Osteoporosis. A prominent cause of back pain in elderly women is postmenopausal osteoporosis, which causes pain from compression fractures of the thoracic vertebrae. Osteoporosis appears to result from an acceleration of the normal decline in skeletal bone mass that begins at age 40. This decline is rapid for the first few years after menopause, then continues at a slower rate. There is considerable evidence that diminished production of estrogen and progesterone, an increased requirement for dietary calcium, and a less physically active lifestyle contribute to this process. Attempts to identify women at high risk for osteoporosis are under way, but to date no simple, accurate method has been found. Prophylactic therapy, including calcium, estrogen, and progesterone started at menopause, can reverse or diminish bone loss in women.[12]

Osteoporosis is extremely common in older people, particularly women, and its prevalence increases with advancing age, rising from approximately 18 percent in the 45–49 age group to 89 percent at age 75 (Table 2). Vertebral fractures, which cause the back pain characteristic of the postmenopausal form of the disease, are the second most common cause of hospitalization for fractures in persons over 65. The main cause of morbidity from osteoporosis is fracture of the femur, which is pri-

Table 2. Prevalence rates of osteoporosis in Michigan women, 1969

Age (years)	n	Osteoporosis (%)
45–49	290	17.9
50–54	309	39.2
55–59	514	57.7
60–64	426	65.5
65–69	299	73.5
70–74	177	84.2
75+	73	89.0
Total	2,088	56.7

Data from Iskrant and Smith.[45]
Based on radiographs of the thoracolumbar spine.

marily associated with the senile form. This occurs in somewhat older persons and has a female–male sex ratio of approximately 2:1, as opposed to the 6:1 ratio for the postmenopausal type.

Idiopathic back pain. In only a small number of persons who have chronic back pain can a structural disease or abnormality be identified. Spondylolisthesis, infections, tumors, and other diseases account for a small fraction of the total. Some low back pain is undoubtedly psychogenic or made worse by psychogenic factors. True malingering is rare and can usually be identified by a proper history and physical examination.

Mechanical factors are undoubtedly important, as back pain in younger people is related to hard physical labor. A relationship has been shown between the physical strength of the worker, the demands of the job, and the incidence of back pain.[13] There is no doubt that those engaged in heavy labor suffer more severe pain and lose more time from work than do those whose work puts fewer demands on the spine.[14] In particular, jobs that involve frequent bending forward, bending and twisting, lifting (especially repeated and heavy lifting), repetitive work, and vibration carry the highest risk. Some influence is exerted by tall stature, extreme obesity, marked scoliosis, and weak muscles.

The management of idiopathic back pain remains empirical and unsatisfactory in part because of the difficulty of classifying the affected persons into etiologically based subgroups.

Gout

Gout is a metabolic disorder that produces joint inflammation as a result of sodium urate crystals deposited in the synovium. It affects more than 1 million people in the United States, the majority of them men. Hyperuricemia may result either from overproduction (in approximately 10 percent) or underexcretion (approximately 90 percent) of urate. Acute gout is characteristically a self-limited disease that usually involves the great toe or another joint of the lower extremity. Chronic gout, which is characterized by urate crystals (tophi) in joints and other soft tissues, develops slowly over many years in about half of the untreated people who have gout. Current therapy, which includes colchicine prophylaxis for acute attacks, probenecid to enhance renal excretion of uric acid, and allopurinol to reduce synthesis of urate, has markedly reduced the prevalence of tophaceous gout. The chief problems in managing gout are proper diagnosis and persuading those with this disorder to take prophylactic therapy for the rest of their lives.

On the basis of HIS data, in the United States an estimated 2,018,000 persons (9 per 1,000) suffer grom gout. For women the frequency is 4.7 per 1,000, and for men, 13.5 per 1,000. These figures are probably too high. In a follow-up examination of individuals who reported they had gout, the diagnosis could not be substantiated in two thirds of those examined.[15] A better figure for the prevalence of gout is approximately 4.0 per 1,000 (5.0–6.6 in men and 1.0–3.0 in women).[11,15]

The prevalence of gout increases with age; it is rare in persons under 17 and most frequent in those 54 years of age and over.[10]

Inflammatory Connective Tissue Diseases

Inflammatory connective tissue diseases, a group of chronic diseases often associated with arthritis and characterized by autoimmunity, vascular injury, and inflammation in connective tissues, affect almost 1 million people in the United States. Systemic lupus erythematosus (SLE), scleroderma, polymyositis, and the several forms of vasculitis can affect multiple organ systems and produce serious disability. Because individually they are fairly uncommon, these diseases are usually not considered major health problems. However, they pose a serious burden for those who are affected. Because of certain common features it is likely that these diseases are closely related and are similar in etiology.

The prevalence rate of SLE in the United States in 1970 was 15–50 per 100,000.[16] Because these figures are higher than those found in the 1950s, the prevalence may be increasing. The prevalence of scleroderma has been estimated as 14 per 100,000.[17] No good data exist for the prevalence of polymyositis or vasculitis.

Juvenile Rheumatoid Arthritis

Although arthritis is generally considered an affliction of the elderly, approximately 100,000 children have some type of chronic joint inflammation.

Hochberg et al.[18] estimated the true prevalence rate of juvenile rheumatoid arthritis at 0.17–0.57 per 1,000 children.

At least four distinct types of chronic arthritis are now recognized in children: (1) a systemic form in young children, often given the eponym Still's disease; (2) a pauciarticular form more common in girls, usually affecting only the lower extremities and associated with iritis and a positive antinuclear antibody test; (3) the adult form of rheumatoid arthritis in which the test for rheumatoid factor is positive; and (4) a second pauciarticular form most common in boys who possess the HLA–B27 gene. The long-term prognosis for these children (except for those who have seropositive rheumatoid arthritis) is relatively good, though they may reach adulthood with considerable residual deformity. Children who have chronic arthritis have very special problems with adjustment in school, acceptance by peers, effects on other family members, and preparation for adulthood.

MORTALITY

Of the 21 million deaths in the United States during the 11-year period 1968–1978, only 63,148 (0.03 percent) were attributed to musculoskeletal and connective tissue diseases: 35,136 (55.62 percent) in white females, 19,068 (30.23 percent) in white males, 6,202 (9.81 percent) in nonwhite females, and 2,742 (4.34 percent) in nonwhite males.[19] In whites, this higher female mortality was most pronounced in the age range 15–44, which generally corresponds to the childbearing years. In nonwhites, this higher mortality in women was present at every age through 54, though it was most marked in ages 15 to 34. The vulnerability of women was greater in nonwhites than whites in these age groups.[19,20]

SLE,[21] scleroderma,[22] and polymyositis,[23] three of the most life-threatening connective tissue diseases, are known to be more prevalent and severe in young black females than in other population groups, a circumstance that probably explains the relatively high mortality rate from the rheumatic diseases in the young nonwhite female population found in this analysis.

THE COSTS OF ARTHRITIS

At present it is impossible to measure precisely the full economic impact of arthritis. Nonetheless, several important assessments exist, and these have been used to project reasonable estimates of the economic consequences.

Approximately 6 percent of all patients hospital-

ized in the United States, more than 2 million persons, were discharged from short-stay hospitals in 1982 with a primary diagnosis of musculoskeletal system or connective tissue disease (ICD-9 CM 710–739).[24] (See Table 3 for the numbers and incidence rate according to sex and age groups.)

The most common complaint reported by patients seeking office-based medical care is musculoskeletal symptoms. According to data from the National Ambulatory Medical Care survey carried out by the NCHS in 1981, approximately 59 million office visits, 10.1 percent of all visits during the one-year period, were for symptoms referable to the musculoskeletal system.[25] The NCHS has estimated that musculoskeletal diseases (ICD-9 CM 710–739) were the principal diagnoses in approximately 42 million visits. This survey did not report the number of persons who sought medical care but rather the number of visits made.

Musculoskeletal pain also accounted for the largest portion (41 percent) of new visits made to physicians because of pain symptoms during the two-year period 1980–1981.[26]

Because of the nature of musculoskeletal disability, direct costs include a unique component—goods and services that do not come from the health sector. Health services include costs of hospitalization and other institutional care, fees to physicians and other health care providers, medications and devices, other professional services, insurance prepayment for federal programs, and administrative costs (assumed in one study to be 4.5 percent of total direct costs). Goods and services from outside the health sector include transportation to and from health care providers, special diets, household help, rehabilitation, and architectural changes necessitated by the illness (assumed in the same study to be 15 percent of total direct health costs).

See Table 4 for direct and indirect costs in 1983 dollars, based on a study by Grazier et al.[27] This study identified indirect costs at only 29 percent, direct costs at 71 percent. Earlier reports in 1973[28] and 1979[29] indicated that indirect costs amounted to as much as two thirds of the total. The explanation for the shift to only one third is not immediately apparent, but it may reflect the rapid increase in the cost of medical care and the smaller proportion of individuals in the work force as the population ages. Woolley et al.[30] projected that the cost of musculoskeletal diseases in the year 2000 would be almost $95.6 billion and that because of certain shifts in the economy, the direct–indirect cost ratio would be approximately 1:1.

A breakdown in the costs according to disease is revealing. The annual costs inflicted by rheumatoid arthritis are approaching $1 billion, osteoarthritis

Table 3. Patients with diseases of the musculoskeletal system or connective tissue (ICD-9 CM 710–739) as first-listed diagnosis discharged from short-stay hospitals, United States, 1982

Patient characteristics	Number discharged (thousands)	Rate per 10,000 population	Average length of hospitalization (days)
Sex			
Male	1,016	91.5	7.0
Female	1,361	114.5	8.2
Age			
<15	78	15.2	5.1
15–44	943	87.9	6.2
45–64	778	175.1	7.7
65	578	215.4	10.7
Total	2,377	103.4	7.7

Data from National Hospital Discharge Survey.[23]

more than $2 billion, other arthritis $2.5 billion, and lumbar disc and back disorders almost $13.5 billion. Osteoporosis, with its attendant complications of fractures, costs approximately $3.8 billion.

The costs of rheumatoid arthritis[31] were the focus of a study of 12 men and 38 women (average age, 48 ± 1.4 years) who had stage III rheumatoid disease. In 1976 dollars, direct costs for the entire group for the year averaged $2,319, though a wide range was reported, hinging principally on the presence or absence of hospitalization during the year. Indirect costs averaged $6,810 ± $1,358 for all subjects. Average total costs were $9,129 for the year. The authors suggested that the functional and employment status of the average person who has stage III rheumatoid arthritis will not be substantially improved by additional medical care. It was therefore concluded that policy options for chronic disease, such as expanded income supplement programs and sheltered workplaces, should be given serious consideration.

The financial burden of arthritis on a family is one of its most serious effects. Indirect costs, primarily loss of income, are three times the direct costs, according to one study,[31] and less than half the cost is

Table 4. Cost of chronic musculoskeletal conditions, United States, 1983 (millions of dollars)

Disease	Direct cost	Indirect cost	Total
Arthritis	7,712	918	8,630
Back pain	12,923	2,950	15,873
Osteoporosis	5,729	415	6,144
Total	26,364	4,283	30,647

Data from Grazier et al.[27]

covered by transfer payments. In another study[24] 180 persons who had had rheumatoid arthritis for six years were found to be earning an average of 60 percent less than they had before becoming ill. Family income had declined about 25 percent, the difference being made up by disability payments and the earnings of a spouse. In 6 percent of families in which a member had rheumatoid arthritis, the employment status of the spouse had changed as a result of the disease.

An individual's ability to function adequately within his or her environment may be severely impaired by chronic arthritis. The most comprehensive data on limitation of activity due to arthritis and related musculoskeletal diseases are derived from the HIS of 1976.[32] Of 30 million people reporting limitation of activity, 3.8 million (approximately 12 percent) were limited by arthritis. The role of arthritis as a cause of disability increased from 5 percent of those under 48 years old who had disabling chronic conditions to almost 20 percent of those over 65. More than half of those limited by arthritis were restricted in their major activity, and one quarter could not carry on their major activity. The many women engaged in housework are especially likely to be limited by arthritis because women are more commonly affected by most forms of arthritis than are men. In all, arthritis was responsible in 1976 for 416 million of the 2,979 million days of restricted activity because of chronic conditions.

ARTHRITIS AND THE QUALITY OF LIFE

Certain elements of the toll exacted by musculoskeletal diseases cannot be easily measured, nor can a price tag be affixed to the resulting human suffering. In an analysis of the psychosocial impact of rheumatoid arthritis on 245 persons between the ages of 21 and 65, Meenan et al.[32] found that 63 percent had experienced at least one major psychosocial change (e.g., marital status, employment) as a result of their disease. Of those surveyed, 83 percent had made significant changes in their leisure activities.

Although much can be accomplished in the treatment of rheumatoid arthritis through a combination of anti-inflammatory and long-acting drugs, physical therapy, and occupational therapy, the overall effects of the disease on functional status tend to be progressive. In a nine-year follow-up study of 75 patients who had rheumatoid arthritis and who were treated by nonspecialists, Pincus et al.[33] found declines of 35–55 percent in several functional indices.

Transportation is one area in which functional impairment can severely restrict the quality of a person's life. On the basis of one study it has been estimated that a third of the persons who have arthritis have some limitation of mobility, that 13 percent require transportation aids, and that 5 percent need a wheelchair.[34]

Although people who have rheumatoid arthritis appear to exhibit certain personality traits (e.g., somatization, depression, and hysteria) that separate them from control populations, they share these traits with people who are afflicted with other chronic diseases.[35,36] Thus there does not seem to be any specific "rheumatoid personality."

The family must make adjustments to accommodate a family member who has arthritis. A child with arthritis places a heavy burden on the mother, who of necessity must reduce the amount of attention she pays to other children and her spouse. Such a family restricts its participation in many group activities because of the affected child's limitations.

The frequency of divorce and separation is somewhat higher in families in which a member has arthritis (18 percent versus a national average of 11 percent, according to Meenan et al.).[32] Sexual problems are commonly encountered by people who have arthritis. The loss of a positive body image may be a serious problem for many, and some forms of arthritis, particularly the systemic connective tissue diseases, are commonly associated with severe lassitude and fatigability, which make the idea of sexual activity unappealing. Finally, physical limitations, especially of the hips and lower back in persons who have ankylosing spondylitis,[37] simply make satisfactory sexual performance difficult or, at best, awkward.

INTERVENTIONS

In 1983 the National Arthritis Advisory Board, in cooperation with the National Institute of Arthritis, Diabetes, Digestive and Kidney Diseases, held a conference on the prevention of arthritis.[38] A review of the preliminary text (the document summarizing the conclusions of this conference is still in preparation) reveals that most of the strategies are recommendations for further research. None of the causes of these diseases are known, and to date very few risk factors (except genes) have been unequivocally identified. At this time we can make only a few recommendations for the large-scale preventive measures that are most likely to reduce these health problems significantly.

Primary Interventions

Osteoporosis. Low-dose cyclic estrogen therapy should probably be prescribed indefinitely for women whose ovaries are removed before age 50 and should be considered for other women at the time of menopause if no contraindications exist. Research to develop practical screening tests to detect women at a high risk for osteoporosis is being done in several centers.

Because the usual daily intake of calcium in the United States (450–550 mg) is below the 1,000–1,500 mg needed by postmenopausal women and elderly people of both sexes, these persons need either to consume more dairy products (three to five 8-oz glasses of skim milk a day) or to take calcium supplements. Low doses of vitamin D may also be desirable for some people because the requirement increases in old age. Weight-bearing exercises are also advised, as there is some evidence they may reduce bone loss. Other substances such as fluorides, calcitriol, anabolic androgen derivatives, calcitonin, thiazides, parathormone fragments, and biphosphonates are being studied as measures for control of osteoporosis, but neither their efficacy nor their roles have been established. Devising ways of reducing the risk of fractures by preventing falls by the elderly needs more emphasis.

The long-term efficacy of a program for the elderly which would include the above elements is impossible to gauge precisely. However, considerable savings in medical costs, premature death, and suffering would almost certainly evolve. We estimate that such a program could reduce costs and hospitalizations for fractures by one third over a 15-year period.

Scoliosis. The key to the successful prevention of scoliosis is early recognition. There is now good evidence that screening programs can identify scoliosis at a stage at which progression can be halted. Because it is not possible to determine at an early stage which curvatures will progress and which ones will not, regular follow-ups are essential.

Some states and school districts now have mandatory screening programs, but only one third of U.S. children are currently screened by such procedures.[39] In addition, inadequate follow-up of children detected in such programs means that many potentially reversible curvatures are not treated. Many children placed in treatment programs do not adequately adhere to the prescribed regimen, the regular wearing of braces. It is understandably difficult to persuade children to wear a contrivance that calls attention to their unique condition. Because scoliosis in its early stages seldom produces symptoms and does not result in gross deformity or handicap, the problem of compliance is especially difficult. A strategy aimed at preventing scoliosis should include the following:

1. Enact legislation in all states to make mandatory scoliosis screening and follow-up programs in the schools.

2. Ensure that children detected in screening programs receive adequate follow-up and treatment.

3. Improve compliance in scoliosis prevention and treatment programs. Parents should be persuaded to monitor their children's compliance, and the children themselves should be motivated to comply more fully.

4. Educate school personnel, health professionals, and church groups to increase their awareness and define their specific roles.

Such efforts, if carried out successfully, could considerably reduce the prevalence of significant scoliosis. Approximately 5% percent of scoliosis patients, or 200,000 individuals, fall into this category. The relationship of back pain to scoliosis continues to be debated. Edgar[40] found that 47 percent of surgically treated patients were pain free, whereas only 13 percent of the untreated patients were. Pain correlated best with the amount of osteoarthritic changes on the concave side of the vertebral curves.

It appears that the greatest benefits of scoliosis prevention fall into two areas: improving psychological health and self-image, and reducing the number who require extensive corrective surgery.

Low back pain. Even though the precise origins of most low back pain have not been delineated, enough evidence has accumulated to indicate that certain factors increase its severity and duration.

Two approaches to the problem of back pain in industry can be expected to reduce the magnitude of the problem:

1. Screen people for jobs in occupations in which the activities are known to increase the severity, the duration, and probably the incidence of back pain. Use a profile of employees (height, weight, strength, abnormal spine curvature) and of jobs (requirements for lifting, twisting, bending, prolonged sitting, repetition, and vibration) to better match the worker to the occupation and reduce the amount of work loss and other morbidity from back pain.

2. Analyze the physical requirements of jobs associated with back pain to make adjustments that reduce physical stress. For example, mechanical lifts, proper positioning of handles, and varying the job pattern to reduce repetition can do much to improve worker efficiency and reduce economic loss due to back pain.

To achieve these two goals, employers must be satisfied that such measures are cost effective. Unions must recognize that the changes are in the workers' interest and should accept some flexibility in rules governing seniority, job security, and promotion patterns. Workers themselves must be convinced that their health and safety are the goals of such plans.

Because the circumstances surrounding individual jobs, plants, and industries vary greatly, the recommended preventive measures for back pain should be accompanied by careful data collection and ongoing analysis to determine which changes effectively reduce pain and disability and to determine other benefits (e.g., savings resulting from less turnover and more overall productivity). Such data would provide an incentive for continuing those measures that are worthwhile and eliminating those of little value. Close involvement of industrial health personnel (physicians, nurses, and others) is an essential ingredient to success.

Of the annual $2 billion in lost work productivity caused by back pain, we estimate that up to 20 percent might be eliminated by this program over a ten-year period.

Secondary Interventions

In diseases for which no effective primary preventive measures exist, the application of secondary measures to reduce morbidity is an attractive alternative. Such measures have the advantage of being focused on a well-defined group of people who are motivated to apply any recommended techniques.

Gout. Primary prevention of gout is not feasible. The most effective interventions increase the treatment compliance of patients who have gout. According to an unpublished study at Johns Hopkins, when a nurse experienced in rheumatology maintained close communication with gout patients the number of acute attacks dropped sharply. Unfortunately, the effort and the expense of such an approach make it impractical for widespread use at this time. Ideally, combining this intervention with compliance measures for other chronic, asymptomatic diseases would make it more cost effective.

Spondyloarthropathies. The frequent association of Reiter's syndrome with sexual activity, the high prevalence of ureaplasma and other urinary tract organisms often found in promiscuous individuals,[41] and the presence of urethritis as the most common initiating symptom of the Reiter's triad indicate that venereally transmitted factors play a key role in producing this syndrome in susceptible persons. Most physicians strongly advise people who have had Reiter's syndrome to reduce the number of their sexual partners and to use a condom, especially when exposed to a new partner.

Tertiary Interventions

Rheumatoid arthritis. Although rheumatoid arthritis itself cannot be prevented and we lack proof that its long-term course can be altered much by treatment, recent evidence has established that the quality of life and the functional disability of people who have this disease can be improved by measures aimed not at medical management of the disease but at social and personal factors affecting a person's ability to work. Meenan et al.[32] and Yelin et al.[42] have pointed out that further efforts to improve medical management of this disease are not likely to enhance job productivity and that any future advances will stem from effecting changes in working conditions.

A program aimed at reducing job-related disability resulting from rheumatoid arthritis should include the following strategies:

1. Persuade employers, unions, and coworkers that it is advantageous to them to create a work environment that enables the rheumatoid arthritis patient to continue working.

2. Allow as much latitude as possible for workers who have rheumatoid arthritis to set their own hours and rest periods and to make recommendations about the design of their immediate working environment.

3. Use experienced designers to modify tools so that as many handicapped employees as possible can remain in their jobs.

4. Provide vocational rehabilitation training for handicapped persons who have physically demanding jobs that cannot be successfully adapted. Efforts should be made to select for training the persons whose intelligence, stability of social life, and motivation make them most likely to benefit.

5. Improve transportation for handicapped workers. Buses should be more accessible and easier to use by people with arthritis. In addition, special driver training, mechanical aids, and car pools can help them overcome what may be their greatest limitation in returning to their jobs.[43]

6. Provide work at home (cottage industry) for people who have rheumatoid arthritis. Although at first glance this approach is attractive, its success would probably be limited. It is difficult for any enterprise to supervise such persons. Most jobs demand considerable interaction among workers; the end product or service is usually a team effort. Also, much of the psychological benefit of working results from the social contact and person-to-person interaction that a job provides.

Although the economic and social consequences of rheumatoid arthritis have been fairly well defined, it is difficult to predict how much our recommended program would ease the burden that society bears for rheumatoid arthritis. We anticipate that in the early stages of the recommended intervention the biggest problem would be mobilizing the cooperation of key groups (employers, unions, vocational rehabilitation counselors). As it became established, the main difficulty would be to enroll affected persons who have little education, who hold jobs that are physically but not intellectually demanding, who are poorly motivated, or who belong to groups (especially recent immigrants and minorities) that are traditionally hard to reach with such efforts. Using figures for current dollars, we estimate that over a ten-year period we could reduce costs attributable to loss of work productivity by approximately 30 percent ($21 million).

Because so many of the people who have rheumatoid arthritis are in their most productive years, the best strategy at this time is to direct our efforts toward this group. If successful, the same approach could then be extended to people who have other rheumatic diseases such as ankylosing spondylitis, osteoarthritis, and SLE. In addition, we need special programs for those who have juvenile arthritis, to enabling them to become active members of society when they reach adulthood.

Osteoarthritis. The successful introduction of total joint arthroplasty resulting from the work of Sir John Charnley has revolutionized the management of osteoarthritis of the knee and hip in the past 20 years. Data indicate that 285,000 of these procedures are performed annually, most of them on people who have osteoarthritis. Although increasing the availability of such surgery might benefit society as well as the affected individuals, the work-related economic benefits of these procedures are limited. Most persons who have severe osteoarthritis of the hips and knees are over 55 and nearing the end of their active working careers. According to at least one study,[44] total hip arthroplasty succeeds only moderately in returning people to work for any length of time.

SUMMARY

Arthritis and related disorders of the musculoskeletal system are the most frequently reported type of impairment affecting the U.S. adult population.[8] Although the various forms of arthritis and related diseases do not cause many deaths, their high prevalence, painful character, and interference with routine mechanical function make them one of the leading health and economic burdens in the United States today. The prevalence of these conditions increases with age, but arthritis and other musculoskeletal problems also affect the health of a significant number of children.

Strategies aimed at reducing this burden should make the most effective medical care available to more of the affected individuals, recognize arthritis and intervene earlier, and assist those affected to live more productive and fulfilling lives.

REFERENCES

1. Wilder CS. Limitation of activity due to chronic conditions: United States, 1974. Rockville, Maryland: National Health Survey, 1977; DHEW publication no. (HRA)77-1537. (Vital and health statistics; series 10, no. 111).

2. Cunningham LS, Kelsey JL. Epidemiology of musculoskeletal impairments and associated disability. Am J Public Health, 1984;74:6.

3. Lawrence RL, Kelsey J, Hochberg MC, et al. Frequency and cost of the rheumatic diseases in the United States (in press).

4. Engel A. Osteoarthritis in adults by selected demographic characteristics: United States, 1960–1962. Washington, D.C.: National Center for Health Statistics, 1966; DHEW publication no. 1000. (Vital and health statistics; series 11; no. 20).

5. Maurer K. Basic data on arthritis—knee, hip and sacroiliac joints in adults ages 25–74 years: United States, 1971–1975. Hyattsville, Maryland: National Center for Health Statistics, 1979; DHEW publication no. (PHS)79-1661. Vital and health statistics; series 11; no. 213).

6. Engel A, Roberts J, Burch TA. Rheumatoid arthritis in adults: United States, 1960–1962. Washington, D.C.: National Center for Health Statistics, 1966; DHEW publication no. 1000. (Vital and health statistics; series 11; no. 17).

7. O'Sullivan JB, Cathcart ES. The prevalence of rheumatoid arthritis: Follow-up evaluation of the effect of criteria on the rates in Sudbury, Massachusetts. Ann Intern Med 1972;79:573.

8. Kelsey JL. Epidemiology of musculoskeletal disorders. New York: Oxford, 1982.

9. Wilder CS. Limitation of Activity due to Chronic Conditions, United States, 1969 and 1970. Hyattsville, Maryland: National Center for Health Statistics, 1973; DHEW publication no. (PHS73-1506). (Vital and health statistics; series 10; no. 80).

10. Collins JG. Prevalence of selected chronic conditions: United States, 1979–81. Hyattsville, Maryland: National Center for Health Statistics, 1983; DHHS publication no. (PHS)86-1583. (Vital and health statistics; series 10; no. 155).

11. Mikkelson WM, Dodge HF, Duff IF, et al. Estimates of the prevalence of rheumatic disease in the population of Tecumseh, Michigan, 1959–60. J Chron Dis 1967;20:351.

12. Christiansen C, Christensen MS, McNair P, et al. Prevention of early postmenopausal bone loss: Controlled two year study in 315 normal females. Eur J Clin Invest 1980;10:273.

13. Chaffin DB. Human strength capability and low back pain. J Occup Med 1974;16:248.

14. Andersson GB. Epidemiologic aspects of low back pain in industry. Spine 1981;6:53.

15. O'Sullivan JB. Gout in a New England town: A prevalence study in Sudbury, Massachusetts. Ann Rheum Dis 1972;31:166.

16. Masi AT. Clinical epidemiologic perspective of systemic lupus erythematosus. In: Lawrence RC, Shulman LE, eds. Epidemiology of the rheumatic diseases. New York: Gower, 1984:145.

17. Michet CJ Jr, McKenna CH, Elveback LR, et al. Epidemiology of systemic lupus erythematosus and other connective tissue diseases in Rochester, Minnesota, 1950 through 1979. Mayo Clin Proc 1985;60:105.

18. Hochberg MC, Lind MS, Sills EM. The prevalence and incidence of juvenile rheumatoid arthritis in an urban black population. Am J Public Health 1983;73:1202.

19. Standardized micro-data transcript. Hyattsville, Maryland: National Center for Health Statistics, 1978; DHEW publication no. (PHS)78-1213.

20. Gittelsohn AM. On the distribution of underlying causes of death. Am J Public Health 1982;72:133–40.

21. Siegel M, Lee SL. Epidemiology of systemic lupus erythematosus. Semin Arthritis Rheum 1973;3:1.

22. Hochberg MC, Lopez-Acena D, Gittelsohn AM. Mortality from systemic sclerosis (scleroderma) in the United States, 1969–1977. In: Myers AC, Black CM, eds: Proceedings of the International Conference on Progressive Sclerosis. New York: Gower, 1985:61–9.

23. Hochberg MC, Lopez-Acena D, Gittelsohn AM. Mortality from polymyositis and dermatomyositis in the United States, 1968–1978. Arthrit Rheum 1983;26:1465.

24. Haupt B. 1982 summary: National Hospital Discharge Survey. Hyattsville, Maryland: National Center for Health Statistics, 1983; DHHS publication no. (PHS)84-1250. (Vital and health statistics; no. 95).

25. Lawrence L, McLemore T. 1981 summary: National Ambulatory Medical Care Survey. Hyattsville, Maryland: National Center for Health Statistics, 1983. DHHS publication no. (PHS)83-1250. (Vital and health statistics, no. 88).

26. Knapp DA, Koch H. The management of new pain in office-based ambulatory care: National Ambulatory Medical Care Survey, 1980 and 1981. Hyattsville, Maryland: National Center for Health Statistics, 1984. DHHS publication no. (PHS)84-1250. (Vital and health statistics, no. 97).

27. Grazier KL, Holbrooks TL, Kelsey JL, et al. The frequency of occurence, impact and cost of musculoskeletal conditions in the United States. Chicago: American Academy of Orthopedic Surgeons, 1984:136.

28. Nuke G, Brooks R, Buchanan W. The economics of arthritis. Bull Rheum Dis 1973;23:726.

29. Rice DP. Scope and impact of chronic diseases in the United States. In: Public Policy & Chronic Disease, a Forum Sponsored by the National Arthritis Advisory Board. Hyattsville, Maryland: National Center for Health Statistics, 1979; DHEW publication no. (NIH)79-1896. (Vital and health statistics: 5–12).

30. Woolley H, Mushkin SJ, Smelker M, et al. Cost of disease and illness in the United States in the year 2000. Public Health Rep 1978;93:493.

31. Meenan R, Yelin E, Henke C, et al. The costs of rheumatoid arthritis. Arthritis Rheum 1978;21:827.

32. Meenan RF, Yelin EH, Newitt M, Epstein WV. The impact of chronic disease: A sociomedical profile of rheumatoid arthritis. Arthritis Rheum 1981;24:544.

33. Pincus T, Callahan LF, Sale WG, et al. Severe functional declines, work disability, and increased mortality in seventy-five rheumatoid arthritis patients studied over nine years. Arthritis Rheum 1984;27:864–72.

34. Michaels RM, Weiler NS. Transportation needs of the mobility-limited. Evanston, Illinois: Northwestern University, 1974.

35. Spergel P, Ehrlich GE, Glass D. The rheumatoid arthritis personality: A psychodiagnostic myth. Psychosomatics 1978;19:79.

36. Lanyon RI. A Handbook of MMPI Group Profiles. Minneapolis: University of Minnesota Press, 1968.

37. Chamberlain MA. Socioeconomic effects of ankylosing spondylitis in females: a comparison of 25 female with 25 male subjects. Int Rehab Med 1983;5:149.

38. Shulman LE, ed. Proceedings of the Prevention Conference on Arthritis. National Arthritis Advisory Board, 1983.

39. Kane WJ. School screening for scoliosis in the USA. In: Zorab PA, Siegler D, eds. Scoliosis 1979. London: Academic, 1980:35.

40. Edgar MH. Long term review of fused and unfused patients with adolescent idiopathic scoliosis. In: Zorab PA, Siegler D, eds. Scoliosis 1979, London: Academic, 1980:181.

41. Ford DK. Non-gonococcal urethritis and Reiter's syndrome: Personal experience with etiological studies during 15 years. Can Med Assoc J 1968;99:900.

42. Yelin E, Meenan R, Nevitt M, et al. Work disability in rheumatoid arthritis: Effects of disease, social and work factors. Ann Intern Med 1980;93:551.

43. Robinson HS, Walters K. Patterns of work—rheumatoid arthritis. Int Rehab Med 1978;1:121.

44. Nevitt MC, Epstein WV, Masem M, et al. Work disability before and after total hip arthroplasty: Assessment of effectiveness in reducing disability. Arthritis Rheum 1984;27:410.

45. Iskrant AP, Smith RW Jr. Osteoporosis in women 45 years and over related to subsequent fractures. Public Health Rep 1969;84:33.

Cancer

Richard Rothenberg, M.D., Philip Nasca, Ph.D.,
Jaromir Mikl, M.P.H., William Burnett, M.D., and
Barbara Reynolds, B.A.

Cancer mortality has increased approximately 250 percent over the past 50 years,[1] and the lifetime probability for developing cancer is now estimated to be one in three. In 1980, the year from which data for this study were drawn, there were an estimated 414,214 cancer deaths in the United States, and 807,364 new cases were diagnosed.

This study reviews the current literature on direct relationships between exposure to risk factors and development of disease in humans. Those data are augmented by reviews of laboratory and animal studies and by "ecologic" studies that compare aggregate population exposure rates with aggregate population disease rates. Finally, consensus estimates were used for ongoing assessment.

It is important to remember that cancer is not a homogeneous entity. In fact, the underlying process—some sort of loss of biological control—may be the only thing many cancers have in common. They are a diverse set of clinical and epidemiologic entities, not a single disease. In the Surveillance, Epidemiology, and End Results (SEER) report of the National Cancer Institute,[2] descriptions of 69 anatomic sites (corresponding to International Classification of Disease rubrics 140–208) are variously combined with 74 histologic types for a total of 1,346 cancer species.

Despite that diversity, a few tumors impose the major part of the public health burden. Four cancers (lung, breast, colon, and prostate) that include only two histologic types (squamous cell and adenocarcinoma) account for 50 percent of the cancers reported to the New York State Registry.[3] Fifteen types of tumors account for 80 percent of reported cases.

We first assessed all 1980 data and then attempted to gauge the central tendency of relative risk estimates reported in a number of studies. In order to do so, we selected studies in which a relative risk was calculated or calculable and examined the data, using a technique called exploratory data analysis.[4] This technique allowed us to define the middle 50 percent of the data for each study and therefore the general domain of the relative risk (RR) for each exposure (such as tobacco use or a specific industrial chemical).

That information was used to calculate the attributable risk (AR) and its range for each exposure according to the standard formula $AR = P_e (RR - 1)/1 + P_e (RR - 1)$.[5] The population exposure rate (P_e) was obtained either from standard source material or from the exposure level reported in control groups. This rate provided an estimate of the proportion of a specific cancer that could be attributed to a given exposure. A summary of the relative and attributable risks for 51 exposures related to these cancers is presented in Table 1.

MAJOR CANCER SITES

The nine major cancer sites chosen for this study—lung, colon, rectum, breast, cervix, pancreas, prostate, bladder, and larynx—accounted for approximately 60 percent of cancer deaths and 62 percent of new cancer cases in the United States in 1980. Information related to cancer incidence, mortality, hospitalization, hospital days, physician visits, years of life lost, hospital costs, physician visit costs, pharmaceutical costs, and institutional care costs was obtained from three sources: the New York State Cancer Registry,[3] the SEER[2] project of the National Cancer Institute, and the National Center for Health statistics (NCHS). A summary of these findings is presented in Table 2.

There are some gaps in data from those sources. The latest NCHS data concerning medical care utilization, for example, are for the years 1981 and 1982. The lack of data for 1980 creates some asymmetry with other base data, but it seems unlikely that the magnitude and direction of results are affected.

Note that the potential years of life lost is calcu-

From the Division of Epidemiology, New York State Department of Health, Albany. Dr. Rothenberg is now at the Centers for Disease Control, Atlanta.

Address reprint requests to Dr. Rothenberg, Centers for Disease Control, Atlanta, GA 30333.

Table 1. Relative and attributable risks for 51 exposures for the major cancer sites: International data from reports published through 1984

Disease	Risk	Number of published studies[a]	Relative risk median (fourth spread)	Estimated population exposure (P_e)	Attributable risk % (fourth spread)
Cervical cancer	Syphilis	2	3.57 (3.56–4.50)	.03[b]	7.2 (7.1–9.5)
	Age at first marriage <20 or 21	16	1.77 (1.67–2.42)		
	Two or more marriages	8	2.18 (1.91–2.80)		
	Onset of coitus <20	5	2.50 (1.89–2.78)		
	Onset of coitus <17	5	2.50 (1.90–3.42)	.275	29.2 (19.8–40.0)
	Two or more sex partners	6	2.76 (2.43–3.68)	.564	49.8 (44.6–60.2)
	Broken marriage	6	2.31 (1.36–3.20)		
	Extramarital sex				
	husband	4	3.80 (3.06–5.51)		
	wife	4	1.77 (1.37–2.43)		
	HSV2	23			
	dysplasia		1.48 (1.27–2.78)	.26	11.1 (6.6–31.6)
	CIS		3.78 (1.88–5.23)		42.0 (18.6–52.4)
	invasive		4.40 (2.03–10.33)		46.9 (21.1–70.8)
	Smoking	13			
	dysplasia		2.32 (1.47–2.67)	.296	28.1 (12.2–33.1)
	CIS		2.27 (1.91–3.32)		27.3 (21.2–40.7)
	invasive		2.07 (1.46–3.75)		24.1 (12.0–44.9)
	Oral contraceptives				
	CIS and dysplasia	14	1.06 (1.30–2.00)	.41	19.7 (11.0–29.1)
Bladder cancer	Smoking (ever versus never)	13			
	males		2.90 (2.05–3.51)	.337	39.0 (26.1–45.8)
	females		1.66 (0.90–2.50)	.298	16.4 (0.0–0.8)
	Coffee drinking (<1 cup/day versus 1+ cups)	13			
	males		1.48 (1.35–1.70)	.814	28.1 (22.2–36.3)
	females		1.30 (1.00–1.90)	.787	19.1 (0.0–41.5)
	Occupation (high-risk occupation versus general population risk)				
	males (<60 years)	13	3.15		23.0 (18.0–33.0)
Pancreatic cancer	Smoking	14	2.10 (1.77–2.60)	.316	25.8 (19.6–33.6)
	High-fat diet	2	2.21	.261	24.0
	Diabetes	8			
	male		5.20 (2.10–8.98)	.0211	8.1 (2.3–14.4)
	female		2.80 (1.65–6.09)	.0259	4.5 (1.6–11.6)
	Coffee	7	1.35 (1.23–2.60)	.80	21.9 (15.5–56.1)
Laryngeal cancer	Cigarettes (ever versus never	16			
	male		9.85 (6.02–13.31)	.337	74.9 (62.8–80.6)
	female		9.0 (7.76–10.5)	.297	70.4 (66.8–73.8)
	Cigars, pipes (ever versus never; males only)	5	3.64 (1.40–7.28)	.1615	29.9 (06.1–50.4)
	Alcohol (more than occasional versus occasional or none)	11	3.26 (2.06–4.50)	.09	16.9 (08.7–24.0)
Lung cancer	Smoking	22	10.85 (4.35–16.0)	.316	75.7 (51.4–82.6)
	Radon	5	20.00 (13.98–24.0)	.006[c]	10.2 (07.2–12.1) (ARE = 95%)
	Asbestos	8	3.25 (2.44–5.19)	.011[c]	2.4 (01.6–04.4) (ARE = 69%)
	Arsenic	11	3.36 (2.65–5.3)	.0024[c]	0.5 (00.4–01.0) (ARE = 70%)
	Chromates	4	14.59 (3.60–37.97)	.011[c]	13.0 (02.8–28.9) (ARE = 93%)
	Coke	15	2.27 (1.97–2.70)	.005[c]	0.6 (0.5–0.8) (ARE = 51.5%)

Table 1. Continued

Disease	Risk	Number of published studies[a]	Relative risk median (fourth spread)	Estimated population exposure (P_e)	Attributable risk % (fourth spread)
Breast cancer	Race (white versus nonwhite)	3	1.19	.83	13.6
	Religion	3			
	Jewish/Catholic		1.14	.0273	0.4
	Jewish/Protestant		1.08	.0273	0.2
	Urban/rural	7	1.27 (1.14–1.37)	.745	16.7 (9.4–21.6)
	Marital status (never versus ever married)	8	1.39 (1.31–1.42)	.052	2.0 (1.6–02.1)
	Benign breast disease (ever versus never)	10	2.61 (1.58–2.90)	.089	12.5 (4.9–14.5)
	Socioeconomic status (12+ years education versus <12 years)	11	1.35 (1.17–1.46)	.681	19.2 (10.4–23.9)
	Age at menarche (age <13 years versus 13+ years)	12	1.17 (0.93–1.57)	.374	6.0 (0.0–17.6)
	Age at natural menopause (age 50+ years versus <50 years)	8	1.37 (1.26–1.39)	.593	18.0 (13.4–18.8)
	Oophorectomy (bilateral) age <40 years)	5	0.27 (0.25–0.36)		d
	Age first pregnancy (age 20+ yr versus <20 yr)	20	1.64 (1.19–1.81)	.649	29.3 (11.0–34.5)
	Nulliparity (yes versus no)	14	2.46 (1.85–3.15)	.182	21.0 (13.4–28.1)
	Prior tumor	7			
	Ovary (yes versus no)		2.45 (1.80–3.55)	.0017	0.2 (0.1–00.4)
	Uterus (yes versus no)		1.40 (1.34–1.50)	.00026	0.0
	Family history (mother or sister versus neither)				
	Young	7	3.15 (2.49–4.56)	.048	9.4 (6.7–14.6)
	Middle age	7	2.28 (1.72–2.49)	.048	5.8 (3.3–6.7)
	Older	8	1.70 (1.24–2.34)	.048	3.3 (1.1–6.0)
	Weight (>60 kg versus <60 kg)	8	1.64 (1.27–2.29)	.6733	30.0 (15.4–46.5)[e]
	Radiation	12	2.69 (2.22–3.92)	f	
Colorectal cancer	Beer	4	1.88 (1.37–2.53)	.05	4.2 (1.8–7.1)
	Cruciferi	1	3.00	.412	45.2
	Cholecystectomy	5	1.70 (1.40–1.90)	g	
Prostatic cancer	Benign prostatic hypertrophy	6	2.65 (1.76–4.50)	.55	47.6 (29.5–65.8)
	Cadmium oxide	6	3.50 (1.70–5.75)	.00004	0 (ARE = 71%)
	Family history	5	3.92 (2.46–5.38)	.04	10.5 (5.5–14.8)

[a] References are listed in original paper, available from the Carter Presidential Library. Each reference may have provided more than one observation of RR.
[b] Historical; current P_e approximately 0.
[c] Based on the total number of industrial workers *potentially* exposed. This is probably an overestimate of those actually exposed to the agent. A total of 26.7 percent AR for all these exposures would appear prima facie on the high side. The range is 12.5–47.2 percent. At the lower end, it may not be unreasonable to attribute 75 percent of lung cancer to smoking and 10–15 percent to these particular occupational exposures. (Information on joint exposure with smoking is not available.)
[d] Protective factor–AR not calculated.
[e] AR in postmenopausal women only.
[f] P_e not available.
[g] Older age groups.

lated by multiplying the number of cancer deaths in an age interval by the difference between the mid-point of that interval and age 65. This yields the years of working life lost, not the total number of years lost. This approach gives proportionally greater weight to diseases that affect young people. Using age 65 as a cutoff point implies that the older a person is at onset of disease, the less the years of

Table 2. Health impact of major cancers, United States, 1980

Cancer Sites	Number of deaths (1980)	Number of years lost before the age of 65	Number of hospital days	Cost (millions of dollars)[a]
Lung	88,459	334,213	3,357	1,598
Colon	46,418	110,455 ⎫	3,225	915
Rectum	10,804	27,273 ⎭		386
Breast	37,518	217,270	2,243	1,265
Cervix	5,457	39,133	565	179
Pancreas	22,988	61,498	524	244
Prostate	22,572	12,650	1,339	519
Bladder	11,000	14,228	482	409
Larynx	3,449	12,475	268	240
				(+281)[b]
Total	248,665	829,195	12,003	6,036
% of all cancer	60	47	57	44

Data from National Cancer Institute[2] and New York State Cancer Registry.[3]
[a] Includes hospital care, physician visits, pharmaceutical costs, and home care.
[b] Nursing home care not included in the individual costs.

life lost "count." The social choice implicit in this method must be kept in mind when assessing the overall costs of cancer.

In this section we describe briefly the most important risk associated with the nine specific cancers selected for study. Figures for relative and attributable risks represent the median values from the studies reviewed.

Exposures implicated in the occurrence of each cancer are considered suitable targets for intervention if (1) there is convincing biologic, clinical, ecologic, and epidemiologic evidence of the exposure's effect; (2) we could evaluate the attributable risk in terms of the strength of the association between exposure and disease and the degree of population exposure; (3) an intervention program would be feasible; (4) proposed interventions would not produce negative effects that would outweigh their benefits. In making our final recommendations, we also considered which exposures affect multiple cancer sites and which may also constitute risks for other leading causes of morbidity and mortality.

Lung

Lung cancer accounts for 15–25 percent of all cancer, 22 percent in men and 8 percent in women. Mortality and incidences have risen dramatically since 1940 for both sexes, but especially for women. Lung cancer mortality rates for women increased by 276 percent between 1952 and 1979, compared with a 167 percent increase for men. That difference in rate increase is unanimously attributed to increasing tobacco consumption by women since 1955. If current trends continue, the mortality rate for lung cancer among women will exceed the rate for breast cancer by the late 1980s.

There has not been a substantial change in the five-year survival rate for lung cancer in the past 20 years, although a slight upward trend has been evident.[6] The five-year survival rate in 1940 was 4 percent; today it is 9 percent.

Smokers have an RR of 10.9 for developing cancer of the lung when compared with nonsmokers (according to 27 studies). Various authors have attributed 83–85 percent of all lung cancers among men and 43 percent of all lung cancers among women to smoking.[7,8] In addition, smoking is recognized as the major risk factor for coronary heart disease, chronic obstructive pulmonary disease, and a variety of other cancers discussed in this paper.

An overwhelming body of evidence implicates smoking in the etiology of lung cancer. In addition, a number of occupational exposures to specific substances have been closely linked to carcinoma of the lung. Such substances include asbestos, arsenic, radon, chromates, and coke oven emissions. In many cases, the risk conferred by those exposures is augmented in persons who also smoke.

Of all environmental or occupational factors, asbestos is probably the most significant. Approximately 2.5 million workers, or 1.1 percent of the U.S. population, were exposed to asbestos in 1981. Work sites where asbestos has been studied include schools and shipyards. The carcinogenicity of asbestos has been documented through numerous studies, and there is evidence that both the duration and the degree of exposure increase the risk for developing cancer of the lung. The effects of asbestos exposure are estimated to be eight to nine times greater in workers who also smoke.

Approximately 1.5 million workers are exposed to arsenic, 95 percent of which is produced as a byproduct of copper and lead ore smelting. There is some controversy about whether arsenic itself elevates the risk for lung cancer or other factors found in the same working environments are at fault. On the average, researchers have found an RR of 3.4 for people who are exposed to arsenic.

There have been only a few studies of the effects of radon, a radioactive gas released by radium in the soil. The RRs vary considerably from study to study, perhaps because of lack of information about smoking history and accurate exposure records, as well as other study limitations. But the low value of 6.5 and the high value of 50 indicate that radon may be a significant risk factor for lung cancer.

Occupational disease associated with chromates has been reported since 1827, when skin disorders were observed among workers exposed to potassium bichromate. Today, approximately 2.5 million workers in the United States are potentially exposed to chromium compounds. Evidence that chromates are linked to cancer of the lung has been found in several human studies, although none of those studies has controlled for smoking status. The median RR is 20, which is high enough to suggest that smoking does not account for all the carcinogenicity observed.

Coke oven emissions consist of a number of potentially carcinogenic gases and particles. In 1978 more than 400,000 workers were employed by 4,400 foundries in the United States, and the RR for lung cancer is estimated to be between 2 and 10.

Interventions aimed at reducing or eliminating unnecessary deaths from lung cancer clearly should target two groups: cigarette smokers and industrial workers who are exposed to hazardous substances. Tobacco consumers are by far the larger and more diverse group. Although smaller numbers of people are subject to occupational exposure, their concentration in a smaller number of industries makes them easy to identify.

Colon and Rectum

Cancer of the lower gastrointestinal tract, from cecum to anus, is the most common neoplastic disease in the United States; in 1980 the number of cases was estimated at 120,438.[2] It is a disease for which the incidence has been increasing while the mortality has remained constant, indicating that advances in diagnosis and treatment have not been matched by improvements in risk identification and reduction.

It is only logical that the bulk of research has been focused on the role of diet, yet despite that emphasis, data on humans are only now emerging. Three generalizations can be drawn from research concerning diet and the risk of colorectal cancer.

First, good ecologic correlations have been found between consumption of both fat and meat and the risk of colon cancer.[9] Second, several plausible biologic hypotheses relate diet to colon cancer:

1. Bile salts, which appear to be increased in patients who have colon cancer, may promote tumor growth when modified by intestinal flora.[10]

2. Indole-containing cruciferous vegetables may inhibit carcinogenesis by inducing arylhydrocarbon hydroxylase activity.[11]

3. Vitamin A influences cell differentiation and acts as an antioxidant.[12]

Third, although some studies suggest important relationships between dietary factors and colorectal cancer, these relationships are often contradictory. As an example, ecologic comparisons have shown higher rates of cancer in geographic areas where high-fat, high-protein diets are eaten than in areas where they are not.[12] Case control studies, however, have generated conflicting findings.

For reasons that are not biologically clear, the consumption of beer has been a fairly consistent risk factor for rectal cancer. According to the most carefully constructed investigation, a prospective study by Pollack et al.,[13] heavy beer drinkers (15 liters or more per month) incurred an RR of 3.

Other events and exposures have also been scrutinized as potential risks for colorectal cancer. Of these, only prior cholecystectomy seems to confer a definite risk, and that is an RR of 1.7 for right-sided colon cancer after surgery.[14] Isolated clusters of colorectal cancer have been reported among wood and carpet workers, but the significance of those observations is unknown. Radiation exposures, source of drinking water, and genetic endowment have all been postulated as factors in the development of colorectal cancer, but none has been satisfactorily explored.

At least one researcher has hypothesized that indole-containing vegetables may protect against the development of colorectal cancer. As noted earlier, there is a plausible biologic pathway through which this may occur. According to a study conducted in Buffalo,[15] an increased risk was associated with lower consumption of cruciferous vegetables: an RR of 3 for persons who never eat them, in comparison with those who eat them more than once a week.

Dietary fiber has also been proposed as a protection against colorectal cancer.[16] Although the hypothesis is attractive, it has yet to be demonstrated in human studies.

The consensus of current estimates attributes approximately 20 percent of colorectal cancer to dietary factors (P. Greenwald, unpublished observations, 1984), but that figure may rise as research results emerge. The highest AR that can be calculated from current information is conferred by the absence of cruciferous vegetables in the diet, and it suggests that meaningful intervention is possible through dietary change.

Breast

Breast cancer is the most common form of cancer among women in the United States, and a woman's lifetime risk for developing cancer of the breast is estimated at 7.2 percent.[17] Over the years, breast cancer incidence rates have shown a slow but steady increase, while mortality has remained fairly constant.

Considerable epidemiologic effort has been devoted to delineating risk factors for cancer of the breast. Most of these have been sociodemographic (e.g., race, religion, geographic location, marital status, socioeconomic status) or related to reproductive and family history (e.g., age at first pregnancy, oophorectomy, parity, age at menopause, disease in a mother or sister). Although some strong associations have been observed, these risk factors are not subject to easy elimination or modification by preventive efforts.

Other possible risk factors for cancer of the breast include benign breast disease, obesity, high-fat diet, and exogenous estrogens such as oral contraceptive and hormone replacement preparations prescribed for menopausal women.

A history of fibrocystic disease (benign breast disease) is associated with a two- to fourfold increase in risk for breast cancer.[18] Recent data suggest that the risk may vary with the type of lesions observed and with the interaction between fibrocystic disease and chemicals, including oral contraceptives, menopausal estrogens, and hair dyes.

Various studies have examined the possible relationship between body size and the risk of breast cancer, and the most consistent relationship has been observed among postmenopausal women.[19] In general, women who weigh more than 60 kg (132 lbs) have approximately twice the risk of lighter women. Additional research is needed to clarify the relative importance of body type, obesity due to dietary habits, and the relative contributions of fat and muscle to total weight in high-risk women.

Prior exposure to high doses of radiation, which has been observed in atomic bomb survivors and women who have undergone radiation therapy,[20] conveys a substantially increased risk for cancer of the breast. Because so few women have undergone such exposure, the impact of this risk on breast cancer incidence appears to be small.

Data from numerous animal studies show that high-fat diets enhance or promote the development of mammary cancer after tumor growth has been initiated by chemicals or x-rays. These experiments also suggest that intake of fat, rather than of total calories, is the important factor in cancer development.

The significance of these findings for humans is as yet unclear. Several case-control studies have shown positive associations between dietary fat and breast cancer risk; ecologic comparisons have shown a strong association between breast cancer rates and dietary fat. Current estimates attribute perhaps 20 percent of breast cancer to dietary fat.

Exogenous estrogens may play a part in breast cancer risk. To date, there is not enough evidence to support either a putative or a protective role for oral contraceptives. However, several studies have suggested that certain subgroups of women (e.g., who have a history of benign breast disease, a family history of breast cancer, or no children, or who began using oral contraceptives before bearing children) may be at increased risk for breast cancer when exposed to oral contraceptives. Other studies have not confirmed those observations. The relationship between estrogen preparations given to menopausal women and breast cancer risk is even less certain, and conflicting findings resemble those for oral contraceptives.

As mentioned, the best-known risk factors for breast cancer—such as family and reproductive history—cannot be changed to prevent the disease. Furthermore, the low AR associated with each factor or group of factors does not appear to justify their use as selection criteria for directed screening programs.

If additional research demonstrates a strong connection between dietary fat intake and breast cancer risk, primary interventions could then be directed at modifying dietary patterns. Despite the current lack of convincing proof, the National Academy of Science has issued interim guidelines recommending that Americans reduce their dietary fat intake from 40 percent of total calories to 30 percent.

In addition, as much as a 30 percent decrease in breast cancer mortality may be possible through secondary prevention programs,[21] including widespread breast self-examination, clinical breast examination, and mammography.

Cervix

Early studies of cervical carcinoma implicated sexually transmitted disease, specifically syphilis,[22] and sexual behavior as risk factors. More recent work, both in clinical epidemiology and molecular genetics, has suggested that herpesvirus type 2 (HSV2) and genital warts caused by human papillomavirus (HPV) may also play important roles in the disease.[23] In addition, cigarette smoking[24] and oral contraceptive use,[25] particularly if exposure takes place at a young age, appear to be independent risk factors for cancer of the cervix.

Much current research focuses on the interrelationship of those risk factors. It is possible that several risk factors may act together to initiate and promote cancerous changes in the cervix, but how this might come about is not yet known.

The evidence is mounting that HSV2 infection brings about changes in cervical tissue that may be associated with carcinoma. It seems clear that HSV2 is capable of transforming cells, but the virus cannot be unequivocally implicated in the occurrence of cervical cancer. Its role may eventually be explained as that of an initiator, promoter, mutagen, or cocarcinogen in the presence of another risk factor.

A link between HPV, which produces genital warts, and cervical cancer is now emerging. One careful microscopic analysis demonstrated the presence of HPV in 73 of 80 patients who had cervical neoplasia, compared with 10 of 80 matched controls.[26] Some investigators have speculated that HPV may help promote cancer after carcinogenic events have been initiated by other factors such as HSV2 or smoking.[27]

Smoking is the best-described risk factor for cervical cancer. The majority of studies have shown that women who smoke have an RR of 2.1–2.3; the RR is 4.8 for those who began smoking at the age of 15 or earlier. The increased risk for early age of exposure indicates that smoking exerts a preferential effect on youthful cervical tissue.

Since their introduction in 1960, steroid contraceptives have been investigated as a possible risk factor for diseases of the female reproductive tract. Researchers have been troubled by problems defining exposure to risk; it is often difficult to determine the consistency and duration of use and the exact steroid preparation used. Another difficulty is evaluating oral contraceptive use in the context of age, socioeconomic status, ethnicity, number of sex partners, age at first coitus, HSV2 infection, smoking, and other risk factors associated with cervical carcinoma.

At least six studies have demonstrated that duration of oral contraceptive use is a factor in development of cervical cancer; three studies, however, have found no such association. A few researchers theorize that what looks like an increased risk of cervical cancer among users of oral contraceptives

may actually be the protective effects of diaphragm use among the women chosen for comparison. In any event, the strong biologic action that oral contraceptives exert on other hormonally sensitive sites indicates to us that we need to know more about their role in cancer of the cervix.

Although our knowledge of risk factors for cervical tumors continues to grow, we have no primary interventions to prevent the development of the disease. We recommend efforts to alter personal behavior concerning the use of tobacco and oral contraceptives.

Fortunately, secondary prevention has a well-established and valuable role in carcinoma of the cervix. An estimated 10–20 percent of invasive cancer of the cervix may be prevented by secondary intervention in the form of widespread Papanicolaou testing (Pap smear). For the past 30 years, invasive cancer of the cervix has been declining in proportion to cancer in situ (which is confined to one place and easier to remove surgically). Although there is some controversy about its cause, many observers attribute this shift to early detection by Pap smear screening.

Pancreas

After having been on the rise for three decades, cancer of the pancreas is now the fourth leading cause of cancer deaths in the United States. It is responsible for 20,000–23,000 deaths per year, or more than 6 percent of all cancer deaths.

Cancer of the pancreas has perhaps the bleakest prognosis of any of the major tumors: the 5-year survival rate has been estimated at 1–3 percent.[6] Short survival, coupled with a cryptic clinical syndrome, has made it difficult to define the etiology of the disease. By the time pancreatic cancer is diagnosed, 90 percent of cases exhibit regional node metastases, and 80 percent have liver metastases.

Four main risk factors—smoking, diabetes, coffee consumption, and a high-fat diet—have been associated with pancreatic cancer in several case-control and prospective studies.

Prospective studies have shown that a person who smokes has close to twice the risk of developing cancer of the pancreas, and estimates of disease attributable to smoking range from 23 to 68 percent. In addition, smokers tend to be diagnosed as having pancreatic cancer about ten years earlier than nonsmokers.

It is not particularly surprising to find that diabetes, which affects the pancreas, appears to be associated with carcinoma of that organ. Diabetic women, when compared with nondiabetic controls, have an RR for pancreatic cancer of approximately

2.8; the comparable figure for men is 5.2. More study is needed, however, to understand the temporal and causal relationships between the two diseases.

Preliminary evidence from the few studies that have focused on the possible relationship between high dietary fat intake and pancreatic cancer suggests than a high-fat diet may increase the risk two-fold. If those findings are confirmed, the AR for a high-fat diet may be in excess of 25 percent—comparable to the risk conferred by cigarette smoking.

Several studies have found no association between coffee drinking and pancreatic cancer; others have reported that coffee consumption may produce an RR of 1.4. Most of the studies so far have suggested that the amount of coffee consumed does relate to the development of cancer of the pancreas. As is true of bladder cancer, the potential importance of observations about coffee as a risk factor is magnified by the estimate that 80 percent of the people in the United States drink coffee.

Again, the most accessible intervention point appears to be promoting smoking cessation programs for persons who smoke and preventing the onset of smoking among young people.

Prostate

Cancer of the prostate is the second leading cause of cancer deaths in American men and was responsible for an estimated 25,000 deaths in 1984. It accounts for approximately 15 percent of tumors in men and more than 90 percent of all male genital cancers.

The incidence and mortality of prostatic cancer increase with age; only 1.1 percent of all cases occur in men younger than 50 years of age. Both incidence and mortality rates are higher in black men than in whites. Five-year survival rates for cancer of the prostate have improved steadily for the past 40 years, and prognosis is most favorable for patients whose carcinoma is localized within the prostatic region. More than 50 percent of all cases are diagnosed as localized, and the five-year survival rate for those tumors is 64–68 percent, compared with 52–56 percent for less localized tumors.

Numerous possible risk factors for prostatic cancer have been studied, yet the etiology of the disease is largely unknown. Controversial risk factors include HSV2, sexual and venereal disease history, marital status, and a high-fat diet. We will focus here on three factors that appear significant: family history, prostatic hyperplasia, and occupational exposure to cadmium oxide.

A wide range of RRs has been calculated for men who have a family history of prostate cancer; the median risk has been calculated as 3.9. When a distinction between close and distant relatives has been made, the risk has consistently been greater if cancer has occurred in close relatives such as siblings or fathers.

Benign prostatic hyperplasia (BPH) is the most common nonmalignant tumor among American men, and it is estimated that more than 50 percent of all men older than 50 years of age have some form of BPH. Like prostatic cancer, the prevalence of BPH increases with age and is higher among black men. Yet the issue of BPH as a risk factor for cancer of the prostate remains controversial: Several authors have reported a strong association between the two; others have found no association. The RR calculated by the researchers who have found an association is 2.7.

Interest in cadmium oxide exposure as a risk for prostatic cancer has been high since 1963, when one researcher found an excessive number of deaths from the disease among workers in a battery factors.[28] More recent research has observed an RR of 3.5 among workers exposed to cadmium oxide in the workplace. Although a significant RR, it has little impact on the overall incidence of prostate cancer because so few workers are exposed.

Neither family history nor benign prostatic hypertrophy is amenable to change through primary prevention efforts. The risks associated with both, however, might be diminished through screening programs. Cadmium oxide exposure is a primary risk that could be reduced through organized efforts to make workplaces less hazardous. That risk could be grouped with other occupational risks for other cancers and addressed as part of a larger prevention program for the workplace.

Bladder

Cigarette smoking has been firmly established as a cause of bladder cancer in men (RR, 2.9) and in women (RR, 1.7). Several investigators have estimated that 39–78 percent of bladder cancer in men can be attributed to cigarette smoking; the comparable figure for women has been estimated at 17–29 percent. Other studies have indicated that there is a relationship between the number of cigarettes smoked and the likelihood of developing cancer of the bladder. Data concerning filter cigarettes are inconsistent: one study found a decreased risk in filter cigarette smokers and one showed no difference.

Occupational exposure to chemicals such as aniline dyes confers an overall risk of 3.2; again, the RR seems to be higher for men than for women. Estimates of the AR for men employed in hazardous occupations range from 18 to 35 percent and appear to vary with age. Among women, only 1–6 percent of bladder cancers can be attributed to high-risk occupations. Having reviewed extensive and complicated data concerning occupational exposure and bladder cancer, we have adopted 23 percent as the proportion of bladder cancer that can be attributed to occupation.

Coffee drinking has been suspected of playing a part in development of bladder tumors, but studies attempting to clarify its role have so far only confused the issue. Although the estimated risks of coffee drinking are small, they could be magnified by the fact that so many Americans drink coffee.

Other factors such as artificial sweeteners, hair dyes, drug use, and diet have been investigated as possible contributors to bladder cancer. None of these has been consistently shown to be related to bladder cancer risk, but we should continue to investigate the possibility that specific subgroups may be at special risk because of personal habits or occupational exposure.

In the meantime, it is clear that the focus of primary intervention for bladder cancer should be encouraging people to give up cigarette smoking and minimizing the exposure to hazardous chemicals in the workplace.

Larynx

Laryngeal cancer is considerably more common in men than in women; the age-adjusted incidence rate for men is 8.5 per 100,000, compared with 1.3 per 100,000 for women. The sex differentials hold true regardless of race. In general, laryngeal cancer incidence and mortality tend to be higher among blacks than among whites, among lower socioeconomic groups, and among urban populations. The patterns probably reflect differences in smoking, alcohol consumption, and occupational exposures rather than true demographic differences. Smoking and heavy alcohol consumption have been clearly implicated in the development of cancer of the larynx. In addition, these two risk factors appear to have a synergistic effect.[29]

Numerous studies have shown cigarette smoking to be the single most important risk factor for laryngeal cancer. The RRs for smokers compared with nonsmokers range from 2.4 to 24.6. There is a linear dose–response relationshp between the number of cigarettes smoked and the RR for the disease, and that relationship appears stronger for people who smoke unfiltered cigarettes than for those who smoke filtered cigarettes.

Heavy alcohol consumption has also repeatedly been shown to be a risk factor for development of laryngeal cancer. Here, too, there is a relationship between the quantity of alcohol consumed and the RR for cancer.

Combined exposure to cigarette smoking and alcohol use seems to confer the greatest relative risk. An RR of 14 was observed for the highest level of smoking after controlling for alcohol use, and a risk of 2.2 was seen for the highest level of alcohol use after controlling for smoking. Subjects who were in the highest exposure categories for both smoking and alcohol consumption had an RR of 22.1, far greater than that for either risk taken alone.

Occupational exposures have also been investigated as risk factors for cancer of the larynx. An increased laryngeal cancer rate has consistently been reported for men whose occupations exposed them to asbestos. Isolating the effects of asbestos exposure has proved difficult, however, because asbestos effects tend to occur in subjects who are also exposed to cigarettes. Work site exposure to other substances, such as nickel and wood dust, may also prove important upon further investigation.

The most provocative recent finding suggests that certain dietary elements may protect against laryngeal cancer. Graham et al.[30] found that men whose diets were low in vitamin A or C had a twofold increased risk for cancer of the larynx in comparison with men whose diets contained large amounts of those vitamins. A dose–response relationship was also observed between laryngeal cancer risk and both vitamins. Those relationships held when the study was controlled for the effects of both smoking and drinking.

The clear roles of smoking, drinking, and the combination of the two in the development of laryngeal cancer provide clear targets for intervention. The ameliorative effects would be most apparent in men, who bear the brunt of this disease. We might be able to further reduce the incidence of cancer of the larynx if we knew more about the possible protective effects of vitamins A and C, an inquiry that seems deserving of more study.

INTERVENTIONS

This review of cancer epidemiology details only a small portion of the ongoing search for risk factors and etiology. In our discussions of cancer sites we have referred to various primary and secondary prevention strategies. At this point we will enlarge on what we mean by prevention and describe interventions that we believe can help reduce the mortality rate of cancer.

Primary prevention refers to measures that do not permit the disease to develop in the first place. *Sec-*

ondary prevention, in the case of cancer, usually means early detection in order to prevent more advanced stages of the disease.

Risks may not be subject to intervention for one or more of the following reasons: there is inadequate proof that a suspected risk leads to the disease in question; the association is strong, but only a very few people are exposed; an intervention program is not feasible, either in terms of implementation or effectiveness; the intervention may have negative health or social consequences that must be considered.

There are, however, a substantial number of risks and potential interventions that should be considered as we attempt to close the cancer gap.

Risk Factors Amenable to Intervention

The risks for seven cancers that should be amenable to public health intervention are listed in Table 3. The conclusion that smoking, alcohol, and occupational exposure to carcinogens are principal factors in cancer deaths should come as no surprise to anyone. Those three risks accounted for approximately 17 percent of all cancer cases in 1980. Smoking alone accounted for 11 percent. Acting alone, alcohol appears to be a powerful carcinogen only for cancer of the larynx. Its more sweeping importance may be its interaction with tobacco. None of the occupational exposures, examined in isolation, appears to reach a substantial part of the population, and their ARs are small. Each, however,

has an enormous AR in those who are exposed, and it would make sense to group them together on a short list of targeted carcinogens in the workplace.

When we say that 17 percent of all cancers in the U.S. in 1980 could be attributed to those three risk factors, we must note that no intervention program can make 136,494 cases of cancer disappear. No deus ex machina will eliminate a risk all at once. The process is gradual, and its effects are even more so. There is a lag of years, even decades, between reduction of a risk and a change in cancer incidence. The important point here is that the figure of 17 percent measures the gap that must be closed: it is the potential for reducing cancer by reducing smoking, alcohol consumption, and a specific group of occupational exposures.

Diet: A Special Case.

There is a steady stream of new data suggesting a strong connection between diet and various forms of cancer. Doll and Peto proposed that 35 percent of all cancer may be attributed to diet.[31] But by no means is all the evidence in. Our concern is that delaying public health interventions until we can prove that diet causes cancer may mean missing a prime opportunity for disease prevention.

Ecologic studies correlating meat and fat consumption with breast and colon cancer in various populations provide by far the most impressive data concerning the diet and cancer link. The National Cancer Institute's review of dietary fat and breast cancer suggests that the RR is 1.5–2 for

Table 3. Health impact of major cancers amenable to intervention, United States, 1980

Cancer sites	Risk factor (AR %)	Number of deaths (1980)	Number of years lost before the age of 65	Number of hospital days (hundred thousands)	Cost (millions of dollars)[a]
Lung	Smoking (75.9)	67,140	253,667	2,548	1,213
	Occupation (12)	10,615	40,106	403	192
Colorectal	Diet (20)	11,444	27,546	645	260
Breast	Diet (20)	7,504	43,454	449	253
Cervix	Smoking (24.1)	1,320	9,431	136	43
Pancreas	Smoking (25.8)	5,931	15,866	135	63
Bladder	Smoking (39.0 M)				
	(16.4 F)	4,347	4,513	153	131
	Occupation (23)	2,530	3,272	111	94
Larynx	Smoking (74)	2,552	9,232	198	178
	Alcohol (16.9)	583	2,108	45	41
Totals		113,966	409,195	4,823	2,468
% of all cancers		28	23	23	18

[a] Includes hospital care, physician visits, pharmaceuticals, and home care.

women whose diets are high in fat. In another important and as yet unpublished study, convincing relationships between dietary fat and a number of tumors, including colon, breast, and lung, have emerged. The epidemiologic data reviewed here suggest a relationship between the low consumption of cruciferous vegetables and dietary fiber and the development of colorectal cancer. In addition, the strong association between beer consumption and rectal cancer has been well-documented. At least 23 major studies of diet and cancer are now in process, all seeking direct evidence of the connection through case control of cohort analyses.

The consensus of current estimates is that 20 percent of colorectal and breast cancer could be prevented if our nation's eating habits could be changed. The actual proportion of some cancers attributable to diet may be much higher; Doll and Peto,[31] for example, estimated that 90 percent of colorectal cancer may be related to diet.

If we adopt a conservative approach and do not attempt to modify dietary habits because all the evidence is not yet clear, we may be permitting a large number of preventable deaths.

Secondary Prevention

The ultimate goal of cancer research is the primary prevention of most forms of cancer. This goal can be achieved only when basic and applied research provides a more complete understanding of cancer etiology and only when we have a better understanding of how to apply that knowledge to the general population. In the interim, secondary prevention can play an important part in closing the cancer gap.

Screening programs are based on the assumption that treating cancer in the early, symptomless stage is more effective than treating more advanced disease. Current scientific evidence indicates that the wider application of available screening techniques can significantly reduce the number of deaths attributable to breast, cervical, and colorectal cancers.

SUMMARY

At least 23 percent of current cancer incidence can be attributed to four important risk factors: smoking, alcohol use, a high-fat diet, and occupational exposure to carcinogens. We estimate that those risk factors account for 113,966 cancer deaths annually (27.5 percent of total cancer mortality), 409,195 years of life lost before age 65, 4,823,000 days of hospitalization, and close to $3 billion in direct health care costs. The estimates have been derived from our study of nine cancer sites: lung, colon, rectum, breast, cervix, pancreas, prostate, bladder, and larynx.

The incidence of tumors of these nine sites, which represent almost two thirds of all cancer, would be reduced by 27 percent if risks from smoking, alcohol use, and occupational exposure were eliminated. The primary sites affected would be the bladder, pancreas, larynx, and lung. In addition, the consensus is that approximately 20 percent of breast and colon cancer would be eliminated if Americans ate less fat and more cruciferous and retinoid-containing vegetables.

The total number of carcinomas attributable to smoking, alcohol, dietary factors, and occupational exposure to carcinogens (182,868), divided by the total number of cancers for 1980 (807,364), yields the figure of 23 percent. This figure represents the minimum percentage of cancer incidence that could be eliminated if those risks were removed. It might be possible to reduce cancer incidence even further if we could address additional risk factors and tumor sites and the possible interaction between risk factors.

Reduction or elimination of specific risk factors is one way of substantially reducing the incidence of cancer. Additional reduction in disease can be brought about through secondary prevention efforts such as early screening and detection programs. For example, a 30 percent decrease in mortality from cancer of the female breast may be attributed to screening by breast self-examination, physician examination, and mammography. Routine cervical cytology screening (Pap smear) may be responsible for preventing 10–22 percent of deaths from cervical cancer. Although accurate estimates are not available for colorectal disease, it awaits confirmation that periodic screening can yield substantial benefits for those tumors as well.

Even though the risks identified here are part of a complex social and economic fabric, there is real potential for effective intervention. For example, consider the economics of cigarette smoking. It has been asserted that a 10 percent rise in price would decrease demand by 4 percent.[32] Another researcher has calculated that doubling the federal excise tax on cigarettes would prevent an estimated 1.5 million adults and 0.7 million teenagers from smoking.[33] The effects of less global strategies, such as counteradvertising or behavior modification, are more difficult to assess.

Interventions aimed at reducing occupational and environmental exposure to specific carcinogens would most likely follow a similar pattern: legislative change, coupled with personal and managerial behavior modification. But those efforts must overcome the inertia from the tremendous social and financial investment of corporation and of individual workers.

Clearly, there are options for intervention, and presumably the array of interventions will increase with increased knowledge of cancer. The risk factors emphasized in this report—smoking, alcohol, dietary habits, and occupational exposures—are attractive targets for action because the benefits of intervention will extend to other human diseases as well. But because these risk factors are woven into the fabric of our lives, we must also look at proposed interventions in their social, economic, and demographic context. Our current understanding of risks for cancer leads us to estimate that effective intervention could eliminate one quarter to one third of the current disease burden.

The authors would like to extend their special thanks to the following individuals who contributed to the development of this review: Patricia Wolfgang, Paul Buckley, Marjory Simmons, Robert Durlak, Patricia Farmer, and Trudi Harris.

REFERENCES

1. Devesa SS, Schneiderman MA. Increase in the number of cancer deaths in the United States. Am J Epidemiol 1977;106:1–5.

2. Surveillance, epidemiology, and end results: incidence and mortality data, 1973–1977. Bethesda, Maryland: National Cancer Institute, 1981; DHHS publication no. (NIH)81-2330.

3. Burnett W. Cancer incidence and mortality by county —New York State, vol. 1. Albany: New York State Department of Health, 1982.

4. Tukey J. Exploratory data analysis. Reading, Massachusetts: Addison-Wesley, 1977.

5. Walter SD. Calculation of attributable risks from epidemiological data. Int J Epidemiol 1978;7:175–82.

6. Devesa SS, Silverman DT. Cancer incidence and mortality trends in the United States: 1935–74. J Natl Cancer Inst 1978;60:545–71.

7. Health consequences of smoking: cancer. A report of the Surgeon General. Rockville, Maryland: Office of Smoking and Health, Public Health Service, 1982; DHHS publication no. (PHS)82-50179.

8. Cancer Facts and Figures 1984. New York: American Cancer Society, 1983.

9. Armstrong B, Doll R. Environmental factors and cancer incidence and mortality in different countries with special reference to dietary practices. Int J Cancer 1975;15:617–31.

10. Wynder EL, Reddy BS. Studies of large bowel cancer: human leads to experimental application. J Natl Cancer Inst 1973;50:1099.

11. Borchert P, Wattenburg LW. Inhibition of macromolecular binding and benzo(a)pyrene and inhibition of neoplasia by disulfiram in the mouse forestomach. J Natl Cancer Inst 1976;57:173–9.

12. Willett WC, MacMahon B. Diet and cancer—an overview. N Engl J Med 1984;310:633–8, 697–703.

13. Pollack ES, Nomura AM, Heilbrun LK, et al. Prospective study of alcohol consumption and cancer. N Engl J Med 1984;310:617–21.

14. Vernick LJ, Kuller LH. Cholocystectomy and right-sided colon cancer: an epidemiologic study. Lancet 1981;2:381–3.

15. Graham S, Dayal H, Swanson M, et al. Diet in the epidemiology of cancer of the colon and rectum. J Natl Cancer Inst 1978;61:709–14.

16. Graham S. Diet and cancer: epidemiologic aspects. Rev Can Epidemiol 1983;2:2–45.

17. Zdeb MS. The probability of developing cancer. Am J Epidemiol 1977;106:6–16.

18. Roberts MM, Jones V, Elton RA. Risk of breast cancer in women with history of benign disease of the breast. Br Med J 1984;288:275–8.

19. Hirayama T. Epidemiology of breast cancer with special reference to the role of diet. Prev Med 1978;7:173–95.

20. Boice JD Jr., Monson RR. Breast cancer in women after repeated fluoroscopic examinations of the chest. J Natl Cancer Inst 1977;59:823–32.

21. Shapiro S, Venet W, Strax P, et al. Ten- to fourteen-year effect of screening on breast cancer mortality. J Natl Cancer Inst 1982;69:349–55.

22. Graham S, Priore R, Graham M, et al. Genital cancer in wives of penile cancer patients. Cancer 1979;44:1870–4.

23. zur Hausen H. The role of viruses in human tumors. Adv Cancer Res 1980;33:77–107.

24. Winkelstein W. Smoking and cancer of the uterine cervix: hypothesis. Am J Epidemiol 1977;106:257–9.

25. Trevathan E, Layde P, Webster LA, et al. Cigarette smoking and dysplasia and carcinoma in situ of the uterine cervix. JAMA 1983;250:499–502.

26. Reid R, Stanhope CR, Herschman BR, et al. Genital warts and cervical cancer: I. Evidence of an association between subclinical papillomavirus infection and cervical malignancy. Cancer 1982;50:377–87.

27. zur Hausen H. Human genital cancer: synergism between two virus infections or synergism between a virus infection and initiating events? Lancet 1982;2:1370–2.

28. Potts CL. Cadmium proteinuria—the health of bat-

tery workers exposed to cadmium oxide dust. Ann Occ Hyg 1965;8:55–61.

29. Rothman KR, Cristina IC, Flanders D, et al. Epidemiology of laryngeal cancer. In: Sartwell PE, ed. Epidemiologic Reviews, vol. 2. Baltimore: Johns Hopkins University Press, 1980; 195–209.

30. Graham S, Mettlin C, Marshall J, et al. Dietary factors in the epidemiology of cancer of the larynx. Am J Epidemiol 1981;113:675–80.

31. Doll R, Peto R. The causes of cancer. J Natl Cancer Inst 1981;66:1191–1308.

32. Warner KE. The federal cigarette excise tax. In: Proceedings of the National Conference on Smoking and Health. New York, November 1981.

33. Harris JE. Increasing the federal excise tax on cigarettes. J Health Econ 1982;1:117–20.

Cardiovascular Disease

Craig C. White, M.D., Dennis D. Tolsma, M.P.H.,
Suzanne G. Haynes, Ph.D., and Daniel McGee, Jr.

Cardiovascular disease (CVD) has been the leading cause of death in the United States since 1940.[1] Heart disease and cerebrovascular disease (stroke) ranked first and third, respectively, among the ten leading causes of death for the years 1940, 1960, 1970, and 1980. Because of the widespread impact that CVD has had on death, illness, disability, and medical costs, the scientific community has devoted considerable time and effort since 1950 toward preventing our nation's number one killer. Epidemiologic studies have identified the major risk factors for CVD. At least 20 large-scale clinical trials have documented the efficacy of intervention in reducing the frequency and severity of most of these risk factors.[2]

Since 1968, deaths from CVD have declined significantly compared with other diseases.[3] The mortality rate from stroke dropped 40 percent between 1968 and 1979, compared with a 12 percent decline in other diseases' mortality rates. Since 1972 stroke mortality has been declining about 5 percent a year, a phenomenal decrease in the history of the disease. Deaths from coronary heart disease (CHD) decreased about 27 percent during the same period. These declines in mortality have been observed in all age groups, for both men and women, and for all races. Although the reasons for the steep decline in mortality rates from stroke and CHD are not specifically known, a 1978 National Heart, Lung, and Blood Institute (NHLBI) conference concluded that changes in coronary risk factors and improvements in medical care both probably contributed to the decline.[4]

Nonetheless, more than half of all deaths in the United States today are attributable to heart and vascular system diseases. We know how to prevent a significant proportion of cardiovascular cases, and yet preventable disease continues to develop. Clearly a gap exists between our knowledge and the successful implementation of prevention measures.

BURDEN OF ILLNESS

Mortality

In 1980, almost 1 million deaths were attributed to major cardiovascular diseases (ICD 390–448). Coronary heart disease was the cause of 565,755 deaths, and cerebrovascular disease accounted for 170,225 deaths (Table 1).[5] The crude death rates per 100,000 persons resulting from CVD, CHD, and cerebrovascular disease were 436.4, 249.7, and 75.1, respectively.[5]

Age-adjusted death rates by race and sex for 1980 demonstrate that men have about twice the risk of dying from major CVD and CHD than do women.[5] Black men are at highest risk of dying from CVD (425.7 per 100,000), followed by white men (336.9 per 100,000), black women (278.3 per 100,000), and white women (179.1 per 100,000). In general, blacks have higher rates of CVD than whites (342.0 versus 248.4), but rates of CHD are almost identical among blacks and whites (150.5 versus 150.6).[5] Thus, men are at higher risk of developing CVD than women, and blacks are at higher risk than whites.

Potential Years of Life Lost

Mortality patterns for CVD can also be expressed in terms of the potential years of life lost before age 65 (Table 1). Nearly 1.8 million years of life lost prematurely result from CVD every year, while CHD accounts for almost 1 million years of life lost prematurely every year, and cerebrovascular disease accounts for nearly 230,000 years lost. Over 70 percent of these years of potential life lost are among men. For both men and women, approximately 75 percent of years of life lost prematurely are accounted for by deaths among individuals 45–64 years of age.

From the Center for Health Promotion and Education, Centers for Disease Control, Atlanta (White, Tolsma, and McGee) and the National Center for Health Statistics, Hyattsville, Maryland (Haynes).

Address reprint requests to Mr. Tolsma, Center for Health Promotion and Education, Centers for Disease Control, 1600 Clifton Road, Atlanta, GA 30333.

Table 1. Morbidity and mortality of coronary heart disease, stroke, and all cardiovascular diseases, United States, 1980

Condition	Mortality	Potential years of life lost before the age of 65	Morbidity
Coronary heart disease	565,755	982,224	5,404,713
Stroke	170,225	229,607	2,101,274
All cardiovascular disease	988,545	1,763,073	23,176,056

Mortality data from NCHS[5]; morbidity data from unpublished data from NCHS 1980 Health Interview Survey. Potential years of life lost were calculated using the midpoint of each age group subtracted from age 65 and multiplied by total deaths in that age group.

Morbidity

One of the major gaps in our knowledge concerns cardiovascular disease morbidity. Currently, periodic measurement of coronary disease, documented by electrocardiogram, is accomplished through National Health and Nutrition Examination Surveys (NHANES). However, no national system has been established to monitor the incidence (new cases) and prevalence (existing cases) of CVD. Currently, the NHLBI is undertaking an effort called ARIC (Atherosclerosis Risk in Communities) to study the development of CVD and to determine the incidence of nonfatal heart attacks in four communities.

Our knowledge regarding the age-, race-, and sex-specific prevalence of chronic conditions in the United States is also minimal. The last comprehensive report on the prevalence of self-reported chronic circulatory diseases was published by the National Center for Health Statistics (NCHS) using 1972 data.[6] Unpublished Health Interview Survey (HIS) data on total numbers of CVD cases were provided by the NCHS for 1980. In this analysis, the measure of morbidity is CVD prevalence. Age- and sex-specific prevalence estimates for 1980 are based on the 1980 HIS data broken into age and sex groups according to the 1972 distributions. All told, approximately 23 million Americans suffered from some form of CVD in 1980.

Costs

Personal health care expenditures for various diseases of the cardiovascular system totaled approximately $32.5 billion in 1980, according to the NCHS.[7,8] More than 70 percent of this amount resulted from heart disease, stroke, and high blood pressure.

Several trends are apparent when expenditures are examined according to the various age, sex, and diagnostic categories. First, heart disease accounts for the largest share, more than 40 percent. Surprisingly, the CVD expenditures for men and women under the age of 65 were similar. However, among persons over age 65, CVD expenditures for women were double those for men. This difference is probably explained by the larger number of surviving older women in the population and the fact that for every circulatory disease category, the per capita personal health care expenditures for women were greater than the comparable figure for men.[7,8]

RISK FACTORS

During the past 30 years, considerable research has been devoted to identifying CVD risk factors. In 1981, Hopkins and Williams[9] identified 246 coronary risk factors suggested in the literature. Of these, six are accepted as standard risk factors for CHD: age, male sex, cigarette smoking, elevated serum cholesterol, elevated systolic or diastolic blood pressure, and glucose intolerance/diabetes. Other risk factors included on some lists as standard include family history, physical inactivity, type A personality, alcohol consumption, and obesity.

Physical activity has become increasingly identified as a significant variable influencing CVD risks.[10] Similarly, a National Institute of Health consensus conference on the health implications of obesity, reviewing the combined data of the eight cohort studies of the U.S. Pooling Project and a recent analysis of the Framingham study, found "increasing risk of coronary artery heart disease with increasing levels of obesity, independent of the other standard risk factors."[11] Obviously, these two issues are also related to each other in terms of intervention strategies. Because physical inactivity and obesity are thought to influence blood pressure, cholesterol levels, and glucose intolerance, the effects of modifying exercise levels and weight control are at least partially reflected in our calculations. However, the logistic equations used for the estimates described in this paper do not lend themselves to independent estimates of exercise and weight control. Both factors likely make substantial additional contributions to attributable risks, and physical inactivity in particular may contribute as much to the risk of CVD illness as any one of the four other standard risk factors.[12]

Some of the other risk factors identified are not modifiable (age, sex, and family history) and were, therefore, considered for purposes of stratifying tabular data only. The modification of type A behavior has not been adequately documented in longitudinal cohort studies, so elimination of this risk factor was not considered in our estimates. Also excluded from these estimates are risks associated with exposure to environmental cardiotoxins—particularly in work settings—such as carbon monoxide, carbon disulfide, nitroglycerine, and nitrates.[13]

METHODS

The population-attributable risk fraction (PARF) is the primary statistic reported in this paper. Simply stated, it is the proportion of total events (e.g., deaths and cases) in a population that could be prevented if a particular risk factor could be eliminated.[14] The PARF can be interpreted from an etiologic viewpoint (i.e., the causal outcomes attributed to a risk factor) or a prevention viewpoint (i.e., the cases that could be prevented).

Risk Factor Assumptions

Four major risk factors for study were identified by the group: smoking, hypertension, elevated serum cholesterol, and glucose intolerance. Numerous prevention paradigms were considered and analyzed to estimate the effect of each risk factor. Although 28 different paradigms were tested, we will present only the seven that best serve to illustrate the relationships:

1. Smoking prevalence is decreased to zero.
2. All systolic blood pressures of 160 mm Hg or greater are reduced to 159 mm Hg.
3. All systolic blood pressures of 140 mm Hg or greater are reduced to 139 mm Hg.
4. All diastolic blood pressures of 90 mm Hg or greater are reduced to 89 mm Hg.
5. All serum cholesterol counts of 260 mg/dL or greater are reduced to 259 mg/dL.
6. All serum cholesterol counts of 220 mg/dL or greater are reduced to 219 mg/dL.
7. All cases of glucose intolerance attain normal glucose levels.

Although many of these risk factors are continuous, they were analyzed in a dichotomous fashion for simplicity of presentation and conceptualization. Any categorical reduction—e.g., systolic blood pressure from 160 mm Hg or greater to 139 mm Hg—is assumed to remove a person from the high-risk category.

PARF Calculations

The PARF estimates presented in this report are based on logistic regression equations originally derived for the Centers for Disease Control Risk Factor Update Project, prepared by Breslow et al.[15] The project team produced multivariate logistic risk equations by combining several prospective studies of CVD, synthesized into a single coherent contingency table by the procedure known as iterative proportionate fitting, or raking.[14] An important advantage of these equations is that it allows our analysis to relate CVD outcomes in the U.S. population to risk estimates based on several independent epidemiologic studies. A disadvantage is that the coefficients selected are not citable to a single study or study population, have not at this point been documented by the project team, and require additional assumptions noted in the project report.[15]

Among the prospective studies considered by the Risk Factor Update Project, the Framingham heart study is the longest-running study of a cohort of white individuals in the country. Established in 1950, the Framingham cohort is still being followed for CVD death. Because of the widespread publication of the Framingham data, the cardiovascular working group compared the equations derived by the project team with the Framingham logistic equations. Overall, the two sets of equations contained a similar list of coronary risk factors. An exception to this rule was the inclusion of an age x smoking interaction term in the Breslow but not the Framingham model.

Another difference was the treatment of the electrocardiogram as a risk indicator. Other investigators have also compared the risk estimates of these two sets of equations. In a recent study to evaluate the scoring systems employed by 41 health risk assessment instruments, Smith and colleagues compared the predicted probability of CHD death to two criterion models, estimates from the Framingham study and the Risk Factor Update Project. The two criterion models produce very similar mean risk estimates for both men and women.[16]

Basically, then, this analysis uses logistic equations based on multiple studies of CVD conducted during the past 20 years which were pooled to yield a new set of equations applying to men and women, whites and blacks, and for myocardial infarction morbidity and mortality as well as for stroke morbidity and mortality. The equations were used to calculate the PARF for each risk factor in the following manner:

1. We programmed each logistic regression equation for age, sex, race, and CVD outcome.

2. We obtained the current distributions of values for blood pressure, serum cholesterol, and smoking prevalence in the United States.

3. We computed the risks of developing CVD for the population based on the current distribution of the risk factor under study (by age, race, and sex), inserting mean population values for other risk factors into the equation.

4. We recalculated the risks of developing CVD, based on the changes noted in the various assumptions.

5. The PARF is represented by the following equation:

$$\frac{I_t - I_o}{I_t}$$

where I_t is the mortality or morbidity in the total population based on current risk factors and I_o is the expected outcome if risk factors were reduced.

6. The PARF was computed for white males, black males, white females, and black females for ages 25–44, 45–64, and 65+ years.

7. The number of deaths and cases in each group was computed by multiplying the 1980 NCHS mortality data and morbidity data by the PARFs and summed to obtain the total.

We made numerous assumptions when applying logistic regression equations in an analysis of this type; these are discussed below. Each assumption represents a limit to the analysis. In making analytic judgments, we often found it necessary to make choices in order to accomplish the purposes of the health policy consultation this paper supported— i.e., to illustrate the magnitude of the burden of CVD illness attributable to generic risk factors.

Assumptions

The logistic equations calculate the burden of coronary heart disease and of stroke separately. In order to represent the overall CVD burden, calculations for the remainder of CVD mortality and morbidity used the coronary heart disease PARFs (step 7, above). Tables 2–6 sum these three categories.

We based these equations on studies initiated more than 20 years ago with follow-up ten years later. If the relationship of CVD risk factors to CVD outcomes is different now, our estimates would not reflect these differences. This concern is not likely to be valid, given the overwhelming, consistent evidence demonstrating that these coronary risk factors are related to CVD, both in the United States and throughout the world. Missing from the Breslow et al. equations are more recently identified coronary risk factors, such as LDL-C and HDL-C (low- and high-density lipoprotein cholesterol), which are now thought to be more powerful predictors of CHD than total cholesterol, and variables that estimate the independent contributions of physical activity and obesity.

Our approach also assumes that a change in one risk factor does not change another risk factor, i.e., that there is no correlation among systolic blood pressure change, serum cholesterol change, or cigarette smoking cessation. This assumption may not be entirely valid, because most epidemiologic studies report modest correlations among the coronary risk factors noted.

Another important assumption made is that the effects reported would occur over a ten-year period. Longer follow-up periods were not available for most of the cohort studies used. Thus, the effect of intervening on the 25- to 44-year-old group reflects the experience of only ten years, not a lifetime, which would add 30 to 40 more years. To estimate the effects over longer periods of time, one must look at the PARF for the 45- to 64-year-old group. In addition, latency periods for risk factor reduction are not built into the equations.

This report is focused on persons over the age of 25, on the assumption that major interventions would likely occur in an adult population for CVD prevention. Major cigarette cessation programs or dietary/obesity programs aimed at young adults could eventually affect the prevalence of risk factors in a cohort as its members grow older, thus affecting the PARF estimates.

Finally, our PARF estimates are presented separately for whites and blacks, males and females, and different age groups on the assumption that each group will be affected differently by various proposals. This assumption is supported by the fact that mortality and morbidity rates are different by demographic group, as is the prevalence of coronary risk factors. (Because cost estimates are available only for men and women under the age of 65 and 65 years of age and over, but not by race, separate estimates by race and age are not presented for medical care costs.)

Prevalence of Coronary Risk Factors

The prevalence of coronary risk factors used in our analysis was derived from several sources of na-

Table 2. Smoking and all cardiovascular diseases: population-attributable risk fractions (PARF), estimates of mortality, death, years of life lost before the age of 65, and morbidity by race, sex, and age, United States, 1980

Event/age group (years)	White men n (estimated)	PARF[a]	Black men n (estimated)	PARF	White women n (estimated)	PARF	Black women n (estimated)	PARF	Total n (estimated)	PARF
Mortality										
<45	3,809	39	1,225	42	661	17	319	17	6,014	33
45–64	37,638	35	6,463	40	5,373	13	1,643	15	51,118	29
65+	61,407	18	8,303	28	33,840	9	1,882	5	105,432	13
Total	102,854	23	15,991	33	39,874	9	3,844	8	162,564	17
Years lost										
<45	119,147	39	44,291	42	26,757	17	11,630	17	201,825	31
45–64	252,168	36	38,779	40	32,239	13	9,859	15	333,045	30
Total	371,315	37	83,070	41	58,996	14	21,489	16	534,870	30
Morbidity										
<45	569,243	28	105,963	33	554,068	19	90,626	19	1,319,901	23
45–64	882,897	24	136,043	32	588,627	15	75,491	18	1,683,057	20
65+	392,373	12	61,952	21	410,210	8	23,830	5	888,366	10
Total	1,844,513	20	303,958	29	1,552,905	13	189,947	14	3,891,324	17

[a] Calculated from data in Table 1. See Methods for details of computation.

tional prevalence data. The population distributions used for systolic hypertension, elevated serum cholesterol, and glucose intolerance were based on the NHANES II Survey. The NHANES II Survey consisted of a stratified sample of the U.S. population conducted between 1977 and 1979. The smoking data used in the analysis were based on data from the Centers for Disease Control/State Behavioral Risk Factors (BRF) Surveys, conducted jointly by the Centers for Disease Control and 28 states and the District of Columbia in 1982. Smoking data from the BRF surveys paralleled data from the NCHS Health Interview Survey and were thus considered to be appropriate for our uses.

DISCUSSION

Smoking

Smoking is now responsible for approximately 350,000 premature deaths annually.[17] Although approximately 130,000 (including about 100,000 lung cancer deaths) of these deaths are caused by cancer, smoking-related deaths from CVD significantly exceed this number. Approximately one third of the adult U.S. population now smokes.[18] Although the prevalence of cigarette smoking has declined over the past 20 years, the actual number of smokers has remained virtually unchanged as a result of population increases, and the average number of cigarettes consumed per smoker has actually increased over this period of time.[19] Of particular concern is the increasing prevalence of smoking among women 20–24 years of age over the last several years.[18] Given the significant relative risk for CVD among smokers and the continued high prevalence of smoking in the population, it is clear that smoking

remains a major risk factor for premature death and morbidity from CVD.

Specific estimates of CVD mortality and morbidity attributable to smoking (PARF) are presented in Table 2. A significantly greater proportion of CVD mortality can be attributed to smoking for men, particularly black men, than for women. This relationship, though less pronounced, is similar for morbidity as well.

PARF generally decreases by about half in all over 64 age groups, except for black men. This reflects a decreased prevalence of smoking in this age group rather than any decrease in the relative risk for smokers with increasing age. The explanations for this trend are numerous. For example, smokers have increased mortality ratios for many diseases, not just CVD, and may have already died from other diseases such as cancer, thus lowering the proportion of smokers in this age group. Furthermore, this difference may to some extent reflect a cohort effect involving persons now 65 years of age who were part of a cohort in which smoking was always less prevalent. In contrast, persons 45–64 years of age are part of a cohort in which tobacco use was broadly accepted socially. Lastly, persons over 64 years of age may have been smokers for years but quit because of health problems; therefore, death from CVD or cancer may in reality still be attributable to smoking. However, PARF would underestimate this latter group because they are not counted as smokers and are assumed to have a lower risk than they actually do. This is clearly true for cancer, which has a long latency period, and it is probably important to our estimates for smoking and CVD.

Overall, 17 percent of all CVD mortality can be attributed to smoking. Most of these deaths occur in

Table 3. High blood pressure and all cardiovascular diseases: population-attributable risk fractions (PARF), estimates of mortality, years of life lost before the age of 65, and morbidity by race, sex, and age, United States, 1980

Event/age group (years)	White men n (estimated)	PARF[a]	Black men n (estimated)	PARF	White women n (estimated)	PARF	Black women n (estimated)	PARF	Total n (estimated)	PARF
Mortality										
<45	817	8	523	18	259	7	191	10	1,790	10
45–64	23,994	23	5,246	33	7,533	18	3,278	30	40,052	23
65+	111,702	33	10,491	35	119,427	31	11,701	33	253,320	32
Total	136,513	30	16,260	33	127,219	29	15,170	31	295,162	30
Years lost										
<45	25,555	8	18,913	18	10,949	7	7,079	10	62,496	10
45–64	160,659	23	31,476	33	45,200	18	19,669	30	257,003	23
Total	186,214	18	50,389	25	56,149	14	26,748	20	319,499	18
Morbidity										
<45	110,714	5	37,703	12	142,731	5	34,585	7	325,733	6
45–64	507,370	14	91,969	22	496,717	13	97,395	23	1,193,450	14
65+	733,779	23	65,896	23	1,104,969	22	112,139	25	2,016,783	22
Total	1,351,863	15	195,568	19	1,744,417	15	244,119	18	3,535,966	15

[a] Calculated from data in Table 1. See Methods for details of computation.

persons over the age of 64. However, because CVD deaths in younger persons are primarily due to smoking, it accounts for a much larger portion of premature death—30 percent of the years lost before the age of 65 resulting from CVD mortality.

Smoking is responsible for 17 percent of CVD morbidity. Among persons younger than 45 years of age, smoking accounts for 23 percent of all CVD morbidity. Gender differences in mortality are markedly reduced when morbidity is measured. While smoking does not seem to be a major cause of CVD mortality among women, it is a significant factor in terms of illness. Of the nearly $33 billion expended annually for CVD, $4.51 billion (14 percent) is attributable to smoking.

Elevated Blood Pressure

We examined the effect of diastolic and systolic blood pressure separately. PARF estimates were substantially lower in all groups when diastolic pressure was used. This may reflect the stronger association of systolic blood pressure with CHD mortality in most epidemiologic studies. Though the relative risk may be greater for elevated diastolic pressure, the number of persons at risk is greater for elevated systolic pressure. For our study purposes, therefore, systolic blood pressure over 139 mm Hg was the risk factor on which our PARF estimates were made.

In general, PARF estimates associating elevated blood pressure with CVD mortality were highest for blacks and among persons over age 64 (Table 3). Overall, 30 percent of CVD mortality is attributable to systolic pressure greater than 139 mm Hg. This percentage was constant across all race and sex groups. A much lower percentage of years of life

lost from CVD mortality is attributable to elevated systolic blood pressure (18 percent). This relates to the fact that such a large proportion of mortality attributable to elevated systolic blood pressure occurs among persons over the age of 64 (32 percent). Compared with smoking, sex-related differences are minimal. Blacks have substantially higher attributable risks than do whites.

Only 15 percent of CVD morbidity is attributable to elevated systolic blood pressure; most of this morbidity attributable to elevated systolic blood pressure is slightly higher among blacks, and sex-related differences are modest. More than 19 percent of the costs associated with CVD are attributable to elevated systolic blood pressure.

Elevated Cholesterol

Numerous epidemiologic studies have established elevated serum cholesterol as a major risk factor for CVD. Although different measures such as blood levels of low-density-lipoprotein cholesterol have been suggested as better predictors for heart disease risk, "lowering blood cholesterol levels will afford significant protection against heart disease risk."[20] However, the serum cholesterol level considered to place one at significant risk for CVD has been questioned, especially because lowering serum cholesterol too far may increase the risk for cancer. Two levels were considered to define the risk of elevated serum cholesterol: ≥260 mg/dL and ≥220 mg/dL. Because serum cholesterol ≥260 mg/dL identified a small portion of cholesterol-related mortality in the population, a level of ≥220 mg/dL was selected for estimating PARF and PAR for high cholesterol in this study.

PARF estimates for CVD mortality associated

Table 4. Cholesterol and all cardiovascular diseases: population-attributable risk fractions (PARF), estimates of mortality, years of life lost before the age of 65, and morbidity by race, sex, and age, United States, 1980

Event/age group (years)	White men n (estimated)	PARF[a]	Black men n (estimated)	PARF	White women n (estimated)	PARF	Black women n (estimated)	PARF	Total n (estimated)	PARF
Mortality										
<45	806	8	353	12	188	5	96	5	1,443	8
45–64	7,830	7	1,196	7	6,599	16	1,677	15	17,303	10
65+	10,632	3	908	3	65,998	17	5,482	15	83,020	10
Total	19,268	4	2,457	5	72,785	17	7,255	15	101,766	10
Years lost										
<45	25,280	8	12,718	12	8,150	5	3,609	5	49,757	8
45–64	52,737	2	7,184	7	39,593	16	10,062	15	109,576	10
Total	78,017	8	19,902	10	47,743	12	13,671	10	159,333	9
Morbidity										
<45	141,489	7	34,918	11	518,218	17	83,535	18	778,160	13
45–64	339,806	9	47,825	11	1,351,942	35	161,627	38	1,901,200	23
65+	233,607	17	24,040	8	1,691,277	34	163,091	37	2,112,014	24
Total	714,902	8	106,783	10	3,561,437	30	408,253	30	4,791,374	21

[a] Calculated from data in Table 1. See Methods for details of computation.

with serum cholesterol ≥220 mg/dL were highest for women over 44 years of age (Table 4). Surprisingly, PARF estimates decrease significantly with increasing age for men. Overall, 15 percent of CVD mortality among women is attributable to elevated serum cholesterol, in contrast to about 4 percent among men. Together these accounted for 101,766 deaths in 1980.

PARF estimates for years of life lost were similar to those observed for mortality, although because of the different age associations with men and women, the overall proportion of life years lost attributable to elevated serum cholesterol was roughly equivalent (9 percent versus 11 percent). Elevated serum cholesterol accounted for nearly 160,000 years of life lost prematurely in 1980, more than 61,000 of which were among women. Differences by race for this risk factor are minimal. The only significant difference is a slightly higher mortality among young black men relative to young white men; the rest of the groups are similar.

A most dramatic and important finding concerns the tremendous number of cases of CVD attributable to elevated serum cholesterol for women over 44 years of age. Approximately 36 percent of CVD morbidity in older women can be attributed to elevated serum cholesterol. This is approximately four times that for men—morbidity among men being roughly parallel to mortality. Racial differences are minimal, analogous to those for mortality. Overall, nearly 4.8 million cases of CVD can be attributed to serum cholesterol ≥220 mg/dL. This disproportionate morbidity among women over the age of 44 is reflected in the proportion of costs related to CVD attributable to elevated serum cholesterol (23 percent).

Table 5. Glucose intolerance and all cardiovascular diseases: population-attributable risk fractions (PARF), estimates of mortality, years of life lost before the age of 65, and morbidity by race, sex, and age, U.S., 1980

Event/age group (years)	White men n (estimated)	PARF[a]	Black men n (estimated)	PARF	White women n (estimated)	PARF	Black women n (estimated)	PARF	Total n (estimated)	PARF
Mortality										
<45	16	<1	12	<1	399	11	174	9	601	3
45–64	820	1	372	2	13,127	31	3,787	35	18,106	10
65+	7,541	2	979	3	146,945	38	13,565	38	169,030	21
Total	8,377	2	1,363	3	160,471	37	17,526	36	187,737	19
Years lost										
<45	488	<1	425	<1	17,548	11	6,544	9	25,004	4
45–64	4,923	1	2,216	2	78,764	31	22,720	35	108,623	10
Total	5,411	<1	2,641	1	96,312	23	29,264	22	133,627	8
Morbidity										
<45	16,181	1	3,870	1	234,024	8	30,592	6	284,667	5
45–64	177,824	5	33,714	8	767,926	20	109,872	26	1,089,337	13
65+	248,986	8	24,388	8	1,217,325	24	132,486	30	1,623,184	18
Total	442,991	5	61,972	6	2,219,274	19	272,950	20	2,997,188	13

[a] Calculated from data in Table 1. See Methods for details of computation.

Table 6. Summary of the impact of the four major risk factors for all cardiovascular diseases: population-attributable risk fractions (PARF), estimates of mortality, years of life lost before the age of 65, and morbidity, United States, 1980

Risk factors	Mortality		Years of life lost <65		Morbidity		Costs[b]	
	n (estimated)	PARF[a]	n (estimated)	PARF	n (estimated)	PARF	Millions of dollars	%
Smoking	162,564	17	534,870	30	3,891,324	17	4,509	14
High blood pressure	295,162	30	319,499	18	3,535,966	15	6,289	19
Cholesterol	101,766	10	159,333	9	4,791,374	21	7,655	23
Glucose intolerance	187,737	19	133,627	8	2,997,188	13	5,239	16

[a] Calculated from data in Table 1 and summarized from Tables 2–5. See Methods for details of computation.
[b] Calculated from NCHS data.[7]

Glucose Intolerance

Although diabetics have long been recognized as being at increased risk for CVD, a more broadly classified group with glucose intolerance has long been a subject of debate. One difficulty in identifying the potential risk for this group lies with the numerous, often quite liberal definitions of glucose intolerance (e.g., laboratory determinations based on casual, nonfasting samples). The Framingham study, for example, used any one of three definitions of glucose intolerance. Despite this broad classification and the large proportion of the population it includes, glucose intolerance does represent a major risk factor for CVD. For purposes of our analysis, relative risk estimates based solely on the Framingham study were used for calculating our PARF estimates.

PARF estimate for CVD mortality from glucose intolerance is of major importance for women, particularly those over 44 years of age. The estimates for men are almost negligible. Although to some extent this difference is related to differences in sex-specific relative risk, the major influence is the prevalence of glucose intolerance among postmenopausal women.[2] Among women, glucose intolerance accounts for 36–37 percent of CVD mortality (Table 5). Women accounted for 95 percent of the 187,737 deaths attributable to glucose intolerance in 1980. PARF estimates for years of life lost are similar to those for mortality, if somewhat lower overall, reflecting the age–risk relationship for mortality with this risk factor. A total of 133,627 years of life lost from CVD can be attributed to glucose intolerance.

PARF estimates for CVD morbidity attributable to glucose intolerance are similar to those for CVD mortality. Men show a slight increase in attributable risk for CVD morbidity associated with glucose intolerance. Overall, glucose intolerance is responsible for nearly 3 million cases of CVD.

A significant proportion of costs from CVD can be attributed to glucose intolerance, primarily as a result of PARF for older women. Nearly 16 percent ($5.24 billion) of all direct health care costs from CVD can be attributed to glucose intolerance.

INTERVENTIONS

Smoking

At the turn of the century, virtually no Americans smoked manufactured cigarettes.[21] However, by the time of the Surgeon General's Report in 1964, the prevalence of smoking in the cohort of men born from 1921 to 1930 was greater than 60 percent.[22] The antismoking campaign that followed the release of this report was accompanied by significant declines in male smoking. Warner and Murt[23] estimated the impact on smoking-related premature deaths during the period 1964–1978 as a result of antismoking campaigns. They estimate that more than 200,000 premature deaths were avoided, saving 4.8 million years of potential life between the age at death and the normal life expectancy at that age.

Efforts to reduce the prevalence of smoking have been numerous and varied. To significantly change health behaviors, it is essential to understand the determinants of such behaviors. Although knowledge is the most obvious factor, appropriate skills are also necessary to facilitate behavior change. The importance of the individual's values, attitudes, and beliefs is sometimes overlooked or ignored, as are the societal factors that strongly influence these personal factors.

To reduce the prevalence of smoking, we propose an effort drawing on each of the following: informational and educational efforts; promotion and increased access to cessation programs; implementation of key public policies; reinforcement of nonsmoking through significant economic incentives; and utilization of existing social systems to establish nonsmoking as a social norm.

Educational and informational programs tend to

focus either on preventing smoking among young people or on public awareness campaigns generally aimed at increasing public knowledge regarding the hazards of smoking. In view of the amount of smoking-related CVD in blacks, special efforts to direct campaigns to blacks are indicated. Although later public information efforts have had a demonstrable impact on public knowledge of smoking risks[24] and remain essential for maintaining public support for smoking cessation, the greatest long-term potential lies with smoking prevention.

The School Health Education Evaluation (SHEE) has provided rigorous evidence of the effectiveness of school-based health education curricula to produce changes in health knowledge, attitudes, and practices. Christenson and colleagues[25] illustrated the robust effect on self-reported smoking practices of one curriculum studied, the School Health Curriculum Project. Extrapolating the results nationwide, they estimate that 146,000 seventh-grade students would delay the onset of smoking each year. However, at present, only a small percentage of the nation's schoolchildren are exposed to quality curricula.

Smoking cessation efforts must cope with the extreme addiction associated with nicotine, a major constituent of tobacco smoke.[26] Nicotine has been called six to eight times more addictive than alcohol, and withdrawal symptoms associated with smoking cessation are quite severe for many persons. Yet more than 33 million Americans have quit smoking since the release of the first Surgeon General's Report.[19] Though the effectiveness of smoking cessation services is difficult to document, many smokers desire such assistance, typically lack adequate access to such services, and often quit smoking when they do gain access. Reasonable estimates of the efficacy of smoking cessation programs range between 25 and 40 percent cessation at 6–12 months' follow-up.[19,27]

Implementing public policy measures could dramatically affect the prevalence of tobacco use in this country. The promotion of tobacco products is a key factor affecting tobacco consumption. Tobacco companies spend $2 billion annually to promote a product which is known to be deadly and addictive. A minimum goal would be to require that advertisements comply with the industry's own codes prohibiting suggestions that cigarette smoking is essential to social prominence or social attraction or portrayals of smokers participating in physical activity requiring stamina or athletic conditioning beyond normal recreation. Many current advertisements do not conform to these codes. Compensatory space for counteradvertisement would be more

effective, as was the case on television before tobacco advertisements were banned. While a total ban on the promotion of tobacco products might not be attainable, the impact of such efforts on initiation of youth smoking and continuation of adult smoking would be undeniable.

The momentum for such restrictions is growing. The American Heart Association has recommended limiting print advertising to black and white statements of fact ("tombstone" advertising), and the American Medical Association has voted to seek a total ban on cigarette advertising—unquestionably the strongest statement on smoking ever issued by the U.S. medical profession.[28] Advertising has already been banned in such disparate countries as Sweden and the Sudan.

To support nonsmoking as a social norm and protect the rights of nonsmokers to a smoke-free environment, restrictions on smoking in public and private places have become increasingly widespread through state and community legislation and corporate, school, and hospital policies. In addition to restricting tobacco use, limiting public access to cigarette sales could reinforce these policies. At minimum, it would be appropriate to eliminate cigarette sales in hospitals, nursing homes, and other health care facilities that deal daily with the consequences of tobacco use, as well as in schools, where health and educational goals are undercut by allowing the use of tobacco products. Totally eliminating cigarette sales from vending machines would help limit consumption by minors, probably serving to reduce overall consumption.

Economic incentives and disincentives are effective tools to help decrease cigarette smoking. Increased taxation of tobacco products serves to drive up cigarette prices, leading to reduced consumption, particularly among the young. Taxation has the added benefit of increasing federal and state revenue.[29] Economic incentives, through decreased premiums for health, life, home, and property insurance for nonsmokers, create a positive financial benefit for not smoking and support the concept of nonsmoking as a social norm. The economic issues associated with tobacco production are understandably sensitive and difficult. Economic hardships among small tobacco farmers seem likely unless they are assisted to make the transition to nontobacco crops.

An additional and often overlooked issue concerns the important roles particular professions and institutions play in smoking intervention. The health care sector is an important setting for smoking cessation activities.[30] Moreover, for the same reasons that nonsmoking policies have special relevance in health care institutions, health workers should recognize their importance as role models and refrain from tobacco use themselves. The educational sector is also essential. Along with restricting tobacco use in schools, cessation aid should be available for all faculty, staff, and students. The importance of teachers as role models should be emphasized; their behavior should reinforce educational efforts, not contradict them.

The work site is an extremely important setting for intervention activities. The 1986 Surgeon General's Report on smoking and health concludes that broadly based health promotion efforts for workers should be encouraged by labor, management, and government.[31] Smoking cessation and education programs should be available for all employees, but especially for workers at high risk of pneumoconiosis. Workplace policies that limit or eliminate smoking would deter smoking and protect nonsmokers. Economic and other incentives would provide valuable reinforcement for cessation activities and nonsmoking behavior.

Clearly no single strategy has been or is likely to be the panacea to the smoking problems. However, a combined effort utilizing all or many of these varied strategies offers the best chance for decreasing smoking in our society. The key is to link smoking cessation activities, made available and affordable for all individuals, with positive reinforcements and public policies supporting nonsmoking as the social norm. Our long-term success lies in coupling efforts aimed at the individual to those with impact on society as a whole.

Elevated Blood Pressure

The risk from hypertension increases as blood pressure levels rise. However, a decade of evidence from epidemiologic and clinical trials has firmly established that elevated blood pressure can be controlled and that cardiovascular risk declines when it is. In its 1984 report, the Joint National Committee on Detection, Evaluation, and Treatment of High Blood Pressure reaffirmed the stepped care approach to drug therapy and summarized its treatment conclusions: "The effectiveness of antihypertensive drugs in reducing elevated pressure is well established. Nonpharmacologic approaches are used both as definitive intervention and as an adjunct to drug therapy."[32]

The committee recommended such interventions as a regular exercise program, weight reduction, dietary modifications to reduce intake of sodium and saturated fats, moderation in alcohol consumption, and avoidance of smoking. The committee also noted that "the recommendations for nonpharmacologic modalities for the management of hypertension . . . may be of value in primary prevention" of high blood pressure.[32]

In light of the consistently high PARFs for blacks as compared with whites, special efforts to reduce risks through health promotion and preventive service programs focused on the needs of minorities are warranted.

Elevated Cholesterol

Elevated serum cholesterol may be reduced by both pharmacologic and nonpharmacologic means.[33] The report of the Consensus Development Conference on Lowering Blood Cholesterol defined elevated cholesterol at levels that place millions of Americans at excess cardiovascular risk. The conference's intervention recommendations included both diet and drug therapy: "The first step in the treatment of high-risk and moderate-risk blood cholesterol levels is diet therapy and caloric restriction for weight normalization in the overweight. Weight loss reduces blood cholesterol. The dietary approach should be to lower total fat, saturated fat, and cholesterol consumption. . . . Drug therapy should be used only after a careful trial of diet modification."[20]

These recommendations are echoed in the Dietary Guidelines for Americans, issued jointly by the U.S. Department of Agriculture and the U.S. Department of Health and Human Services.[34]

A variety of societal measures could help lower the population's mean cholesterol and blood pressure levels. Examples include reducing sodium and saturated fat levels in processed foods, both in the marketplace and in restaurants and fast food outlets; labeling salt, fat, cholesterol, and calorie contents in food products; and offering wide access to opportunities and facilities for exercise.

Glucose Intolerance

The principal means of reducing the prevalence of glucose intolerance is through reduction of overweight.[35] Because weight control is essentially energy balance, the fundamental behavioral modifications required to achieve weight loss are either dietary modifications, increased energy expenditure through physical activity, or both. Various approaches to weight control have been proposed. Although initial weight loss is usually achieved by these approaches, long-term maintenance of the desired weight has proved more difficult.[36] Because overweight children are more likely to be overweight adults than are thinner children, early intervention would plausibly be a key strategy for primary prevention. Despite a wave of pessimism in the 1970s, recent examples of effective programs for youth do exist.[37] Nevertheless, weight control measures targeted at persons already diagnosed with glucose intolerance are also essential components of appropriate care.

SUMMARY

Despite nearly two decades of decreasing mortality rates for heart disease and stroke, CVD continues to constitute an enormous human and economic burden on the nation. CVD was responsible for 984,780 deaths in 1980, as well as an estimated 1.8 million potential years of life lost before the age of 65, 50.7 million hospital days, 900 million disability days, and $33 billion in medical care expenditures.

By any of several measures of the burden of illness (Table 6), a significant percentage of cardiovascular disease is attributable to several known modifiable risk factors. Consequently, intervention strategies that result in reducing smoking, elevated blood pressure, and cholesterol and correcting glucose intolerance can be expected to maintain and extend the recent positive trends for CVD. Table 6 documents the gap between today's level of CVD and what might be accomplished through full application of individual and societal measures to reduce risk. While no interventions can be 100 percent effective, it is clear that much room remains for additional actions to close the gap.

The authors gratefully acknowledge the counsel provided by *Closing the Gap* consultants Manning Feinleib, M.D., Dr.P.H., Mary Jane Jessee, M.D., Daniel L. McGee, Sr., Ph.D., Jeffrey M. Newman, M.D., Leonard Syme, Ph.D., H. A. Tyroler, M.D., and Laurence Watkins, M.D.

REFERENCES

1. Levy RI, Moskowitz J. Cardiovascular research: decades of progress, a decade of promise. Science 1982;217: 121–9.

2. Kaplan NM, Stamler J, eds. Prevention of Coronary Heart Disease. Philadelphia: Saunders, 1983.

3. Feinleib M, Havlik RJ, Thom TJ. The changing pattern of ischemic heart disease. J Cardiovasc Med 1982;7:139–48.

4. Havlik RJ, Feinleib M, eds. Proceedings of the Conference on the Decline in Coronary Heart Disease Mortality. Bethesda, Maryland: Department of Health, Education and Welfare, 1979; DHEW publication no. (NIH)79-160.

5. Advance report of final mortality statistics, 1980. Hyattsville, Maryland: National Center for Health Statistics, 1983; (Vital and health statistics; series 32; no. 4).

6. Prevalence of chronic circulatory conditions. Hyattsville, Maryland: National Center for Health Statistics, 1974; DHEW publication no. (HRA)75-1521. (Vital and health statistics; series 10; no. 94).

7. Hodgson TA, Kopstein AN. Health care expenditures for major diseases in 1980. Health Care Fin Rev 1984;5:1–12.

8. Hodgson TA, Kopstein AN. Letter to the editor. Health Care Fin Rev 1984;6:128–30.

9. Hopkins PN, Williams RR. A survey of 246 suggested coronary risk factors. Atherosclerosis 1981;40:1–52.

10. Siscovick DS, LaPorte RE, Newman JM. The disease-specific benefits and risks of physical activity and exercise. Public Health Rep 1985;100:180–8.

11. Health implications of obesity. Bethesda, Maryland: National Institutes of Health, 1985; Consensus Development Conference Statement, vol. 5, no. 9.

12. Powell KE, Thompson PD, Casperson CJ, Kendrick JS. Physical activity and the incidence of coronary heart disease. Ann Rev Public Health 1987;8:253–87.

13. Leading work-related diseases and injuries—United States cardiovascular diseases. Morbid Mortal Weekly Rep 1985;34:219–22.

14. Deubner DC, Tyroler HA, Cassel JA, et al. Attributable risk, population attributable fraction of death associated with hypertension in a biracial population. Circulation 1975;52:901–8.

15. Breslow L, Fielding J, Afifi AA, et al. Risk Factor Update Project—final report. Atlanta, Georgia: Centers for Disease Control, 1984.

16. Smith KW, McKinlay SM, Thorington BD. The validity of health risk appraisal instruments for assessing coronary heart disease risk. Am J Public Health 1987;77 1:419–24.

17. The health consequences of smoking: chronic obstructive lung disease. A report of the Surgeon General. Rockville, Maryland: U.S. Public Health Service, 1984; DHHS publication no. (PHS)84-50205.

18. Health, United States, 1985. Washington, D.C.: US Government Printing Office, 1985; DHHS publication no. (PHS)86-1232.

19. Health consequences of smoking. A report of the Surgeon General. Washington, D.C.: US Government Printing Office, 1979; DHEW publication no. (PHS)79-50066.

20. Lowering blood cholesterol to prevent heart disease. Bethesda, Maryland: National Institutes of Health, 1985; Consensus Development Conference Statement, vol. 5, no. 7.

21. The health consequences of smoking for women. A report of the Surgeon General. Rockville, Maryland: U.S. Public Health Service, 1980.

22. The health consequences of smoking: cancer. A report of the Surgeon General. Rockville, Maryland: U.S. Public Health Service, 1982; DHHS publication no. (PHS)82-50179.

23. Warner KE, Murt HA. Premature deaths avoided by

the antismoking campaign. Am J Public Health 1983;73: 672–7.

24. Health promotion data for the 1990 objectives. Estimates from the National Health Interview Survey of Health Promotion and Disease Prevention: United States, 1985. Hyattsville, Maryland: National Center for Health Statistics, 1986; DHHS publication no. (PHS) 86-1250. (Vital and health statistics; no. 126).

25. Christenson GM, Gold RS, Katz M, Kreuter MW. Preface to results of the school health education evaluation. J School Health 1985;55:295–6.

26. Pollin W. The role of the addictive process as a key step in causation of all tobacco-related diseases [Editorial]. JAMA 1984;252:2874.

27. Wynder EL, Hoffman D. Tobacco and health. N Engl J Med 1979;300:894–903.

28. Okie S. AMA votes to seek ban on cigarette advertising. Washington Post 1985 Dec 11.

29. Warner KE. Cigarette taxation: Doing well by doing good. J Public Health Policy 1984;5:312–9.

30. Mason JO, Tolsma DD. The importance of individual health promotion. West J Med 1984;141:772–6.

31. The health consequences of smoking: cancer and chronic lung disease in the workplace. A report of the Surgeon General. Rockville, Maryland: U.S. Public Health Service, 1985; DHHS publication no. (PHS)85-50207.

32. National High Blood Pressure Coordinating Committee, 1984 Report. Arch Intern Med 1984;144:1045–57.

33. Lipid Research Clinics Program. The Lipid Research Clinics coronary primary prevention trial results. I. Reduction in incidence of coronary heart disease. JAMA 1984;251:351–64.

34. Nutrition and your health: dietary guidelines for Americans. 2d ed, Hyattsville, Maryland: USDA, Human Nutrition Information Service, and Rockville, Maryland: DHHS, FDA, Consumer Inquiries, 1985. (Home and Garden Bulletin No. 232).

35. Herman WH, Teutsch SM, Geiss LS. Diabetes mellitus. Diabetes Care 1985;4:391–405.

36. Foreyt JP, Scott LW, O'Malley MP, Gotto AM. Diet modification: an example of behavioral medicine. Natl Forum 1980;60:9–13.

37. Mellin L. Shapedown: weight management program for adolescents. San Francisco: Balboa, 1984.

Dental Disease

Michael E. Fritz, D.D.S., Ph.D., and
Douglas G. Rundle, D.M.D., M.P.H., M.S.

Dental caries and periodontal diseases continue to be the most prevalent dental diseases, despite the strides made by the dental profession in combating these problems during the last two decades. Because of their impact on American society, the prevention of caries and periodontal disease should be a part of any community health program. The Harvard University School of Public Health takes a six-pronged approach to community health: aging, maternal and child health, mental health, innovation in health care delivery, health promotion, and health science evaluation. In fact, the treatment of caries and periodontal disease has a role in each one of these six disciplines.

The definitions of caries and periodontal disease in the dental literature have changed over the years. For that reason, relating older to more recent data on the epidemiology of these two health problems can be difficult.

DENTAL DISEASE IN THE UNITED STATES

Dental Caries

Dental caries (dental decay), described as the most prevalent chronic disease, is characterized by the destruction of tooth enamel and dentin as a result of the action of microorganisms that colonize tooth surfaces at an early age and remain indigenous to the mouth throughout life. These bacteria adhere to the tooth surface in a film (dental plaque) and have the ability to ferment sugars and other carbohydrates and convert them to acids. The acids, in turn, attack the tooth surfaces with which they are in contact, causing a loss of mineral substance. Caries appear initially as softened or chalky areas in the enamel. If left untreated, they may progress to cause a substantial loss in the tooth structure, which eventually leads to loss of the tooth itself.

From the Emory University School of Dentistry, Atlanta.

Address reprint requests to Dr. Fritz, Emory University, School of Dentistry, 1462 Clifton Road, Atlanta, GA 30322.

Periodontal Diseases

Gingivitis. Gingivitis, or inflammation of the gums, is characterized by edema of the gum tissue and destruction of the connective tissue fibers holding the gum tissue in position. The disease is a result of interaction of tissues with microorganisms that colonize the gingival sulcus area and the tooth. The microorganisms, however, are thought to differ from those involved in dental caries. The disease process for gingivitis is not as well substantiated as that for dental caries. Gingivitis is most frequently seen in young adults. There is some discussion at present as to whether gingivitis, if left untreated, progresses to a more advanced form of disease called periodontitis, which involves the destruction of the bone holding the teeth in position. Some studies indicate that many forms of gingivitis do not make the transition to periodontitis. Indeed, they appear to be two distinct clinical entities.

Periodontitis. Periodontitis is an inflammation of the periodontium, which consists of the cementum of the teeth, the periodontal ligament that holds the teeth to the bone, and the alveolar bone itself. The disease is characterized by bone loss directly or indirectly as a result of action of microorganisms or their by-products. It is thought that the microorganisms causing the various types of periodontitis are different from those of both caries and gingivitis. If periodontitis is not treated, in many cases the bone is irreversibly lost around the teeth, and the teeth become loose and exfoliate.

Presently, most patients with periodontitis are adults over the age of 35.

Gathering Data on Dental Diseases

Dental caries. Three extensive studies of dental caries were consulted in the preparation of this paper. The first, the National Health and Nutrition Examination Survey (NHANES I), measured nutritionally related general health status for a probability sample representative of the civilian noninstitutionalized population of the United States.[1] This report contained the national estimates of decayed, missing, and filled teeth among people 1–74 years of age by sex, age, race, and other selected demographic characteristics.

Second, the National Dental Caries Prevalence Survey, designed by the National Caries Program in cooperation with the National Center for Health Statistics, was specifically formulated to provide prevalence data for all children 5–17 years of age enrolled in public or private schools.[2]

Third, we used the Rand Health Insurance Experiment (HIE).[3] This study involved six sites across the United States, which were chosen to represent an urban–rural mix and to reflect variations in the amount of stress on the ambulatory medical care systems. This smaller sample was used as a basis of comparison.

Periodontal Diseases. The primary source of data in the present report was the NHANES I survey. This group of examinees, 18–74 years of age, were given a 10-minute oral examination, and no X rays were taken. Russell's Periodontal Index[4] was used to measure the clinical signs of past or present periodontal disease activity. Green and Vermillion's Oral Hygiene Index (OHI-S) was used to determine the examinee's oral hygiene status.[5] There are no data for the group between 1 and 17 years of age that can be used for a national evaluation of periodontal disease.

Obtaining a precise estimate for the prevalence of periodontal disease is difficult. Signs of periodontal diseases are much more subjective than caries. Also, the periodontal diseases are characterized by exacerbation and remission, which makes it difficult to determine the state of the disease process at any particular time. Most important, there is no uniform way to detect the disease in a large population. Dental X rays would be helpful in detecting bone-destroying periodontal disease, but they also increase the time required for examination markedly and are less suitable for studies of large populations. In the future it may be possible to sample crevicular fluid in the gingival sulcus (between the gum and the tooth) to determine whether the disease is active. Probe measurements have serious limitations.

THE SCOPE OF THE PROBLEM: PREVALENCE AND INCIDENCE

Dental diseases are chronic and affect people's quality of life and how they perceive themselves in their environment. In this report we describe the specific health problems involved, examine their effects on the quality of life, time lost from work, and costs, and consider possible intervention strategies.

Dental Caries

Children of low-income families continue to be five times more likely to have untreated decayed teeth than those from high-income families. About 73 million people use nonfluoridated central water supplies, and 37 million people live in communities that have no central water supply. The children in these communities could be benefiting from a school-based fluoride system.

The incidence of caries in persons 5–17 years of age decreased dramatically in the last decade. According to all studies, the DMFS index (decayed, missing, and filled surfaces) is positively correlated with age. Also, the DMFS in females is consistently higher than for males. Persons between the ages of 18 and 74, however, are likely to remain a significant problem in the future.[6] As shown in Table 1, both the NHANES I study of 1971–1974 and the HIE of 1974–1976 showed a cumulative effect with advancing age. Not shown in the table is that the highest prevalence of decay alone occurred in those 12–17 years of age. The number of missing teeth increased after age 18, and the highest prevalence of filled teeth was in people 18–44 years of age.

The need for restorative dentistry will increase in the population between the ages of 45 and 75 as a result of the greater numbers of people in this age group who now keep their teeth and the larger number of teeth per person.

Previous studies have shown that black children and adolescents have fewer caries than whites, although this may reflect socioeconomic status and access to diagnostic services rather than a true difference.[7]

The occurrence of caries is inversely related to socioeconomic status, but data regarding urban–rural differences are conflicting. The most recent study of the National Dental Caries Prevalence Survey showed that without adjusting for fluoridation, the nonurban group had a DMFS level approximately 80 percent higher than the urban group.[2]

Periodontal Disease

About 60 percent of the population over the age of 45 who still have their teeth suffer from periodontal disease, yet a recent statewide study shows that less than 2 percent of dental practice involves periodontal treatment.[8]

Periodontal disease is the primary cause of tooth loss after age 35 (Table 2). In 1971 an estimated 23

Table 1. Age-specific prevalence and incidence of dental caries (decayed, missing, or filled teeth), United States, 1971–1974

Age	Mean annual prevalence	Mean annual incidence
<1	N/A	N/A
1–4	1.0	1.0
5–9	1.0	1.0
10–14	2.7	1.7
15–19	6.2	3.5
20–24	10.7	4.5
25–34	15.4	4.7
35–44	19.2	3.8
45–54	19.9	0.7
55–64	21.1	1.2
65+	22.2	1.1

Data from National Center for Health Statistics[10] and U.S. Public Health Service.[1]

million Americans were missing all their teeth.[9] This condition, called edentulism, increases dramatically with age. At the time of the NHANES I survey, almost one third of adults aged 35 or older were edentulous, and more than one half of those 65 and over had lost all their teeth.[10]

The average periodontal index (PI) rises more than threefold for both men and women 18–74 years of age. Average OHI-S scores also rise with age, but more sharply for men than for women. Men have approximately a 22 percent higher prevalence of moderate to severe disease (one or more pockets) than women, and they experience almost a 30 percent higher prevalence of severe disease (four or more pockets). Periodontal disease is inversely related to education and income, with education having the slightly stronger relationship.

When black and white adults of similar educational levels are compared, the differences in disease severity disappear. The prevalence and severity of disease appear to be slightly greater among individuals living in rural areas than among their urban counterparts. Although the prevalence and

Table 2. Age-specific rates of periodontal disease, United States, 1971–1974

Age	Mean annual prevalence (%)	Mean annual incidence (%)
0–17	N/A	N/A
18–24	6.5	6.5
25–34	13.9	7.4
35–44	26.4	12.5
45–54	34.7	8.3
55–64	41.4	6.7
65+	50.9	8.5

Data from National Center for Health Statistics.[10]

severity of periodontal disease do not differ by geographic region for adults, they do for children and youths. Specifically, persons 6–17 years of age living in the South have slightly higher PI scores than their counterparts in the Northeast, Midwest, and West.

Bacterial plaque is the major cause of periodontal diseases. The plaque associated with periodontal disease appears to differ from that associated with dental caries. Accumulation of plaque is promoted by many factors, adding to the risk of periodontal disease, most notably poor oral hygiene. In addition, cigarette smoking and other local factors (e.g., faulty occlusion or poorly prepared restorations) can promote the retention of bacteria and hence periodontal disease. Furthermore, people with altered immune systems, such as diabetics or those with inflammatory bowel disease, have been shown to be more predisposed to periodontal disease.

From 1962 to 1974, there was no apparent change in the percentages of patients with periodontal disease in every age group older than 35. Some overall improvement was noted in both oral hygiene status and gingivitis, with the major changes occurring in young adults.[11] However, in the future an increase in periodontal disease can be expected in people 55–74 years of age.[12] The fact that more people retain their teeth, coupled with the increasing number of older people, has resulted in a net rise in the number of elderly patients who have advanced periodontal disease. Because of this trend,[12] no decline in the percentage of advanced periodontal disease among those 55–74 years of age is expected until the year 2000.

THE COSTS OF DENTAL DISEASE AND DISABILITY

The primary factors associated with time lost from work seem to be oral health status, the cost of work loss to employees and employers, and access to dental care. In 1979 acute dental conditions led to 19.4 days of restricted activity and 3.5 workdays lost per adult person.[13] When acute and chronic conditions were combined, there were 20.5 days of restricted activity and five workdays lost per employed adult. Thus, the 6.8 million acute dental conditions reported resulted in 31.5 million days of restricted activity and 6.0 million workdays lost. In 1981, 6.7 million workdays were lost. A detailed review of several sources indicates that these data may well be a gross underestimate.[13]

From 1974 to 1980, the number of dental visits per person has remained roughly constant, although the number of people who have never visited a dentist decreased. This was especially true for the black population, which experienced a 50 percent reduction in the number of people who had never visited a dentist.

After a period of stability in the 1970s, the estimated number of visits to a dentist has increased from 366 to 436 million per year.[13] Approximately 90 percent of dentists' time is occupied by treatment of caries and periodontal disease and their sequelae. In 1984 approximately 0.5 percent of the U.S. gross national product was generated by the treatment of caries and periodontal disease, including sales of medications and toothpaste.[8,14]

Estimates of total time expended on dental visits range from 549 to 654.5 million hours (69–82 million workdays).[13] These estimates include travel, waiting, and visit time.

Bailit estimates that 16–19 million workdays were lost to dental services in 1979.[13] We estimate that caries and periodontal disease and their sequelae accounted for 90 percent of these (15–16 million workdays lost).

Overall, we estimate that the costs of dental services in 1982 were $19.5 billion, of which $18.7 billion was in the private sector. Over-the-counter medications probably added $3 billion to $4 billion to this figure.

INTERVENTIONS

The prevention of caries and periodontal disease requires multiple strategies which will suit the nature of the problem as well as the populations at risk. We next consider control measures for the etiologic categories of agent, host, and environment.

Strategies Focused on the Agent

Dental caries is an infectious disease which begins when the human infant acquires cariogenic flora, about the time the teeth erupt. Many different bacterial pathogens are involved in periodontal disease. Although no practical antimicrobial strategy presently exists for either caries or periodontal disease, several alternatives have potential benefit for the future.

The ideal procedure for elimination of dental caries would be prevention; that is, immunizing the infant before he or she has had sufficient contact with a carrier to contract the disease.[9]

Another method would reduce the amount of cariogenic organisms by using antibiotic rinses in the mouth of an infant or in the mouths of people close to the infant. Chlorhexidine has had limited success in children and adolescents, but it has

unresolved problems such as tooth discoloration. It has only recently been approved for commercial distribution in the United States.[9,15]

Periodontal destruction occurs during relatively brief bursts of disease activity. If the active phases of these diseases could be detected, the specific groups of organisms associated with different forms of periodontal disease could be identified and treated with chemotherapeutic and antibiotic agents.[6,16]

Short-term use of antibiotics may be helpful in controlling caries in difficult cases and reducing the severity of gingivitis. However, most authorities discourage long-term use because of the development of drug resistance, the proportional increase of resistant oral flora, and the risk of hypersensitivity reactions.[9,15]

Some of these disadvantages may be overcome if low doses of tetracycline or metronidazole are delivered locally in hollow fiber devices placed subgingivally.[17] However, this method is time consuming and labor intensive and alters the flora only in those pockets in which the hollow fibers are placed.

Culturing microflora sampled from designated diseases in gingival sites can help to direct antimicrobial therapy. If combined with other nonsurgical therapy, specific antibiotic coverage may be needed for only two-weeks at a time, thus reducing the risk of adverse effects.[16,18]

Plaque control is effective in preventing both caries and periodontal disease. Enzyme preparations may break down the plaque matrix, leading to the dispersion of the plaque, but clinical results have been disappointing. No preparation completely inhibits plaque formation, and they are unpleasant to use and cause local adverse effects. Despite continued research, their future as plaque control agents is not optimistic.[9,15]

A variety of other antimicrobial agents, including modified phenol compounds, fluorides, iodides, and peroxides, show a varying degree of effectiveness against plaque. Evidence suggests that stannous fluoride, because it is retained well by the teeth and has antibacterial properties, may be both an effective antiplaque and antigingivitis agent. Compounds of potassium iodide may be effective in low concentrations, but even small amounts are too toxic for general use. Peroxides have been shown to have some effect in reducing supragingival plaque. Slow-release devices supplied with antiperiodontitis agents attached to the teeth may play an important role in periodontal disease prevention in the future.[19,20]

Although antiseptics may play a future role in

supportive therapy, they do not replace the careful removal of plaque by the patient, hygienist, and dentist.

Strategies Focused on the Host

Host resistance to caries can be enhanced either by making teeth more resistant to decay or by increasing the amount or quality of the saliva. However, no practical intervention strategy presently exists that can alter hosts enough to prevent or control periodontal diseases in large populations.

Fluorides can make teeth more resistant to decay if consumed during tooth formation (systemic application) or if placed directly onto teeth (topical application). Fluoride molecules reorganize the enamel crystal into a more caries-resistant structural form and can actually arrest lesions through remineralization and antimicrobial actions. These benefits extend to adults as well as children.

Community water fluoridation. Fluoridation of water supplies has proved the most cost-effective community-wide means of preventing tooth decay. No direct action is required of an individual, yet tooth decay is reduced by 50–70 percent among children who consume optimally fluoridated water from birth. The benefits have been shown to continue well into adulthood, as long as the individual remains in a community with water fluoridation.[7] However, approximately 100 million Americans are deprived of the benefits of either optimally adjusted or naturally fluoridated water. Of these, about 73 million lack fluoridation because of the political success by antifluoridationists and the constraints of limited budgets of local governments. Effective water fluoridation systems require constant maintenance of equipment, training of waterworks personnel, and close monitoring of fluoride levels in the water.[21] The other 37 million live in areas that lack central water systems.[19,21–23]

School water fluoridation. Areas that lack a central water supply may choose to fluoridate school water supplies. The cost is low, the method requires no active participation on the part of the individual, and it targets a group especially prone to tooth decay. Presently, over 550 schools in 11 states are fluoridating their water. The reduction in tooth decay achieved by this method has been approximately 30–40 percent,[9,19,22,23] yet many school systems have not implemented water fluoridation, largely for political and economic reasons.

Self-applied fluoride in the schools. Because most children attend grade school regularly and many also attend preschool or day care facilities, the school setting is a logical place for administering self-applied fluorides. New tooth decay can be reduced 20–50 percent by once-a-week fluoride mouth rinsing and 30–40 percent by the daily use of a fluoride tablet in school.[22–25] Today, an estimated 12 million children benefit from such programs. These programs are usually well accepted by school systems because the procedure is quick, inexpensive, and easy for children of all ages to learn and carry out. In addition, lay personnel can supervise the process with minimal training. Such programs require and deserve continued financial and political commitment.

Self-applied fluoride in the home. Toothpastes with fluoride have long been available to help reduce tooth decay, and their use is recommended for everyone. Regular use can reduce children's tooth decay by 15–20 percent.[9,19,22,23] Supervision of young children may be required to ensure proper brushing and prevent them from swallowing the toothpaste and ingesting an excessive amount of fluoride.

Professionally applied topical fluoride. Fluoride can be applied to teeth by a dentist or dental auxiliary. After the teeth have been thoroughly cleaned, a fluoride solution may be painted on the teeth or a fluoride gel applied in a mouth tray. To be effective for caries-prone children, the procedure should be done at least semiannually. Although professionally applied fluorides will reduce tooth decay by 30–40 percent, they are more expensive than other methods.[9,19,24]

Slow-release devices. Compact intraoral slow-release appliances have been designed to bathe the mouth continuously with fluoride at low concentrations. One form is a tablet-shaped fluoride reservoir having an outer diffusion-limiting membrane. If clinical trials prove successful, fluoride slow-release devices may be the caries-preventive method of choice for use with caries-susceptible individuals, dental patients undergoing orthodonic treatment, and individuals who are mentally or physically handicapped. These devices will require professional application and maintenance, however, thus raising the initial costs.[9]

Screening. Regular oral examination and screenings serve to identify caries and periodontal disease at an early stage. High-risk groups can then be targeted for prompt secondary preventive therapy, thus preventing unnecessary further destruction and loss of teeth. The most important finding of the recent National Preventive Dentistry Demonstration Program was that it was not possible to eradicate decay or periodontal disease in an institution-based, highly comprehensive preventive program and that the cost of such a program for all children would be prohibitive, approximately $55 per child.[25] On a national level, comprehensive preventive services sponsored by public funds could cost $750 million for children and $1.6 billion for adults, based on need alone.[19]

A more rational approach may be to combine the use of an institution-based dental surveillance and education program and referral of targeted, high-risk groups with our current private practice delivery system. A reimbursement system that includes adequate financial incentives and optimal preventive coverage would encourage the expansion of appropriate preventive services provided by the private practitioners.[6,19] At the present time reliable, cost-effective technology to identify the target high-risk groups for treatment needs adequately is not available. Greater efforts in applied research are needed to develop the technology and clinical decision-making skills required of health care providers.

Strategies Focused on the Environment

An important area for intervention is the oral environment, which supports the microorganisms involved in the carious process and the pathogenesis of peridontal disease. Possible interventions include diet modification, oral hygiene, professional dental care—including plaque removal—tooth sealants, and surgical and nonsurgical therapies.

Frequent consumption of sugar-containing snacks that are readily retained on the tooth surfaces is closely related to high caries activity. Discontinuing the practice of eating sticky sweets between meals can reduce caries as much as 90 percent. This strategy may be effective in the long run, but extensive efforts would be required to achieve long-lasting changes in eating habits.[9,26]

Routine daily brushing and flossing by the patient is the sine qua non in caries prevention and periodontal therapy. These mechanical approaches for controlling dental plaque formation are the most easily applied methods now available to the patient and dental provider.[27-29] However, it is difficult to teach people to brush and floss correctly and regulary without supervision. Formal classroom instruction in dental health for children without the provision of dental treatment has failed to produce long-term behavioral changes. More effective strategies might involve parental reinforcement and media campaigns directed toward parents and teenagers.

The regular removal of plaque can successfully control new and recurrent caries and periodontal disease in children and adults. However, the frequency with which the procedure must be performed to be effective makes this method of caries and periodontal disease prevention much more expensive than other more primary preventive methods.

The procedures used include scaling, planing, and root curettage. Scaling is the general term for the removal of bacteria, bacterial products, and calculus; root planing refers to procedures used to smooth the root surface and correct defective restoration margins; curettage involves the removal of material from the gingival pocket and root surface, including treatment to destroy bacteria or toxic products. Their combined purpose is to alter the local environment associated with periodontal inflammation and thereby to control the destructive effects of the disease.[18]

In the United States in 1984, the total cost of providing professional prophylaxis, including scaling, root planing, and curettage, was approximately $100–$125 per capita.[29] The total price of such services to the individual consumer is approximately $150–$175 per person per year. Such treatment results in cleaner teeth and therefore a diminished incidence of caries, a decrease in gingival inflammation, and a decrease in loss of attachment tissues.

Adhesive tooth sealants have been developed to exclude bacteria and food constituents from the pits and fissures of teeth, where fluoride-based techniques are less effective. If such pits and fissures remain sealed, the occlusal tooth surface remains caries-free in a very high percentage of cases. The sealants remain in place for over four years in 85–95 percent of teeth so treated.[9,24,30] However, the use of sealants is often given a low priority in large public health programs because of the technical and financial commitments required for their application.

These commitments could be reduced by targeting high-risk age groups and individuals. Four sealants per child at ages 6 and 12 could cost approximately $35 if performed by dental auxiliaries and result in a 65 percent reduction in occlusal surface caries.[2,19,25] An even higher reduction in total surface caries, 85–90 percent, may be achieved by the combined use of systemic and topical fluorides and sealants.[2] Substantial savings can be realized if dental auxiliaries apply the sealants, instead of dentists.

Studies comparing the clinical effectiveness of surgical and nonsurgical periodontal therapy[20,28,29,31-35] have found that the time and resources required were large and similar for both modalities.

Prevention Priorities

Measures to ensure that children and adults receive the full benefits of fluoride, consume highly cariogenic foods infrequently, and follow an effective plaque control regimen have a synergistic effect on the prevention of dental caries (Table 3) and periodontal disease (Table 4), thus reducing the need for and cost of extensive dental care. Priority should be given to interventions as follows:

1. Community water fluoridation must be given the highest priority as a public health measure for preventing tooth decay. School and institutional water fluoridation is the second most practical, cost-effective measure.

2. In fluoridated areas, combined preventive regimens of professional prophylaxis, topical fluoride, hygiene instructions, and adhesive sealants could reduce new caries by 80–90 percent. In nonfluoridated areas, giving students daily fluoride tablets from preschool through eighth grade and weekly fluoride mouth rinsing in grades 9–12 could result in a caries reduction of 20–40 percent.

3. Regular and thorough brushing can help con-

Table 3. Criteria for prevention of dental caries

Intervention	Ages affected (years)	Annual cost per patient ($)	Effectiveness (%)	Practicality as a public health measure	Priority[a]
Community water fluoridation	All	.20–.40[b]	50–70	Excellent	1
Institutional water fluoridation	4–18	1.20–1.50	30–40	Good	2
School fluoride supplements					
At home	0–14	4–15	0–50	Poor	6
In school	4–18	4–8	20–40	Fair	3
School fluoride mouth rinse program	4–18	6–8	30–40	Fair	3
Topical fluoride treatment prophylaxis (professionally applied)	4–20 (20+ on incidence)	30–40	20–40	Poor	8
Toothbrushing with fluoride toothpaste					
In school	4–18	0.25[c]	20	Fair–poor	12
At home	All	10	20	Fair	12
Daily self-application of fluoride gel in custom trays	All	30–60	80	Poor	13
Control of detrimental school foods	4–18	NA	NA	Fair	7
Adhesive tooth sealants	6–12	3–10[d]	65	Poor	9
Labeling of sweets (FTC)	All	NA	NA	Fair	10
Regular dental visits	All	8–12[e]	NA	Always recommended	5
Dental health education and promotion	All	12†	NA	Fair–poor	4
Influence of mass media re news events	All	Negligible	NA	Fair	11

[a] 1, highest priority
[b] Per capita
[c] Per treatment
[d] Per tooth
[e] Per visit

Table 4. Criteria for prevention of periodontal disease

Intervention	Ages affected (years)	Annual cost per patient ($)	Effectiveness (%)	Practicality as a public health measure	Priority[a]
Dental health education	All	12	NA	Fair depending on access and if combined with treatment	3
Personal plaque control (brushing, flossing, etc.)	All	10	Fair if regular	Fair depending on individual motivation and dexterity	2
Quarterly professional prophylaxis and oral hygiene instruction	All	30–100	80	Fair if manpower available	1
Nonsurgical periodontal (scale, root plane, antibiotics)	35	100 by auxiliary 240 by dentist	90	Poor due to lack of resources	4
Combined surgical/ nonsurgical therapy	35	600 moderate cases 1000 advanced cases	90	Poor due to lack of resources	5

[a] 1, highest priority

trol plaque and, therefore, caries and early periodontal disease. The use of a fluoride dentifrice can reduce caries by 20 percent.

4. Fluorides professionally applied after a thorough professional cleaning can result in a reduced caries incidence of 35 percent if performed at last semiannually. If prophylaxis is thorough, performed four times a year, and accompanied by health education, there could be a substantial reduction in the development of new caries and periodontal disease in children and adults.

5. Because solid information is lacking on the costs and effectiveness of interventions available for the prevention and control of established periodontal disease, allocating large resources for a major effort in this area may not be advisable at the present time, particularly for adults. When effective methods become available, large-scale commitments would be warranted.

6. Vigorous health promotional efforts to prevent periodontal disease and caries may be effective if all appropriate health care professionals and gatekeepers are utilized. Health promotion is most effective when combined with access to treatment. The American Dental Association and the American Academy of Periodontology are now launching campaigns in the major media to inform the public about the prevention of caries and periodontal disease. High-quality, well-targeted media campaigns by pharmaceutical companies, health/business coalition groups, health care franchises and corporations, and health insurance companies may provide unexpected but effective increases in consumer awareness. The cost-effectiveness of such measures is presently unknown.[6]

Constraints on Available Interventions

Although specific strategies are known to prevent or control dental caries and periodontal diseases, they are not available to all Americans. The American Dental Association has noted that only one third of the US population receives complete dental care, and almost one half of children under the age of 12 have never been to a dentist for treatment.[6] The United States does not have a dental care program for children, let alone any type of national preventive program. Some of the barriers to comprehensive preventive dentistry services are listed below:

1. Economic incentives are lacking in private practice and in institutions such as schools, nursing homes, and the workplace.

2. Reimbursement by third-party payers is not properly designed for prevention.

3. Governmental support of existing cost-effective measures and research is decreasing.

4. Because dental diseases are not life threatening, they are not given the priority of other major health problems.

5. Clinical decision analysis techniques for the effective application of preventive measures have not been developed.

6. State dental practice laws severely limit the duties auxiliaries can perform.

Recommendations

Legislation. Americans who live in high-risk areas, nursing home patients, the medically and physically compromised, and the indigent should receive the full benefit of caries and periodontal disease preventive services. Such services could be institutionally based or contracted privately. Expanded use could be made of Medicare funding, health maintenance organizations, and Veterans Administration dental facilities for the elderly. In addition, there should be political, financial, and technical assistance to support the expansion of community and institutionally based water fluoridation, as well as supervised fluoride rinse programs.

Regulation. Federal, state, and local governments have the responsibility of integrating dental health services into basic insurance plans, to allow preventive dentistry as part of Medicaid, and to expand Medicare. Legal constraints on the use of auxiliaries to provide preventive services (such as brushing on sealants) could be reduced.

Education. Dental and other health professionals, particularly pediatricians, family physicians, and nurses, should teach patients about the causes and prevention of dental diseases and demonstrate preventive methods.

Planning and Research. New and more rigorous evaluations are needed. Dental and allied health professionals must participate at all levels of the planning process. Promising techniques such as antimicrobial rinses should be more rapidly refined and transferred to the marketplace for public and private use. Such transfers require public and private commitments to research and development.

CONCLUSION

We need to integrate what we already know about dental caries and periodontal diseases and to incorporate oral health into related programs, particularly those that reach people at greatest risk and in greatest need of dental care. We must recognize and attend to the barriers to the diffusion of known interventions. We should incorporate our intervention strategies into ongoing and future horizontal community health projects.

The authors express their appreciation to Drs. William Allen, Future of Dentistry Committee, American Dental Association; Howard Bailit, Columbia University School of Public Health; O. R. Butler, Georgia Dental Association; Peter DeGrazia, American Association of Dental Examiners; Chester Douglass, Harvard School of Dental Medicine; Anne Hanse, Georgia Dental Association; Charles R. Jerge, Department of Dentistry, Wake Forest University; Robert Mecklenburg, Chief Dental Officer, U.S. Public Health Service; Kent Nash, American Dental Association; Richard Schoessler, American Dental Association; Philip A. Swango, National Institute for Dental Research; and Raymond P. White, Jr., Robert Wood Johnson Foundation.

REFERENCES

1. Decayed, missing and filled teeth among persons 1–74, United States 1971–74. Hyattsville, Maryland: National Center for Health Statistics, 1981; DHHS publication no. (PHS)81-1678. (Vital and health statistics; series 11; no. 223).

2. The prevalence of dental caries in United States children, 1979–1980: the National Dental Caries Prevalence Survey. Hyattsville, Maryland: National Center for Health Statistics, 1982; DHHS publication no. 82–2245.

3. Spolsky VW, Kamberg CJ, Lohr KN, et al. Measurement of Dental Health Status. Santa Monica, California: The Rand Corporation, 1983.

4. Russell AL. A classification and scoring for prevalence surveys of periodontal disease. J Dent Res 1956;35:350–9.

5. Greene JC, Vermillion JR. The simplified oral hygiene index. J Am Dent Assoc 1960;61:172–9.

6. Strategic plan: report of the American Dental Association's Special Committee on the Future of Dentistry. Chicago: American Dental Association, 1983.

7. Burt B. The epidemiology of oral diseases. In: Striffler DF, Young WO, Burt B, eds. Dentistry, dental practice and the community. 3rd ed. Philadelphia: Saunders, 1983.

8. Bawden JW, DeFriese GH, eds. Planning for dental care on a statewide basis: the North Carolina Dental Manpower Project. WK Kellogg Foundation series on Issues in Dental Health Policy, Durham, North Carolina: Duke University, 1981.

9. National Institute of Dental Research. Challenges for the eighties. Bethesda, Maryland: National Institutes of Health, 1983; DHHS publication no. (NIH)85-860.

10. Basic data on dental examination findings of persons 1–74 years, US, 1971–1974. Hyattsville, Maryland: National Center for Health Statistics, 1979; DHEW publication no. (PHS)79-1662. (Vital and health statistics; series 11, no. 214).

11. Douglass C, Gillings D, Sollectio W, et al. National trends in the prevalence and severity of the periodontal diseases. J Am Dent Assoc 1983;107:403–12.

12. Douglass C, Gillings D, Sollecito W, et al. The potential for increase in the periodontal diseases of the aged population. J Periodontol 1983;54:12.

13. Bailet HL, Beazoglou T, Hoffman W, et al. Work loss and dental disease. Special report of the National Preventive Dentistry Demonstration Program. Princeton: Robert Wood Johnson Foundation, 1982, no. 1.

14. DeFriese GH, Baker BO. Assessing dental manpower requirements: alternative approaches for state and local planning. Cambridge, Massachusetts: Ballinger, 1982.

15. Hull PS. Chemical inhibition of plaque. J Clin Periodontol 1980;7:431.

16. Klavan B, ed. International Conference on Research in the Biology of Periodontal Disease. Chicago: University of Illinois, 1977.

17. Lindhe J, Heijl L, Goodson JM, et al. Local tetracy-

cline delivery using hollow fiberdevices in periodontal therapy. J Clin Periodontol 1979;6:141.

18. National Institute of Dental Research. Surgical Therapy for Periodontitis. J Periodontol 1982;53:475–501.

19. Division of Health Care Services, Institute of Medicine, Washington, D.C. Public policy options for better dental health: report of a study: Academy Press, 1980.

20. Knowles JW, Burgett FG, Nissle RR, et al. Results of periodontal treatment related to pocket depth and attachment level: eight years. J Periodontol 1979;50:225.

21. Centers for Disease Control. Promoting health/preventing disease—objectives for the nation. Washington, D.C.: U.S. Government Printing Office, 1980.

22. Horowitz AM, Horowitz HS. School-based fluoride programs: a critique. J Prev Dent 1980;6:89–94.

23. Preventive Dentistry for Massachusetts. Boston, Massachusetts: Department of Public Health, 1978:1–32.

24. Miller AJ, Brunelle JA. A summary of the NIDR community caries prevention demonstration program. J Am Dent Assoc 1983;107:265–9.

25. Special report of the National Preventive Dentistry Demonstration Program. Princeton: Robert Wood Johnson Foundation, 1983, no. 2.

26. Gustafsson BE, Quensel CE, Lanke LS. The Vipcholm Dental Caries Study: the effect of different levels of carbohydrate intake on caries activity in 436 individuals observed for 5 years. Acta Odont Scand 1954;11:207–31.

27. Axelsson P, Lindhe J. Effect of controlled oral hygiene procedures on caries and periodontal disease in adults. J Clin Periodontol 1978;5:133–51.

28. Axelsson P, Lindhe J. The effect of a plaque control program on dental plaque, gingivitis and caries in school children. J Dent Res 1977;56:142.

29. Rundle D. A cost-effective analysis of surgical and non-surgical periodontal therapy [Thesis]. Boston, Massachusetts: Harvard, 1983.

30. National Institutes of Health. Dental sealants in the prevention of tooth decay. Proceedings of the Consensus Development Conference. J Dent Educ 1984;48:126–31.

31. Bellini HT, Johansen JR. Average time required for scaling and surgery in periodontal therapy. Acta Odont Scand 1973;31:283–8.

32. Ekanayaka A, Sheiham A. Estimating the time and personnel required to treat periodontal disease. J Clin Periodontol 1978;5:85–94.

33. Rosling B, Nyman S, Lindhe J, et al. The healing potential of periodontal tissues following different techniques of periodontal surgery in plaque-free dentitions. J Clin Periodontol 1976;3:233–50.

34. Lindhe J, Westfelt E, Nyman S, et al. Healing following surgical and non-surgical treatment of periodontal disease. J Clin Periodontol 1982;9:115–28.

35. Hill RW, Ramfjord SP, Morrison EC, et al. Four types of periodontal treatment compared over two years. J Periodontol 1981;52:655–62.

Depression

Alan Stoudemire, M.D., Richard Frank, Ph.D.,
Mark Kamlet, Ph.D., and Nancy Hedemark, B.S., M.P.H.

The term "depression" as used here is "major depression" as defined by the American Psychiatric Association.[1] It is a serious psychiatric disorder characterized by a pervasive dysphoric mood disturbance and the loss of pleasure and interest in life. The mood disorder is prominent and is usually associated with symptoms such as appetite disturbance, weight changes, sleep disturbance (especially insomnia), agitation, decreased energy, fatigue, hopelessness, feelings of guilt and worthlessness, difficulty concentrating, decreased sexual drive, and suicidal thoughts or attempts. The syndrome in its most severe forms may be subtyped as either psychotic (delusions and paranoia may be present) or melancholic (a severe form of the illness that includes extreme depression, emotional and social withdrawal, anhedonia, early-morning awakening, anorexia, weight loss, and obsessional guilt).

Mood disturbances that are caused primarily by organic mental disorders or are a side effect of medication are not classified as depression. Major depression is differentiated from transient mild episodes of dysphoria that are a common reaction to stressful events (adjustment reactions). Major depression is also distinguished from dysthymic disorder (depressive neurosis), a chronic (persisting for at least 2 years) low-grade dysphoria that is a relatively stable personality trait and that is not characterized by a profound disruption in mood or biological functioning. Major depression is also distinct from symptoms of demoralization commonly caused by stressful environmental conditions such as poverty and low socioeconomic status.[2,3]

CAUSES AND HIGH-RISK GROUPS

The precise etiological factors in the pathogenesis of depression have not been elucidated. They are probably a combination of biological/genetic vulner-

From the Emory University School of Medicine (Stoudemire) and School of Public Health (Hedemark), Atlanta, the Johns Hopkins School of Hygiene and Public Health, Baltimore, (Frank), and the Carnegie-Mellon University, Pittsburgh, (Kamlet).

Address reprint requests to Dr. Stoudemire, Emory University Clinic, 1365 Clifton Road, Atlanta, GA 30322.

ability, psychological/emotional trauma, and acute sociological/environmental stressors. Those who appear to be at high risk for the development of depression include: (1) persons with first-degree relatives who suffer from alcoholism, sociopathy, or depression[4,5]; (2) persons who are under extreme stress and those who have suffered losses (divorce, separation, bereavement, job loss)[6]; (3) persons who have histories of early parent loss and childhood bereavement; and (4) persons who have major medical illnesses.

In addition, certain demographic characteristics appear to increase the risk for depression. The risk is relatively greater for women than men, for younger persons than older ones, for the separated and divorced, and for the socioeconomically disadvantaged.[7] The amount of social support available (i.e., family, confiding relationships, financial resources) also seems to be an important buffer, as the lack of such support tends to increase vulnerability to depressive illness.[8] Depression is a common phenomenon in the recently bereaved.[9] Physical illness is often associated with depressive symptoms, particularly in patients who have chronic pain, have suffered a stroke, have cancer, or are undergoing renal dialysis.[10] The children of the mentally ill (especially those who have schizophrenia and affective disorders) are also at greater risk of developing behavioral, intellectual, cognitive, and mood disturbances.[11]

EPIDEMIOLOGY

The epidemiology of psychiatric disorders is relatively crude and incomplete, compared with the epidemiological data available for medical illnesses such as cancer and infectious diseases. Part of the difficulty lies in problems with case identification, symptom measurement, and standardization of psychiatric diagnoses. In addition, statistics regarding prevalence of depression are often based on institutional or hospital cases rather than cases in the general community.

Surveys that measure symptoms of depression yield higher rates than do studies in which carefully structured interviews and standard diagnostic criteria are employed. For example, Weissman and Myers[12] reviewed five community surveys conducted around 1970 and reported estimated prevalence of 16–20 percent for "depression." In a later review, Boyd and Weissman[13] examined 11 studies and reported the prevalence of depression to be 9–20 percent. To what extent these studies measure or reflect episodes of major depression (versus minor depressive episodes) is unclear, but such high percentages point to the relative frequency of depressive symptoms (or symptoms of demoralization) that may be germinal to more severe depressive episodes.

Preliminary data from a research project conducted by the Epidemiologic Catchment Area of the National Institute of Mental Health indicate that the most common psychiatric diagnoses for women are phobias and major depression; for men, the predominant psychiatric diagnosis is alcohol abuse/dependence.[14] According to these data, the six-month prevalence for major depression is between 1 and 3 percent, with a higher frequency for women than for men.

Morbidity figures show a marked discrepancy between men and women (Table 1). For men, the number of cases and the rate per 100,000 for a six-month period are only one third what they are for women.[14] (12-month figures are not available.) We have calculated that the total number of cases in a six-month period, based on a 1980 population base, is approximately 4,757,779.

The rates of depression for the medically ill are higher than the rates from community surveys. Although reports vary considerably, most studies place prevalence figures between 12 and 32 percent.[10] Certain populations, such as patients with chronic renal disease, appear to be at higher risk. Depression rates for cancer patients appear to be in the range of 17–25 percent,[10] and as many as one third of patients who have cerebrovascular accidents will have a depressive episode during the year following the stroke.[15]

It appears that only approximately 18–25 percent of patients who have clinically significant depressive symptoms ever see a mental health professional for treatment. More than 80 percent, however, may see a general physician, and nearly 60 percent receive psychotropic drugs.[12]

THE MORTALITY OF DEPRESSION

We have summarized the mortality of depression based on an assumption that 60 percent of patients who commit suicide have a clinically significant depression as the primary psychiatric disorder (Table 2). The balance of suicides are considered to be the result primarily of other psychiatric disorders such as alcoholism, personality disorders, schizophrenia, and drug abuse.[16,17] Based on data from the National Center for Health Statistics, we estimate that 16,111 deaths in 1980 were secondary to depression. Since suicides are significantly underreported, this estimate may be too low; the total may exceed 20,000 deaths a year.

COSTS OF DEPRESSION

There are two major components of the cost of an illness to society: direct costs, which are incurred as a result of treatment, and indirect costs, which are due to lost productivity from morbidity and mortality.

Direct costs derive from hospitalization, physician and other provider services, pharmaceuticals, and rehabilitation. We estimate that affective disorders resulted in approximately 565,532 hospital admissions and 7,056,981 outpatient vistis to psychiatrists in 1980.[18] The direct costs are summarized in Table 3.

Indirect costs result from the loss of productivity due to illness-related morbidity and mortality. Age- and sex-specific rates for total days and work days lost because of depression are shown in Table 4. These morbidity data have been used to calculate the fulltime earnings and household value that are

Table 1. Major depression in men and women: age-specific morbidity, United States, 1980

Age (years)	Cases among men		Cases among women	
	n[a]	Per 100,000	n[a]	Per 100,000
18–24	286,020	1,900	733,458	4,900
25–44	680,936	2,200	1,810,601	5,700
45–64	317,410	1,500	700,260	3,000
65+	30,915	300	198,178	1,300
Total	1,315,281	1,698	3,442,497	4,035

Adjusted to 1980 population data base.
[a] Six-month period prevalence, extracted from ECA project data of the NIMH.[14]

Table 2. Suicides secondary to depression, United States, 1980

Age (years)	n	Per 100,000
<1–4	0	
5–9	2	0.01
10–14	83	0.46
15–19	1,078	5.10
20–24	2,065	9.69
25–29	1,937	9.92
30–34	1,615	9.20
35–39	1,290	9.24
40–44	1,071	9.18
45–49	1,021	9.20
50–54	1,153	9.85
55–59	1,136	9.78
60–64	938	9.30
65 +	2,722	10.65
Total	16,111	7.11

Data (rounded) from NCHS Detail Data Tape[37] and based on the assumption that 60 percent of suicides are due primarily to depressive illness. Adjusted to 1980 population data base.

lost as a result of depression.[18] These indirect costs appear in Table 5.

The indirect costs of mortality are based on the estimated years of life lost because of suicides. From the number of suicides assumed to be primarily the result of depression (see Table 2), we estimated that 377,768 years of life were lost before age 65 and 734,973 years of major activity were lost in 1980. Using sex-specific estimates of discounted lifetime earnings and a 6 percent discount rate, the total indirect mortality cost of depression is estimated at $4.2 billion.[18] (The 6 percent discount rate is the rate at which future dollars are discounted into present dollars.)

The total direct and indirect costs of depression are therefore estimated to be $16.3 billion annually. Details of these cost calculations may be found elsewhere.[18]

IMPACT ON QUALITY OF LIFE

Severe depression is a debilitating illness that usually leads to withdrawal from social, work, and family activities, decreased motivation, feelings of hopelessness, low self-esteem, pessimism, and self-blame. Withdrawal from family relationships can result in separation, divorce, and parent–child problems. Irritability, anger, and withdrawal can cause depressed patients to become isolated in their misery as others are driven away by their despair.

Depression may lead to poor work performance, absenteeism, and unemployment. The cognitive impairments (difficulty in concentrating and

Table 3. Affective disorders: inpatient and outpatient care

Setting	Days/visits[a]	Costs[b]
Inpatient care		
General hospital psychiatric units	260,368	$ 72,845,982
General hospitals outside psychiatric units	1,367,417	382,576,152
Community mental health clinics	505,260	141,361,642
State and county	3,085,929	212,242,612
Private psychiatric	1,014,800	152,025,240
V.A. psychiatric	1,169,080	166,792,780
V.A. general		
Residential treatment centers	465,673	58,016,354
Other	105,469	21,093,834
Nursing homes	2,132,230	62,516,983
Total inpatient care		$1,269,471,579
Outpatient care		
Psychiatrists	7,056,981	234,257,000
Psychologists	7,226,104	219,252,800
Other physicians	6,199,329	175,716,580
Social workers	956,452	28,693,559
Total outpatient		$ 657,919,939
Other direct costs		
Psychotropic drugs		138,378,780
Non-health care costs		47,555,230
Total other		$ 187,984,066
Total direct costs		$2,113,325,528

From Stoudemire et al.[18]
[a] Estimated number of hospitalizations is based on an assumed average stay of 14.1 days (1979 Hospital Discharge Survey, NCHS). This figure is likely to be low for most settings.
[b] Inpatient care is based on an average cost of $279.78 per day.

Table 4. Age- and sex-specific rates for total days lost because of depression, United States, 1980

Age (years)	Men	Women	Total
Days lost			
18–29	9,292,702	32,524,460	41,817,162
30–49	34,847,638	85,977,502	120,825,140
50–54	16,262,231	39,493,987	55,756,218
Total days lost			218,398,520
Work days lost			
18–29	7,434,162	17,237,963	24,672,125
30–49	27,878,110	68,782,002	96,660,112
50–54	13,009,784	21,595,190	34,604,974
Total work days lost			155,937,211

Data from The Manpower and Training Report of the President.[38]

memory loss) can resemble a form of dementia (depressive pseudodementia) that may sometimes lead to nursing home placement. Depressed patients have a high rate of physical complaints, especially pain, headaches, insomnia, and digestive problems. Severe depression can cause paranoia, delusions, and even violent behavior. The most directly lethal component of the depressive syndrome is suicide. Depression that develops as a result of physical disease only exacerbates the stress of an illness such as cancer, stroke, or chronic renal disease, and depression is often the factor that most prohibits recovery and rehabilitation.

Depression also burdens the family, especially if the patient's behavior is not recognized as secondary to a mood disturbance. Depressed patients are often intolerable to live with; they may appear self-pitying, pessimistic, irritable, angry, and overly sensitive. Some self-treat with alcohol and drugs. The depressed person tends to be self-absorbed, withdrawing into an emotional shell and offering little emotional support to others. Depression leads to loss of income, either from days lost from work or from discharge because of hospitalization or poor work performance.

There is strong evidence that the children of depressed patients are affected adversely. As noted in a review by Goodman,[11] the children of mentally ill parents (including depressives) get lower grades, have more symptoms of anxiety–depression, and have more problems with social–interpersonal functioning and classroom behavior. Depressed mothers have been found to be less effective, becoming either withdrawn and unavailable or overly involved in the lives of their children.[19] A family history of depression apparently increases the likelihood of depression in the offspring. In addition, a family history of suicide greatly increases the risk of suicide in the offspring.[20]

INTERVENTIONS

Primary prevention is successful when an illness is well understood, the etiology is identified precisely,

Table 5. Indirect morbidity costs from lost work years for depression, United States, 1980

Age (years)	Days of full-time employment	Days of home employment	Total costs ($)
Men			
18–29	20,367		216,751,649
30–49	76,378		2,075,047,925
50–54	35,643		1,065,412,201
Women			
18–29	47,227	41,880	886,551,730
30–49	188,444	47,110	4,079,102,479
50–54	59,164	49,037	1,705,362,329
Total cost			10,028,000,000

Data from The Manpower and Training Report of the President.[38]

and the pathways of transmission and the susceptibility of the host are established.[21] Efforts to decrease the incidence of an illness are therefore directed toward removing the cause, interrupting transmission of the disease, or enhancing host resistance.

Planning primary intervention is problematic when these concepts of preventive medicine are applied to the broad range of disorders that have been termed psychiatric (e.g., alcoholism, depression, anxiety disorders, personality disorders, psychosomatic disorders) because there is no consensus on the etiology of any of them. Experience has shown that primary prevention efforts in psychiatry have proved effective only when an infectious or toxic agent has been clearly identified as the cause of an illness (e.g., organic mental disorders such as neurosyphilis or lead encephalopathy). Because most psychiatric disorders appear to result from complex interactions of biogenetic, developmental, and sociological factors, identifying a precise cause is usually difficult. For example, even though genetic factors appear to act in the transmission of and vulnerability to schizophrenia, depression, and alcoholism, it is difficult to control for the developmental, environmental, and cultural factors that also play a role in the etiology of these disorders.

Despite the relative obscurity of the primary causes of the chief mental illnesses (schizophrenia, depression, alcoholism), primary prevention strategies are not impossible. Primary prevention is an effort to decrease the incidence of cases by "anticipating a disorder," thereby intervening before the development of symptoms that indicate psychopathology.[22] Strategies that might be used include identifying populations that are at high risk for a psychiatric disorder and applying preventive measures. It should be noted that the per-case averted costs of prevention increase tremendously with the base population. Thus, fine definitions of high-risk groups are critical.

Secondary prevention involves early treatment to decrease the length of the illness, thus decreasing prevalence. Secondary prevention implies that elements and symptoms of the disorder are already operating, but that morbidity and mortality can be reduced or eliminated by early identification. Screening to detect germinal cases is part of secondary prevention. The assessment of risk is part of this phase because screening efforts are best applied in populations in which the disorder is most likely to occur. Thus, primary and secondary treatment strategies for depression may be appropriate insofar as high-risk populations can be identified for screening. In addition, instruments for detecting

symptoms of the illness have been developed, and the effectiveness of some treatments is relatively well established.

The primary problem with screening is targeting and reaching those groups of patients most likely to be affected. The most feasible sites for screening and case detection are schools and primary medical care settings. Nursing homes, churches, and general hospitals are other possibilities. Community screening may not be practical, but organized outreach and support organizations such as those that have been developed for the bereaved and for victims of rape and child abuse are realistic in the community setting.

It is difficult to estimate how particular interventions would affect overall mortality, morbidity, disability, and health care costs. Measuring the success of an intervention depends on clinical, epidemiologic, and economic information that is simply unavailable. For example, to evaluate the impact of a screening program for depressive symptoms in a primary medical setting, we need to know (1) the prevalence of the disorder among patients being treated in the setting, (2) the efficacy and accuracy of screening, (3) the difference in outcome due to improved recognition, (4) the cost of screening, (5) the reduction in indirect costs (i.e., costs of lost productivity) due to early treatment of identified cases, and (6) the increase in direct (treatment) cost resulting from more patients receiving treatment. Little of this information exists. Despite the lack of data with which to carefully evaluate the cost-effectiveness of screening for depression, a number of high-risk groups can be targeted for potential intervention studies.

High-risk populations that might be targeted for the prevention of depression include (1) patients who have chronic or acute medical illnesses such as cancer, stroke, and chronic renal disease; (2) children of the mentally ill; (3) the recently bereaved, especially the surviving spouse, children of deceased parents, and parents of deceased children; (4) persons undergoing an inordinate degree of stress such as separation, divorce, or unemployment; and (5) children detected through school screening as having early signs of cognitive, academic, emotional, and behavioral problems.

The educational setting is one area in which persons could be identified for early interventions. A number of studies have shown that efforts to promote psychological development in children decrease emotional problems and enhance academic performance.[23-25] Although numerous psychoeducational approaches exist, they may be broadly categorized as values clarification; psychological education; skills training in coping, in human relations (interpersonal), in making decisions, and in communication; and moral education programs. Models for early interventions attempt to evaluate the cognitive and emotional status of children and to tailor interventions to each person's vulnerability. Reports of the early outcome of well-developed programs in the Portland public school system[26] and the Head Start program[27] are positive, indicating decreases in subsequent academic and behavioral problems.

Any intervention relating to prevention of depression, however, is inevitably met by one main obstacle—the general public's misinformation or lack of information about the causes, manifestations, and treatment of depression. Mental illness, including depression, is commonly viewed as a sign of moral or spiritual weakness, a failure to cope, and a sign of being crazy. Resistance and embarrassment thus prevent many persons from seeking appropriate help. Better public education would decrease the stigma of the illness and increase the numbers of those who seek and receive treatment.

Because the majority of Americans receive their mental health care[28] through the general medical sector rather than the mental health sector, general medical and primary care settings are strategically an important potential source of better case detection in high-risk groups. According to one study, depression and anxiety accounted for approximately 87 percent of patient visits to general physicians for psychiatrically related problems.[29] Other studies have yielded similar results, indicating that the majority of patients who visit physicians for emotional problems are suffering from depression, or a mixture of anxiety and depression.[30–32] As many as 26.7 percent of patients with emotional disorders in the primary care setting meet research diagnostic criteria for depressive disorders; major depressive disorder accounts for 21.7 percent of the diagnoses.[33]

Several studies indicate that despite the fact that general medical physicians see a large percentage of psychiatrically ill patients, these physicians often either overlook the disorder, undertreat, or inappropriately treat depressive illness. Physicians too often prescribe minor tranquilizers (benzodiazepines) or inadequate doses of antidepressants.[34,35] They often treat the superficial symptoms of depression—using tranquilizers for anxiety, analgesics for pain, and sedatives for insomnia—while leaving unexplored the core mood disturbance and the underlying marital, family, and other interpersonal conflicts.

More than half the persons who commit suicide visited a physician within six months of death. Such a high figure raises the question: How many of these deaths could have been prevented by better recognition? More than half of those in one sample who committed suicide by overdose had received a prescription less than a week before dying or had an unlimited prescription for a lethal amount of the pharmaceutical sustances ingested.[36] Based on these data, a strong case can be made for making the diagnosis and treatment of depression a core part of the curriculum in medical student and primary care residency training programs.

SUMMARY

Historically, the efficacy of psychiatric therapies has been difficult to assess, and the recidivism of psychiatric patients is well known. Major depressive illness is the exception; efficacy of treatment has been well demonstrated. The disorder tends to be episodic, and the majority of cases remit with appropriate treatment. It is thus unfortunate that depression continues to bear a stigma when our current knowledge provides treatment to reverse this disorder effectively—both by curing it and by potentially preventing it.

Depression is a relatively common but serious disorder that carries with it a significant economic and health burden for our society. The negative impact is exacerbated by the stigma that prevents affected persons from seeking treatment and keeps families and professionals, who could best identify affected persons, from recognizing the signs of depression. Further studies specifically focusing on the effects of early intervention in high-risk populations, as well as the cost-effectiveness of screening programs, may help to decrease the morbidity, mortality, and social costs associated with this form of mental illness.

The authors thank the following consultants to the psychiatric disorders section of the "Closing the Gap" health policy project: Drs. Morton Silverman, National Institute of Mental Health; Robert E. Roberts, University of Texas Health Sciences Center; Sherryl Goodman, Emory University; Ricardo Munoz, University of California, San Francisco; Milton Weinstein, Harvard University School of Public Health; Myrna Weissman, Yale University; and Mr. Don Eddings, Centers for Disease Control.

REFERENCES

1. Diagnostic and statistical manual of mental disorders. 3rd ed., rev. Washington, D.C.: American Psychiatric Association, 1987.

2. Dohrenwend BP, Shrout PE, Egri G, et al. Nonspecific psychological distress and other dimensions of psychopathology. Arch Gen Psychiatry 1980;37:1229–36.

3. Roberts RE, Vernon SW. The Center for Epidemiologic Studies Depression Scale: its use in a community sample. Am J Psychiatry 1983;140:41–6.

4. Winokur G. The natural history of the affective disorders (manias and depressions). Semin Psychiatry 1970;2:451–63.

5. Andreason NC, Winokur G. Secondary depression: familial, clinical or research perspectives. Am J Psychiatry 1979;136:62–6.

6. Lloyd C. Life events and depressive disorder reviewed. Arch Gen Psychiatry 1980;37:541–8.

7. Hirschfeld RMA, Cross CK. Epidemiology of affective disorders. Arch Gen Psychiatry 1982;39:35–46.

8. Aneshensel CS, Stone JD. Stress and depression. Arch Gen Psychiatry 1982;39:1392–6.

9. Clayton PJ, Halikas JA, Maurice WL. The depression of widowhood. Br J Psychiatry 1972;121:71–8.

10. Stoudemire A. Depression in the medically ill. In: Cavenar JO, ed. Psychiatry, vol. 2. New York: Lippincott, 1985:1–8.

11. Goodman SH. Children of disturbed parents: the interface between research and intervention. Am J Community Psychol 1984;12:663–87.

12. Weissman MM, Myers JK. Rates and risks of depressive symptoms in a United States urban community. Acta Psychiatr Scand 1978;57:219–31.

13. Boyd JH, Weissman MM. Epidemiology of affective disorders. Arch Gen Psychiatry 1981;38:1039–46.

14. Myers JK, Weismann MM, Tischler GL, et al. Six-month prevalence of psychiatric disorders in three communities: 1980–1982. Arch Gen Psychiatry 1984;41:959–67.

15. Robinson RG, Price TR. Post-stroke depressive disorders: a follow-up of 103 patients. Stroke 1982;13:635–41.

16. Robins E, Murphy GE, Wilkinson RH, et al. Some clinical considerations in the prevention of suicide based on a study of 134 successful suicides. Am J Public Health 1959;49:888–99.

17. Monkoff K, Bergman E, Beck A, et al. Hopelessness, depression and attempted suicide. Am J Psychiatry 1973;130:455–9.

18. Stoudemire A, Frank R, Kamlet M, Hedemark N, Blazer D. The economic burden of depression. Gen Hosp Psychiatry 1986;8:387–94.

19. Weissman M, Paykel E, Klerman G. The depressed woman as mother. Soc Psychiatry 1972;7:98–108.

20. Roy A. Family history of suicide. Arch Gen Psychiatry 1983;40:971–4.

21. Spiro HR. Prevention in psychiatry: primary, secondary and tertiary. In: Kaplan H, Freedman A, Sadock B, eds. Comprehensive textbook of psychiatry, 3rd ed. Baltimore: William and Wilkins, 1980:2859–74.

22. Goldston SE. An overview of primary prevention programming. In: Klein DC, Goldston SE, eds. Primary prevention: an idea whose time has come. Rockville, Maryland: National Institute of Mental Health, 1977:23–40.

23. Barclay JR. Primary prevention and assessment. Personnel Guid J 1984;62:475–8.

24. Barclay JR. Primary prevention in schools. Personnel Guid J 1984;62:443–95.

25. Baker SB, Swisher JD, Nadenicheck PE, et al. Measured effects of primary prevention strategies. Personnel Guid J 1984;62:459–63.

26. Sheldon C, Morgan CD. The child development specialist: a prevention program. Personnel Guid J 1984;62:470–4.

27. Lazar I, Darlington R, et al. Lasting effects of early education: a report from the Consortium for Longitudinal Studies. Soc Res Child Dev 1982;47:1–151.

28. Regier DA, Goldberg ID, Taube CA. The de facto US mental health services system. Arch Gen Psychiatry 1978;35:685–93.

29. Marks JN, Goldberg DP, Hillier VF. Determinants of the ability of general practitioners to detect psychiatric illness. Psychol Med 1979;9:337–53.

30. Hesbacher P, Rickels K, Downing RW, et al. Assessment of psychiatric illness severity by family physicians. Soc Sci Med 1978;12:45–7.

31. Goldberg ID, Krantz G, Locke BZ. Effect of a short-term outpatient psychiatric benefit on the utilization of medical services in a prepaid group practice medical program. Med Care 1970;8:419–28.

32. Goldberg D, Steele JJ, Johnson A, et al. Ability of primary care physicians to make accurate ratings of psychiatric symptoms. Arch Gen Psychiatry 1982;39:829–33.

33. Katon W, Kleinman A, Rosen G. Depression and somatization: a review. Am J Med 1982;72:127–35.

34. Keller MB, Klerman GL, Lavori PW, et al. Treatment received by depressed patients. JAMA 1982;248:1848–55.

35. Keller MB, Lavori PW, Endicott J, et al. Treatment of depression. JAMA 1983;249:1824.

36. Murphy GE. The physician's responsibility for suicide. I. An error of commission. Ann Intern Med 1975;82:301–9.

37. Detail Data Tape. Hyattsville, Maryland: National Center for Health Statistics, 1980 (unpublished data).

38. The manpower and training report of the president. Washington, D.C.: 1980.

Diabetes Mellitus

William H. Herman, M.D., Steven M. Teutsch, M.D., M.P.H., and Linda S. Geiss, M.A.

Diabetes mellitus is a heterogeneous group of disorders characterized by abnormally high blood glucose levels.[1] This disease occurs when the body does not make enough insulin or when the cells cannot use the available insulin. The condition may first appear as an acute metabolic crisis or as a chronic illness.

There are 5.5 million people in the United States who have diabetes, and there may be an equal number who are undiagnosed. Our discussion will be limited to persons with diagnosed diabetes. Although there are many types of diabetes, three predominate: type I or insulin-dependent; type II or non-insulin-dependent; and gestational diabetes.

Type I, or insulin-dependent, diabetes mellitus typically develops during childhood but may occur at any age.[1] It is more common in people who have certain genetic markers, and it appears to have an autoimmune basis. People with type I diabetes have little or no circulating insulin and are dependent on injected insulin to sustain life. Approximately 435,000 Americans now have type I diabetes. This number remains fairly constant, because each year, type I diabetes develops in 19,000 Americans, and 19,000 Americans who have type I diabetes die (Figure 1).

Type II, or non-insulin-dependent, diabetes mellitus affects more than 5 million people in the United States, primarily adults, and tends to run in families.[1] This type of diabetes is more common in women and in races other than white. Of those who have type II diabetes, 60–90 percent have a history of being overweight. People who have type II diabetes may have normal, elevated, or depressed insulin levels. Many of these cases can be managed with diet therapy, weight control, and exercise, although some patients are treated with oral hypoglycemic agents or insulin. Every year type II, which is the most common form of diabetes, develops in 586,000 Americans, and 304,000 Americans who have type II diabetes die (Figure 1).

In a woman who has gestational diabetes, high blood glucose levels are first identified during pregnancy.[1] This type of diabetes is more common in older women, who often are overweight, have family histories of diabetes, and have had several pregnancies. Gestational diabetes develops in approximately 86,000 women each year in the United States.

Diabetes may be associated with diabetic ketoacidosis (a life-threatening complication caused by inadequate insulin) and, in those treated with insulin or oral hypoglycemic agents, hypoglycemic coma. With time, diabetes may cause complications in pregnancy, accelerate atherosclerotic cardiovascular disease, and cause blindness, renal failure, neuropathy, and amputations. These acute and chronic complications of diabetes contribute directly to the morbidity, mortality, and cost of diabetes in the United States.

Diabetes also exacts a large, though less quantifiable, psychosocial toll from affected persons and their families.[2] Treatment necessitates strict dietary management, daily exercise, urine or blood testing, and daily therapeutic decisions. These exigencies demand major alterations in lifestyle and may result in emotional disequilibrium, lowered self-esteem, and interpersonal conflicts. Living with the fear of life-threatening complications can also generate denial, hostility, anxiety, and depression.

Diabetes has traditionally been regarded as an incurable disease, but recent evidence shows that much can be done to prevent type II diabetes and delay or prevent the complications of all types of diabetes. Yet the incidence and prevalence of the disease continue to be too high because of the gap between knowledge and practice. We present here the scope of the problem and our recommendations for closing that gap.

RISK FACTORS FOR DIABETES

Age, sex, and race. The highest incidence of type I diabetes occurs in children 10–14 years of age.[3] By

From the Division of Diabetes Control, Center for Prevention Services, Centers for Disease Control, Atlanta.

Address reprint requests to Dr. Teutsch, Division of Diabetes Control, Centers for Disease Control, 1600 Clifton Road, Atlanta, GA 30333.

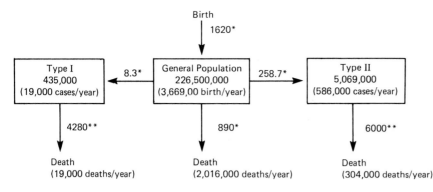

* rate per 100,000 general population per year
** rate per 100,000 diabetic population per year
( ) indicates number of new cases per year

contrast, the incidence and prevalence of type II diabetes increase dramatically with age.[4] The rate of gestational diabetes also increases as maternal age increases.[5–7]

The incidence of type I diabetes is similar for boys and girls.[3] The incidence and prevalence of reported type II diabetes, however, are 1.8 and 1.4 times greater in women than in men.[4]

The incidence and prevalence of type I diabetes are slightly higher in whites than in other races.[4,8–10] By contrast, the prevalence of type II diabetes is higher in races other than white and is extremely high in Hispanics (relative risk (RR), 3.1) and native Americans (RR, 10.8).[11–14] Race does not independently affect the incidence of gestational diabetes.[5]

Genetic and familial factors. People with certain genetic markers or human leukocyte antigens (HLAs) are at increased risk for developing type I diabetes. In whites, type II diabetes is not associated with any specific HLA types. The risk of type II diabetes in the siblings of patients who have type II diabetes is, however, up to six times that of the siblings of normal, age-matched persons, and the risk of type II diabetes in the children of these patients is approximately twice that of other children.[15] Women who have family histories of diabetes are also at increased risk of gestational diabetes.[5]

Obesity. Obesity is not associated with the development of type I diabetes, but it is an important risk factor both for type II diabetes and for gestational diabetes. Studies comparing the siblings of patients with type II diabetes with controls have found that the prevalence of diabetes is approximately twice as high among the nonobese siblings of diabetic patients as among the nonobese siblings of controls. Among the obese siblings of diabetic patients, the prevalence of diabetes is approximately three times that among nonobese siblings.[16] This finding and the observation that the body's

ability to tolerate glucose improves in approximately 75 percent of obese hyperglycemic patients who lose weight suggest that obesity is as important as familial factors in the development of type II diabetes.[17,18] Obese women in all age groups, compared with nonobese women, have a twofold increased risk for gestational diabetes.[5]

Inactivity. Inactivity, though not related to the pathogenesis of type I diabetes, does contribute directly to type II diabetes. Exercise helps maintain glucose control; inactivity reduces the body's ability to handle glucose.[19] Because inactivity often accompanies and contributes to obesity, which is itself a risk factor for type II diabetes, exercise may also reduce the risk of type II diabetes by lessening obesity.

Gestational diabetes. When the National Diabetes Data Group criteria for the diagnosis of gestational diabetes are used, women who have gestational diabetes are at significantly increased risk of developing overt diabetes later.[1] In one group of 752 women who had gestational diabetes, all but 2 percent reverted to normal glucose tolerance postpartum.[20] On follow-up, however, 60 percent of the women who had gestational diabetes developed overt diabetes during the next 16 years.[7] The impact of gestational diabetes on infact morbidity is unclear.

INCIDENCE AND PREVALENCE OF DIABETES

According to the National Health Interview Survey (HIS) conducted by the National Center for Health Statistics (NCHS), approximately 2.4 percent of the U.S. civilian, noninstitutionalized population reported that they have diabetes.[2] According to another NCHS prevalence survey, the Health and Nutrition Examination Survey (HANES), during the period 1976–1980, 3.2 percent of the adult population who had no history of diabetes did have diabeticlike responses to oral glucose tolerance tests.[12]

Some have interpreted these data to mean that for every person in the United States who is diagnosed as having diabetes, there is another person whose diabetes is undiagnosed. Because the characteristics, morbidity, mortality, and costs of diabetes in this undiagnosed population are unknown, we have limited our discussion to diagnosed diabetes as estimated by the HIS.

Each year in the United States an estimated 605,000 new cases of diabetes occur, an incidence rate of 267 cases per 100,000 population (Figure 1). Females have a higher incidence (337 per 100,000) than males (191 per 100,000). The incidence increases with age: The rate is 14 cases per 100,000 among persons less than 25 years of age and 907 cases per 100,000 among persons 65 years of age or older.

Separate figures for the incidence and prevalence of type I and type II diabetes are not available from the HIS. The prevalence of type I diabetes for all age groups in the general population is estimated at 160 per 100,000 population.[21] Type II diabetes accounts for 93–97 percent of diabetes cases; thus, the estimated incidence and prevalence of this type of diabetes in the U.S. population are 259 per 100,000 and 2,368 per 100,000, respectively.

Before 1980 the failure to apply uniform criteria for the diagnosis and classification of gestational diabetes caused much confusion about its incidence. Using the National Diabetes Data Group criteria, in the United States gestational diabetes occurs in approximately 2.4 percent of all pregnancies.[1,7,22] Thus, diabetes is associated with approximately 86,000 pregnancies each year.

COSTS

During 1980 diabetes was the primary diagnosis in 1.7 percent of the 575.7 million office visits made to private physicians in the United States,[23] and 2.9 percent of all visits involved a diagnosis of diabetes. Diabetes was also the first-listed discharge diagnosis for 666,000 hospitalizations, accounting for almost 7 million hospital days. It was listed as one of seven discharge diagnoses for 2.25 million hospitalizations and was related to 24.6 million hospital days. People with diabetes were 2.3 times more likely to be hospitalized than age-matched people without diabetes in the general population.[24]

In 1977, there were 189,600 diabetics living in U.S. nursing homes, that is, roughly 15 percent of nursing home residents. At that time the prevalence of diabetes in people over 65 living in nursing homes was 2.1 times that in the general, noninstitutionalized population over the age of 65.[25]

The total direct cost of these office visits, hospitalizations, nursing home stays, and medications for diabetes in the United States is estimated at $7.9 billion per year (Table 1).

Employed people who have diabetes average 10.8 days lost from work per person per year—twice that of age-matched people who do not have diabetes.[26] This accounts for an estimated annual total loss of 37,500 work years by employed people with diabetes, 53,000 work years by women with diabetes who keep house, and 116,300 work years by people with diabetes who are unable to work.[27]

Diabetes as an underlying cause of death before age 65 accounts for 145,000 years of life lost in the United States every year. When examined as one of multiple causes of death, diabetes annually accounts for 411,000 years of life lost before age 65. When underlying cause of death data are multiplied by a factor of 10 to reflect the true mortality of people who have diabetes, diabetes is annually associated with 1,450,000 years of life lost before age 65.[28]

These indirect costs of diabetes have been estimated to amount to approximately $10 billion per year.[29]

THE MORTALITY AND MORBIDITY OF DIABETES

Because people die of the complications of diabetes rather than the disease itself, diabetes as the underlying cause of death is underreported, particularly on death certificates of older people who have mul-

Table 1. Estimated direct and indirect costs of diabetes mellitus, United States, 1980

	Millions of dollars
Direct costs:	
Physician office visits	652
Hospitalization	6,157
Nursing home care	663
Insulin and oral hypoglycemic agents	380
Total	7,852

	Thousands of person-years lost
Indirect costs:	
Disability	
Employed persons with diabetes mellitus	37.5
Homemakers with diabetes mellitus	53.0
Unemployed because of diabetes mellitus	116.3
Premature mortality	1,450.0

tiple chronic conditions. For this reason, the mortality rate of diabetes is underestimated in the data. However, it is clear that mortality rates of people who have diabetes are higher than those of the general population.[30] The risk of premature death is greater for people who were younger when diabetes developed than for those who were older when it developed. In general, the life expectancy at diagnosis for a person who has type I or type II diabetes is one third shorter than that of a person of the same age who does not have diabetes.

The principal causes of death, as shown in Figure 2, correlate with the major causes of morbidity (Figure 3). Persons who develop diabetes before the age of 20 are 23 times more likely to die of renal disease than people of the same age in the general population.[31] Cardiovascular disease accounts for about three fourths of the deaths of persons who develop diabetes after the age of 40 and was responsible for at least 1,538,000 illnesses in 1980 (Figure 3).

Risk Factors

Age, sex, and race. The rates of end-stage renal disease and hospitalization for ketoacidosis are highest in the diabetic population under 45 years of age.[32-34] The rates of congenital malformations increase as maternal age increases.[35] The rates of atherosclerotic cardiovascular disease and amputation also increase dramatically with age.[36] The incidence of diabetic blindness is highest in persons over 65 years of age.

Sex appears to be a risk factor for many of the

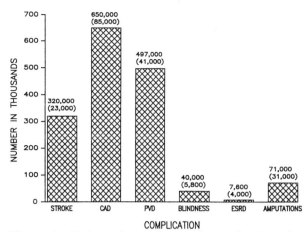

Figure 3. Estimated prevalence of complications from diabetes, United States, 1980 (1976 NHIS[32,34,50,52,54]) Prevalence above bar, incidence in parentheses. CAD, coronary artery disease; PVD, peripheral vascular disease; ESRD, end-stage renal disease.

complications of diabetes. For example, women are hospitalized for diabetic ketoacidosis 1.1 times more often than men.[33,37,38] Among diabetics, the incidence of stroke and diabetic blindness is higher in women than in men. And although the incidence of coronary heart disease and peripheral vascular disease is higher in diabetic men, the additional risk for stroke, coronary heart disease, and peripheral vascular disease is actually greater for women than for men.[36] Amputations are 1.4 times more frequently on diabetic men than on diabetic women.

Race can also be a factor in the development of diabetic complications. For example, compared with white diabetic patients, diabetics who are of races other than white have a death rate from diabetic ketoacidosis which is three times as high, and more than twice the incidence of blindness. Black diabetics have three times the incidence of end-stage renal disease and twice the incidence of amputations when compared with diabetic whites. Perinatal mortality rates are three times higher among the offspring of black diabetic women than of white diabetic women. The prevalence of atherosclerotic heart disease, however, is approximately the same in whites and in blacks.

Types and duration of the disease. The type of diabetes a person has is an important contributing factor when considering diabetic complications. For example, the hospitalization rates for diabetic ketoacidosis are higher for persons who have type I diabetes than for those who have type II diabetes. (Ketoacidosis does occur in type II diabetes, however, during episodes of infection, dehydration, or stress.[1]) People who have type I diabetes are 15 times as likely than those who have type II diabetes

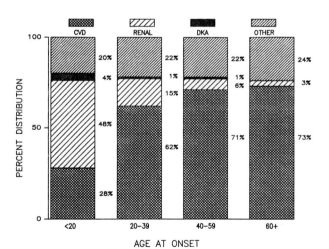

Figure 2. Percentage distribution of principal causes of death among patients with diabetes, by age at onset, Joslin Clinic, 1956–1962. CVD, Cardiovascular disease; DKA, diabetic ketoacidosis. (Modified from Entmacher et al.[52])

to develop end-stage renal disease.[39] On the other hand, persons who have type II diabetes have higher rates of atherosclerotic cardiovascular disease and amputations compared with those who have type I diabetes. More complications and higher morbidity associated with pregnancy (including serious congenital malformations) occur in women who have overt diabetes than in women who have gestational diabetes.[35,40,41]

The duration of diabetes also contributes to complication rates. For example, the rates of diabetic retinopathy and diabetic nephropathy increase dramatically the longer patients have diabetes.

Hypertension. Hypertension is a leading risk factor for atherosclerotic cardiovascular disease and for diabetic end-stage renal disease. Hypertension also contributes to amputations to the extent that it contributes to peripheral vascular disease. The studies done to date, however, have generally not been focused on the impact hypertension has on cardiovascular outcomes in diabetic patients.

The 1976 HIS showed that in all age groups over the age of 20, diabetics report a higher prevalence of hypertension than do nondiabetics. According to community studies, the prevalence of hypertension in diabetic patients is approximately twice that of age- and sex-matched controls.[42,43] Although the strength of the association between diabetes and hypertension diminishes after controlling for obesity, the association remains statistically significant.[44] Black diabetics are 1.2 times as likely as white diabetics to suffer from hypertension; according to some studies, diabetic men are slightly more likely than diabetic women to suffer from hypertension.[45]

Cigarette smoking. Cigarette smoking is an important risk factor for atherosclerotic cardiovascular disease and amputations to the extent that tobacco contributes to peripheral vascular disease. A diabetic person is as likely as a nondiabetic to be a smoker; in the 20- to 44-year age group, however, diabetics are 1.1 times as likely to be smokers than are nondiabetics.[43] No definitive studies have been done on the impact smoking has on persons who have diabetes.

Hyperlipidemia. Hypercholesterolemia (high blood cholesterol) is a risk factor for atherosclerosis and for amputations to the extent that it contributes to peripheral vascular disease. Estimating the prevalence of hyperlipidemia in diabetics has been difficult because hyperglycemia may produce or intensify hyperlipidemia, and improving glycemic control may mitigate the condition.[46] However, levels of serum cholesterol are generally somewhat higher in diabetics, and the levels of triglyceride are considerably higher.[47]

Hyperglycemia. Suboptimal control of blood glucose levels (glycemic control), often associated with acute disease or stress, may lead to diabetic ketoacidosis. Hyperglycemia is a leading risk factor for adverse outcomes of pregnancy in diabetic women. Although hyperglycemia probably accelerates atherogenesis, the mechanism and degree of this effect are unknown.[48-50] Higher blood glucose levels appear to be associated with a higher prevalence of diabetic microvascular disease, and poor glycemic control contributes to amputations to the degree that its predisposes the patient to peripheral neuropathy and infection.

Complications

Diabetic ketoacidosis (DKA). Diabetic ketoacidosis, an acute metabolic complication of diabetes, arises as a result of an absolute or relative deficiency of circulating insulin. Characterized by malaise, dry mouth, thirst, nausea, vomiting, frequent urination, lethargy, and eventually coma, it is associated with high blood glucose levels and metabolic acidosis.

According to the NCHS National Hospital Discharge Survey, in 1980 the annual incidence of ketoacidosis in the U.S. population who had diabetes was 13.6 per 1,000 males and 15.6 per 1,000 females.[33] Approximately half of all episodes of diabetic ketoacidosis occur in people who have type I diabetes and half in people who have type II, but the rates are higher in persons who have type I diabetes (13.4 per 1,000 diabetic person-years) than in those who have type II (3.3 per 1,000 diabetic person-years).[38]

Approximately 20 percent of cases of diabetic ketoacidosis occur as a first manifestation of diabetes.[37,38] Approximately 9 percent of all people hospitalized with this condition die.[37,38] These deaths usually occur among older diabetic patients who have other acute, nonmetabolic diseases such as stroke, heart attack, and pneumonia. The mortality associated wtih uncomplicated diabetic ketoacidosis is approximately 1 percent.[38]

Adverse outcomes of pregnancy. Each year more than 10,000 babies are born to women who have overt diabetes; approximately 86,000 are born to women who have gestational diabetes.[6] Infants of diabetic mothers have disproportionately high rates of hypoglycemia, macrosomia (large body size), and respiratory distress syndrome.[40,41] Pregnant women who have overt diabetes are more likely to carry malformed (RR, 3–4) or nonviable (RR, 10–45) fetuses.[35,50]

Cerebrovascular disease. Strokes are more common in diabetics.[51] According to the 1976 HIS, the RR of stroke in diabetics over the age of 20 is 2.7. Even after hypertension, increasing age (both important risk factors for stroke), and other factors are accounted for, the incidence of stroke remains approximately twice as high among diabetics as among nondiabetics.[36]

Coronary heart disease. Angina pectoris, myocardial infarction, and sudden death are more common among people who have diabetes.[51] According to the 1976 HIS, the crude age-adjusted prevalence rate for heart attack is 2.5 times higher among diabetics over the age of 20 than among nondiabetics. According to one study, cardiovascular disease accounted for as much as 71 percent of deaths in patients who developed diabetes after age 40[51] (Figure 2). After age, hypertension, and smoking are controlled for, the incidence of coronary heart disease still remains approximately twice as high among diabetics as among nondiabetics.[36]

Peripheral vascular disease. Diminished arterial perfusion of the legs, which is common in people who have diabetes, can lead to symptoms such as pain in the legs with exercise (intermittent claudication). When combined with other factors, diminished arterial perfusion can lead to skin ulcers, gangrene, and amputations.

The apparent frequency of peripheral vascular disease depends on the measurement technique used. When peripheral pulse deficits were used as diagnostic criteria, the incidence of peripheral vascular disease among residents of Rochester, Minnesota, over the age of 30 was 2.13 per 100 person-years for men and 1.76 per 100 person-years for women. The prevalence of peripheral vascular disease in this same population was 10 percent.[52] The comparable figure for the nondiabetic population is approximately 2.6 percent.[53]

The prevalence of this type of vascular disease increases dramatically with increasing age,[52] and hypertension and smoking are again leading contributors to the condition in diabetics. The prevalence of peripheral vascular disease also increases with the duration of diabetes. In people who have had diabetes for more than ten years, the rates are twice as great as in those who have had diabetes for less than ten years.[52]

Amputations. Peripheral neuropathy, vascular disease, and infection predispose people who have diabetes to gangrene and amputations. Compared with the rest of the population, people who have diabetes have a 16-fold increased risk for lower extremity amputations. Indeed, 50 percent of lower extremity amputations performed in the United States are done on people who have diabetes. Approximately 31,000 American diabetic patients have lower extremity amputations each year.[55]

Diabetic eye disease. In Americans 20–74 years of age, diabetes is the leading cause of new cases of legal blindness (corrected visual acuity less than 20/200 in the better eye). Approximately 5,800 Americans become blind each year as a result of diabetes, and approximately 39,500 Americans are blind because of diabetes.[34] Compared with the rest of the population, people who have diabetes are at a sixfold increased risk for blindness.[34,55]

In type I and type II diabetes, 87 percent and 33 percent of legal blindness, respectively, is caused at least in part by diabetic retinopathy.[56] After 15 or more years of diabetes, 40 percent of people who have type I diabetes develop proliferative retinopathy, as do about 15 percent of those who have type II diabetes.[58] Without treatment, 20–50 percent of people who have proliferative retinopathy become blind within five years.[59] In persons who have type II diabetes, glaucoma and cataracts are more important causes of blindness.

Diabetic renal disease. Compared with the rest of the population, people who have diabetes are at a 17-fold increased risk for end-stage renal disease. Death caused by renal disease is about 23 times as common in people who have type I diabetes as in the age-matched general population. Diabetes is currently the second leading cause of this disease in the United States, accounting for approximately 25 percent of new cases annually.[60] Approximately 4,000 Americans who have diabetes develop end-stage renal disease each year, and approximately 7,600 Americans are now receiving therapy for it.[32] Approximately 11 percent of patients on renal dialysis have diabetes.

Diabetic neuropathy. Diabetic neuropathy, one of the most common and debilitating complications of diabetes, encompasses a large group of syndromes with a wide range of manifestations. Problems in definition, classification, and diagnosis, as well as uncertainty about this complication's pathophysiology, natural history, and prognosis, have, however, made it virtually impossible to quantify its incidence, prevalence, and cost.

Diabetic peripheral neuropathy, the most common form, usually affects the feet and legs. In general, it is progressive and irreversible. The concomitant lack of sensation may result in unperceived traumatic joint damage or minor trauma, leading to secondary infection, gangrene, and amputation.

A second major type of diabetic neuropathy is visceral or autonomic neuropathy, which usually occurs in conjunction with peripheral neuropathy. It commonly affects the cardiovascular, gastrointestinal, and genitourinary systems. Painless myocardial infarction is more likely, and increased morbidity and mortality may result from delayed diagnosis. Bladder paralysis and urinary retention often develop, which may in turn contribute to ascending renal infection and end-stage renal disease.

Neuropathy may also cause male impotence and retrograde ejaculation. Although asymmetric mononeuropathy is often extremely painful, the prognosis is usually favorable.

INTERVENTIONS

Diabetes has been a model for chronic disease intervention programs, and important strides have been made in implementing these interventions. The programs have taken advantage of the skills and contributions of many critical groups, including consumers and health care professionals, representatives for academia, voluntary agencies, labor, industry, third-party payers, and government.

In 1974 Congress passed the National Diabetes Mellitus Research and Education Act (PL 93-354) and established the National Commission on Diabetes. Also established were the National Diabetes Advisory Board, the National Diabetes Data Group, the National Diabetes Information Clearinghouse, the Diabetes Research and Training Centers, and the Centers for Disease Control, Division of Diabetes Control. Standard definitions and classifications of diabetes have been developed and adopted, and many facts about the epidemiology of the disease have been clarified and compiled.[1,61] Guidelines for diabetes screening,[62] national standards for patient and professional education,[63] standards of care for the prevention and treatment of five complications of diabetes,[64] and a diabetes program handbook[65] have been developed and disseminated.

The Centers for Disease Control, the State Diabetes Control Programs, and other voluntary and professional organizations are translating the consensus of what constitutes quality diabetes care into community practice. State programs have implemented outpatient education and training programs and demonstrated that they are cost effective. Third-party reimbursement for outpatient education has been obtained in several states.[66] In addition, the Centers for Disease Control have helped to develop innovative approaches to translate effective interventions directly into community practice.

Health departments are coordinating diabetes control with related programs (particularly for hypertension, maternal and child health, and native American health). States are developing networks to ensure that diabetic patients who have hypertension are adequately treated and that diabetic

women of childbearing age are identified and their blood glucose levels controlled before conception and throughout gestation. Coordination of community resources and voluntary organizations, including smoking cessation and weight reduction programs, has also been established.

The systematic application of existing knowledge and resources has done much to reduce the morbidity, mortality, and cost of diabetes in the United States, but much more remains to be done. Interventions can prevent people from developing diabetes (primary prevention) and can prevent the development of complications in people who have diabetes (secondary prevention). See Table 2 for a summary of the interventions and the estimated number of preventable cases.

Primary Intervention

Prevention of obesity may reduce the incidence of type II diabetes by one half and gestational diabetes by as much as one third.[18,67] The prevalence of undiagnosed glucose intolerance may also be significantly reduced by preventing obesity. Because weight control has been so difficult to achieve in the general population, however, most efforts focus on secondary prevention.

Secondary Intervention

Although much is known about how to prevent the complications of diabetes, this information has too often not been communicated to health care providers or patients, or has been communicated but not acted upon. Improved education and self-management skills could reduce the incidence of diabetic ketoacidosis by as much as 70 percent and could prevent approximately 50,000 hospitalizations each year.[68-70] According to preliminary data, improved glycemic control before conception and throughout gestation could prevent approximately 500 life-threatening congenital malformations each year in the offspring of women who have overt diabetes. Improved diagnosis and management of pregnant diabetic women would also significantly reduce maternal morbidity and mortality and the incidence of neonatal hypoglycemia, macrosomia, and respiratory distress syndrome.[35,40,41,50]

According to one study, physicians check the blood pressure of their diabetic patients only 67 percent of the time. Only approximately 75 percent of diabetic patients who have hypertension are being treated for it, and only about half of them have adequately controlled blood pressure.[43] Detection and control of hypertension among diabetics

Table 2. Estimated potential impact of interventions for diabetes, United States

Problem	Intervention	Preventable (%)	Preventable cases/year
Type I diabetes	—	—	—
Type II diabetes	Obesity control	50	293,000
Gestational diabetes	Obesity control	33	28,000
	Primary interventions		
Peripheral vascular disease	Hypertension control	60	24,000
Stroke	Hypertension control	85	19,000
Coronary heart disease	Hypertension control Smoking cessation Lipid control	45	38,000
	Secondary interventions		
Ketoacidosis	Glycemic control Education	70	52,000
Serious congenital malformation	Glycemic control Education	70	500
Blindness	Education Laser photocoagulation	60	3,480
End-stage renal disease	Hypertension control	50	2,000
Amputations	Education Hypertension control Smoking cessation Glycemic control	50	15,000

could reduce the incidence of stroke by 75–95 percent, the incidence of coronary heart disease by 25–50 percent, and the incidence of peripheral vascular disease by 30–60 percent.

Over a million people who have diabetes continue to smoke cigarettes.[43] If they would stop smoking, the incidence of stroke in that population could be reduced by 5 percent, the incidence of coronary heart disease by 10 percent, and the incidence of peripheral vascular disease by 30 percent.[36]

Fewer than half of all diabetic patients are examined annually for diabetic retinopathy.[71] Prompt diagnosis and appropriate laser photocoagulation therapy for people who have proliferative diabetic retinopathy could reduce the incidence of severe visual loss by approximately 60 percent.[59] For persons who have diabetic nephropathy, aggressive antihypertensive therapy could reduce the rate of progression by more than 50 percent and delay or prevent the development of diabetic end-stage renal disease.[72,73] Foot care programs could reduce the rate of amputation by more than 50 percent in people who have neuropathy and peripheral vascular disease.[68–70] Psychosocial and peer support can ease

the emotional burdens of diabetes and improve the quality of life for diabetic patients and their families.[3]

Specific Strategies

Adopting healthful behaviors and lifestyles is an important personal intervention for reducing the burden of diabetes in the United States. Health can be promoted as enhancing the feelings of well-being, energy, power, and status. People can be encouraged to adopt lifestyles that incorporate healthy diets and regular exercise and to eschew cigarette smoking. Such promotional efforts should be redoubled in populations at high risk for diabetes—i.e., people who have family histories of diabetes, women who have histories of gestational diabetes, and persons who are black, Hispanic, or native American.

Comprehensive health curricula in schools can emphasize the principles of health maintenance. School lunches and athletic programs can teach by example and reinforce healthful behaviors. Children can be taught how to make decisions, to be responsible for their own actions, and to understand and resist peer pressure and advertising. Business, labor, and the media can be enlisted to promote healthy diets, exercise, and nonsmoking. Parents and public figures can be encouraged to act as role models to promote healthful behaviors.

People who have diabetes should be encouraged to view themselves as a population that has a disproportionate number of risk factors for adverse health outcomes; they should thus be encouraged to adopt healthful lifestyles, to control their obesity and hypertension, to stop smoking, and to control their lipid and blood glucose levels. Efforts to achieve these ends should be intensified in populations at high risk for the complications of diabetes. People who have diabetes also need to be encouraged to understand diabetes and to cope with its daily demands and predictable crises. They must be aware of the potential complications of diabetes and of appropriate prevention, treatment, and rehabilitation strategies. Access to education, dietary and social support systems, and medical care is vital. If these services do not exist, they should be established. If access to these services is restricted, all barriers, including financial ones, should be removed.

Measures must also be taken to ensure that people who have diabetes receive the best medical care available. In general, such care necessitates a team approach. Health care providers need to establish consensus about appropriate interventions and therapies and to develop formal systems to actively disseminate and implement those strategies, taking care to recognize and focus on high-risk populations.

Diabetic ketoacidosis, adverse pregnancy outcomes, blindness, and amputations are no longer the inevitable correlates of diabetes. Thus the practitioner must ensure that diabetic patients have the knowledge and skills necessary for self-care. Hypertension, diabetic pregnancies, diabetic retinopathy, nephropathy, and foot disease should be diagnosed promptly and treated appropriately.

It is critical that our society continue to promote public health, fund diabetes research, and support the translation of research findings into clinical practice. Food, alcohol, and tobacco policies, regulations, subsidies, and tax supports could promote the public health of the nation. Food stamps, for instance, could be used to encourage people to use foods low in fat and simple sugars. Those who administer and fund programs should ensure that health programs (e.g., for mothers and children, native Americans, migrant workers, veterans, and senior citizens, as well as health insurance programs) meet the current standards of diabetes care.[63,64]

Appropriate changes in lifestyle may result from economic incentives provided by employers and insurers. For example, third-party coverage for outpatient educational programs and preventive services such as prepregnancy counseling, glucose monitoring equipment, and eye examinations may help patients take advantage of such services. Accreditation bodies may also foster improved diabetes care by formally recognizing centers of excellence for diabetes, which could serve as referral sources for education and care.

With the cooperation of people who have diabetes, voluntary organizations, practitioners, professional organizations, educators, hospitals, accreditation bodies, health departments, labor, industry, insurers, media, and government, much can be done to close the gap between what is now, and what can be.

We are grateful for the assistance of Robert M. Anderson, Ed.D.; Nina Berlin; Jerry L. Brimberry; Fred A. Connell, M.D., M.P.H.; John K. Davidson, M.D., Ph.D.; Larry C. Deeb, M.D.; Allan L. Drash, M.D.; James B. Field, M.D.; J. William Flynt, M.D.; Richard F. Hamman, M.D., D.P.H.; J. Michael Lane, M.D.; Alice R. Ring, M.D.; Andrew T. Sumner, Sc.D.; Karl E. Sussman, M.D.; and Judith Wylie-Rosett, Ed.D.

REFERENCES

1. National Diabetes Data Group. Classification and diagnosis of diabetes mellitus and other categories of glucose intolerance. Diabetes 1979;28:1039–57.

2. Hamburg BA, Lipsett LF, Inoff GE, Drash AL. Behavioral and psychosocial issues in diabetes. In: Proceedings of the National Conference. Bethesda, Maryland: US Government Printing Office, 1979; National Institutes of Health, publication no. 80-1993.

3. LaPorte RE, Fishbein HA, Drash AL, et al. The Pittsburgh insulin-dependent diabetes mellitus registry: the incidence of IDDM in Allegheny County, Pennsylvania (1965–1976). Diabetes 1981;30:279–84.

4. Carter Center of Emory University. Closing the gap: the problem of diabetes in the United States. Diabetes Care 1985;8:391–406.

5. Mestman JH. Outcome of diabetes screening in pregnancy and perinatal morbidity in infants of mothers with mild impairment of glucose tolerance. Diabetes Care 1980;3:447–52.

6. O'Sullivan JB, Harris MI, Mills JL. Diabetes in pregnancy. In: National Diabetes Data Group. Diabetes in America: Diabetes data compiled 1984. Bethesda, Maryland: National Institutes of Health, 1985; NIH publication no. 85-1468; chap. 20.

7. O'Sullivan JB. Establishing criteria for gestational diabetes. Diabetes Care 1980;3:437–9.

8. Fujimoto WY. Diabetes in Asian Americans. In: National Diabetes Data Group. Diabetes in America: diabetes data compiled 1984. Bethesda, Maryland: National Institutes of Health, 1985; NIH publication no. 85-1468; chap. 10.

9. Sievers ML, Fisher JR. Diabetes in North American Indians. In: National Diabetes Data Group. Diabetes in America: Diabetes data compiled 1984. Bethesda, Maryland: National Institutes of Health, 1985; NIH publication no. 85-1468; chap. 11.

10. Young W, Murphy S, Marcus P, et al. Prevalence of diabetes and incidence of related acute complications in Denver area school-age children. Proceedings of the sixth annual CDC Diabetes Control Conference. Atlanta: Centers for Disease Control, 1983.

11. Bennett CG, Tokuyama GH, Bruyers PT. Health of Japanese Americans in Hawaii. Public Health Rep 1963;78:753–62.

12. Harris M. The prevalence of noninsulin-dependent diabetes mellitus. In: National Diabetes Data Group. Diabetes in America: diabetes data compiled 1984. Bethesda, Maryland: National Institutes of Health, 1985; NIH publication no. 85-1468; chap. 6.

13. Knowler WC, Pettitt OJ, Savage PJ, et al. Diabetes incidence in Pima Indians: contributions of obesity and parental diabetes. Am J Epidemiol 1981;113:144–56.

14. Wheeler FC, Gollmar CW, Deeb LC. Diabetes and pregnancy in South Carolina: prevalence, perinatal mortality, and neonatal morbidity in 1978. Diabetes Care 1982;5:561–5.

15. Kobberling J, Tillil H. Empiric risk figures for first-degree relatives of non-insulin dependent diabetics. In: Kobberling J, Tattersall R, eds. Serono Symposium no. 47: the genetics of diabetes mellitus. New York: Academic, 1982:201–9.

16. Baird JD. Is obesity a factor in the aetiology of non-insulin dependent diabetes? In: Kobberling J, Tattersall R, eds. Serono Symposium no. 47: the genetics of diabetes mellitus. New York: Academic, 1982:231–41.

17. Savage PJ, Knowles WC. Diet therapy for type 2 (noninsulin-dependent) diabetes mellitus: can new approaches improve therapeutic results? Clin Nutr 1984;54:69–87.

18. Newburgh LH. Control of the hyperglycemia of obese "diabetics" by weight reduction. Ann Intern Med 1942;17:935–42.

19. Lipman RL, Raskin P, Love T, et al. Glucose intolerance during decreased physical activity in man. Diabetes 1972;21:101–7.

20. O'Sullivan JB, Mahan CM. Criteria for the oral glucose tolerance test in pregnancy. Diabetes 1964;13:278–85.

21. LaPorte RE, Tajima N. The prevalence of insulin-dependent diabetes. In: National Diabetes Data Group. Diabetes in America: diabetes data compiled 1984. Bethesda, Maryland: National Institutes of Health, 1985; NIH publication no. 85-1468; chap. 5.

22. Centers for Disease Control. Diabetes and pregnancy. Diabetes Control Prog Update 1983;4(March):1–5.

23. National Ambulatory Medical Care Survey, public use data tapes. Hyattsville, Maryland: National Center for Health Statistics, 1980.

24. Sinnock P. Hospital utilization for diabetes. In: National Diabetes Data Group. Diabetes in America: diabetes data compiled 1984. Bethesda, Maryland: National Institutes of Health, 1985; NIH publication no. 85-1468; chap. 26.

25. National Center for Health Statistics. 1977 national nursing home survey. Curr Pop Rep 1982;917:25.

26. Drury TF. Disability among adult diabetics. In: National Diabetes Data Group. Diabetes in America: diabetes data compiled 1984. Bethesda, Maryland: National Institutes of Health, 1985; NIH publication no. 85-1468; chap. 28.

27. Entmacher PS, Sinnock P, Bostic E, Harris M. Economic impact of diabetes. In: National Diabetes Data Group. Diabetes in America: diabetes data compiled 1984. Bethesda, Maryland: National Institutes of Health, 1985; NIH publication no. 85-1468; chap. 32.

28. Herman WH, Sinnock P, Brenner E, et al. An epidemiologic model for diabetes mellitus: incidence, prevalence, and mortality. Diabetes Care 1984;7:367–71.

29. Platt WG, Sudovar SG. The social and economic costs of diabetes: an estimate for 1979. Ames, Iowa: Miles Laboratories, 1979.

30. Kessler II. Mortality experience of diabetic patients: a 26-year follow-up study. Am J Med 1971;70:715–24.

31. Geiss LS, Herman WH, Teutsch SM. Diabetes and renal mortality in the United States. Am J Public Health 1985;75:1325–6.

32. Eggers PW, Connerton R, McMullan M. The Medicare experience with end-stage renal disease: trends in incidence, prevalence, and survival. Health Care Fin Rev 1984;5:69–88.

33. National Hospital Discharge Survey, public use data tapes. Hyattsville, Maryland: National Center for Health Statistics, 1980.

34. Vision Problems in the U.S. New York: National Society to Prevent Blindness, 1980.
35. Day RE, Insley J. Maternal diabetes mellitus and congenital malformations: survey of 205 cases. Arch Dis Child 1976;51:935.

36. Kannell WB, McGee DL. Diabetes and cardiovascular disease: the Framingham study. JAMA 1979;241:2035–8.

37. Faich GA, Fishbein HA, Ellis SE. The epidemiology of diabetic acidosis: a population-based study. Am J Epidemiol 1983;117:551–8.

38. Johnson DD, Palumbo PJ, Chu CP. Diabetic ketoacidosis in a community-based population. Mayo Clin Proc 1980;55:83–8.

39. Rettig B, Teutsch SM. The incidence of end-stage renal disease in type I and type II diabetes mellitus. Diabet Nephropathy 1984;3(Feb):26–27.

40. Karlson K, Kjellmer J. The outcomes of diabetic pregnancies in relation to mother's blood sugar level. Am J Obstet Gynecol 1972;112:213.

41. Peterson J. Goals and end-points in management of diabetic pregnancy. In: Camerini-Davalos RA, Cole HS, eds. Early diabetes in early life. New York: Academic, 1975.

42. Christlieb AR. Hypertension: The major risk factor in juvenile-onset insulin-dependent diabetes. Diabetes 1981;30(suppl 2):90–6.

43. Halpern M, Dodson DL, Beasley J. Diabetes in Michigan: 1980 survey results. Ann Arbor, Michigan: Department of Public Health. Chronic disease reports; no. 4, 1983:30–8.

44. Barrett-Connor E, Criqui MH, Klauber MR, et al. Diabetes and hypertension in a community of older adults. Am J Epidemiol 1981;113:276–84.

45. Horan MJ. Diabetes and hypertension. In: National Diabetes Data Group. Diabetes in America: diabetes data compiled 1984. Bethesda, Maryland: National Institutes of Health, 1985; NIH publication no. 85-1468; chap. 17.

46. Bennion LJ, Grundy SM. Effects of diabetes mellitus on cholesterol metabolism in man. N Engl J Med 1977; 296:1365–71.

47. Wilson DE, Schriebman PH, Day VC, et al. Hyperlipidemia in an adult diabetic population. J Chron Dis 1970;23:501–6.

48. Epstein FH. Glucose intolerance and cardiovascular disease. Triangle 1973;12:308.

49. Garcia MJ, McNamara PM, Gordon T, et al. Morbidity and mortality in diabetics in the Framingham population: sixteen-year follow-up study. Diabetes 1974;23: 105–11.

50. Fuhrmann K, Reiher H, Semmler K, et al. Prevention of congenital malformations in infants of insulin-dependent diabetic mothers. Diabetes Care 1983;6:219–23.

51. Kannell WB, McGee D, Gordon T. A general cardiovascular risk profile: the Framingham study. Am J Cardiol 1976;38:46–51.

52. Entmacher PS, Root HF, Marks HH. Longevity of diabetic patients in recent years. Diabetes 1964;13:373–7.

53. Melton LJ, Macken KM, Palumbo PJ, et al. Incidence and prevalence of clinical peripheral vascular disease in a population-based cohort of diabetic patients. Diabetes Care 1980;3:650–4.

54. Nilsson SE, Nilsson JE, Frostberg N, et al. The Kristianstad survey II. Acta Med Scand 1967;469(suppl):1–40.

55. Most RS, Sinnock P. The epidemiology of lower extremity amputations in diabetic individuals. Diabetes Care 1983;6:87–91.

56. Kahn HA, Hiller R. Blindness caused by diabetic retinopathy. Am J Ophthalmol 1974;78:58–67.

57. Klein R, Klein BK. Diabetes and vision. In: National Diabetes Data Group. Diabetes in America: diabetes data compiled 1984. Bethesda, Maryland: National Institutes of Health, 1985; NIH publication no. 85-1468; chap. 13.

58. Klein R, Klein BK, Syrjala SE, et al. Wisconsin epidemiologic study of diabetic retinopathy: relationship of diabetic retinopathy to management of diabetes: preliminary report. In: Friedman EA, L'Esperance FA Jr, eds. Diabetic Renal–Retinal Syndrome, vol. 2. New York: Grune & Stratton, 1982:21–41.

59. Diabetic Retinopathy Study Research Group. Photocoagulation treatment of proliferative diabetic retinopathy: clinical application of diabetic retinopathy study findings: DRS report no. 8. Ophthalmology 1981;88:583–600.

60. Herman WH, Teutsch SM. Kidney diseases associated with diabetes. In: National Diabetes Data Group. Diabetes in America: diabetes data compiled 1984. Bethesda, Maryland: National Institutes of Health, 1985; NIH publication no. 85-1468; chap. 14.

61. Diabetes data compiled 1977. Washington, D.C.: US Government Printing Office, 1978; DHEW publication no. (NIH) 78-1468.

62. Herron CA. Screening in diabetes mellitus: report of the Atlanta workshop. Diabetes Care 1979;2:357–62.

63. National Diabetes Advisory Board. National standards for diabetes patient education programs. Diabetes Care 1984;7:31–5.

64. National Diabetes Advisory Board. The prevention and treatment of five complications of diabetes: a guide for primary care practitioners. Washington, D.C.: US Government Printing Office, 1983; DHHS publication no. (HHS) 83-8392.

65. Diabetes Program Handbook. Atlanta: Centers for Disease Control, 1983.

66. Sinnock P, Bauer DW. Reimbursement issues in diabetes. Diabetes Care 1984;7:291–6.

67. Kempner W, Newborg BC, Perchel RL, et al. Treatment of massive obesity with rice/reduction diet program: An analysis of 106 patients with at least a 45 kg weight loss. Arch Intern Med 1975;135:1575–84.

68. Davidson JK, Alogna MT, Goldsmith M, et al. Assessment of program effectiveness at Grady Memorial Hospital. In: Steiner G, Lawrence PA, eds. Educating Diabetic Patients. New York: Springer, 1981:329–48.

69. Miller LV, Goldstein J. More efficient care of diabetics in a country hospital setting. N Engl J Med 1972;286: 1388–91.

70. Runyan JW. The Memphis chronic disease program. JAMA 1975;231:264–7.

71. Herman WH, Teutsch SM, Sepe SJ, et al. An approach to the prevention of blindness in diabetes. Diabetes Care 1983;6:608–13.

72. Mogensen CE. Antihypertensive treatment inhibiting the progression of diabetic nephropathy. Acta Endocrinol 1980;94(suppl 238):103–11.

73. Parving HH, Andersen AR, Smidt UM, et al. Early aggressive antihypertensive treatment reduces rate of decline in kidney function in diabetic nephropathy. Lancet 1983;1:1175–9.

Digestive Diseases

Richard S. Johannes, M.D., M.S., Stephen N. Kahane, M.D.,
A. I. Mendeloff, M.D., M.P.H., John Kurata, Ph.D., M.P.H., and
Harold P. Roth, M.D., M.S.

Diseases of the digestive system affect every person sooner or later, whether as a transient ailment or as a life-threatening illness. All diseases that interrupt the processing of nutrients have the potential to inflict damage, and those that are chronic and severe exact an enormous toll both from the individual affected and from society.

This report focuses on the digestive diseases responsible for the highest mortality (colorectal cancer and cirrhosis) and the greatest morbidity (gallbladder disease, peptic ulcer disease, diverticular disease, and inflammatory bowel disease). According to the National Center for Health Statistics (NCHS), in 1980 over 2.3 million people were admitted to hospitals with one of these six diseases (Table 1).[1] Gallbladder, peptic ulcer, and diverticular disease were the most frequent diagnoses.

The NCHS reported that 171,600 deaths occurred in 1977 from malignant and nonmalignant digestive diseases (Table 2).[2] The estimated direct and indirect costs of mortality from digestive diseases in the same year totaled more than $11 billion.

THE SCOPE OF THE PROBLEM

Colorectal Cancer

Ranking second among cancer deaths, colorectal cancer was responsible for 88,947 deaths in 1977, a rate of 19.6 per 100,000 population (18.9 per 100,000 for men, 20.2 per 100,000 for women).[2]

A better understanding of the pathogenesis of colon cancer has evolved in the past few years. Morson's work on the colonic polyp has revolution-

From the Johns Hopkins School of Medicine (Johannes and Kahane) and School of Public Health and Hygiene (Mendeloff), Baltimore, Maryland, the Department of Family Medicine, University of California, Irvine (Kurata), and the Epidemiology and Data Systems Program, National Institute of Diabetes, Digestive and Kidney Diseases, Bethesda, Maryland (Johannes and Roth).

Address reprint requests to Dr. Johannes, Blalock Bldg., Rm. 928, Johns Hopkins Hospital, 600 North Wolfe Street, Baltimore, MD 21205.

ized thinking about colon cancer.[3] Most experts now believe that more than 98 percent of all colon cancer originates in preexisting colonic polyps. If one assumes the adult population has a polyp prevalence of 40 percent and that the attack rate for colon cancer is 90 per 100,000 population, then the malignancy-to-polyp ratio would be approximately 0.1 percent. Although proof of the polyp-to-cancer sequence is lacking, three pieces of convincing evidence favor this hypothesis. First, small nests of cancer-bearing tissue are rarely found within otherwise normal mucosa; when such nests are found, they are almost always within polyps. Second, patients who have polyps tend to have a higher rate of cancer. Third, in experimental animals, carcinogens often produce lesions that progress through a stage that looks much like the dysplastic lesions of humans.[3]

Recently, a National Institute of Health (NIH) panel of experts concluded that a minimum of 85 percent of cancers arise in preexisting polyps. The interval between polyp detection and malignant transformation is five to ten years. Size, one of the chief determinants in the detection of polyps, is also an important factor in the assessed risk of malignancy.[3]

Gilbertson demonstrated that careful surveillance and removal of polyps can reduce the expected cancer incidence rate for the population by as much as 85 percent over a period of 25 years.[4] It has been recognized that early detection—when the tumor is in Dukes' class A rather than class C—will reduce mortality. According to studies in recent years, the tendency toward earlier detection of cancers has been increasing.[5] Unfortunately, whether this has translated into a greater number of survivors is unknown.

Colorectal cancer can be compared with cervical cancer in that (1) there is a known preexisting lesion, (2) there is a long lag time before malignant transformation, (3) there are effective methods for detecting persons at risk, and (4) treatment of the lesion reduces or eliminates the risk. Unlike the Pap

Table 1. Hospital admission rates for digestive diseases, United States, 1980

Disease	Total admissions	Sex Male	Female
Gallbladder disease	645 (1,053)	180 (321)	456 (714)
Colorectal cancer	241 (519)	120 (267)	122 (253)
Cirrhosis	98 (644)	55 (394)	42 (250)
Peptic ulcer disease	611 (3,903)	287 (2,045)	14 (45)
Inflammatory bowel disease	173 (1,232)	74 (516)	99 (716)
Diverticular disease	360 (3,120)	111 (1,172)	248 (1,984)
Total	1,228 (10,571)	827 (4,815)	1,293 (6,058)

Data from National Center for Health Statistics.[1]
The initial rates per 100,000 population represent primary admitting diagnoses; the numbers in parentheses represent secondary diagnoses.

smear for cervical cancer, the methods for detecting colonic polyps are not inexpensive or easy to apply to large populations. Furthermore, only a small percentage of polyps undergo malignant transformation. Although size, histopathologic type, and degree of dysplasia provide clues to help determine which polyps are most likely to become malignant, a full examination by fiber optic endoscopy with biopsy is necessary to establish these facts. The compiled data from Correa et al.[6] suggest a prevalence rate for polyps of 28.5 percent in those 40–59 years of age and a rate of 37.8 percent in people over 60 years old. Because polyps are common in the adult population, finding them is not as great a problem as removing them. Following these patients for recurrence presents an added difficulty.

The methods for searching out polyp-bearing adults at risk include fecal occult blood testing (FOBT), flexible and rigid sigmoidoscopy, barium enema study, and colonoscopy. Colonoscopy, which can also be used to remove polyps nonsurgically, is now being widely performed on outpatients. However, it is expensive both in time and in dollars.

Studies are now in progress to assess the risk of recurrent polyps and to determine the best overall screening procedures for colonic cancer. According to data from David Eddy at Duke University, the cost–benefit curve is much flatter than was originally anticipated.[7] The data were analyzed using decision analysis, which is a formal method of describing a complex interaction of events, each of which carries its own probability of occurrence.

The benefit is greatest if FOBT is used in conjunction with colonoscopy and/or barium enema. Little apparent benefit is derived from screening before age 45. A similar but more simplistic model for determining the cost of the program showed that the overall cost must be similar to today's costs of treating colonic cancer. If the cost of fiber optic endoscopies decreased approximately 30 percent or if the false-positive rate of the FOBT were reduced to under 5 percent, the cost of a surveillance program would be justified on economic grounds alone.

Diet is the second important risk factor in colorectal cancer. Much of the interest in this area was stimulated by Burkitt, who linked low levels of fiber in the diet with increased risk of colorectal cancer.[8] Although it is generally accepted that some degree of risk is associated with a diet low in fiber, the magnitude of risk is difficult to assess. In addition, data are now available that question the concept of diet-related risks. For example, the work of Naraise et al.[9] showed similar levels of dietary fiber in Japan and in Great Britain, dispelling the theory that high fiber levels were responsible for the lower colorectal cancer rates in Japan that had been reported earlier by Armstrong et al.[10] Nonetheless, until additional studies are done, it is prudent to advocate greater amounts of fiber in the American diet.

Table 2. Social and economic costs of digestive diseases, United States, 1977

Disease category	Deaths	Person-years lost before age 65	Estimated direct and indirect costs (millions of dollars)
Nonmalignant disease	68,700	12,807,000	5,943.9
Malignant disease	102,900	14,448,000	5,191.2
Total	171,600	27,255,000	11,135.1

Data from National Center for Health Statistics.[2]

The best data may come from the study of Seventh-Day Adventists in Loma Linda, California, because the gradient of fiber and cancer risk is measurable in this population.

Gallbladder Disease

By all accounts, gallbladder disease is a major health problem both in the numbers of people affected and in the number of hospital admissions that result (Table 1). The full Medicare review of the state of Maine for 1977–1978 showed that gallbladder surgery accounted for more procedures than any other single disease.[11] The cost for that year—$520,894—accounted for slightly more than 19 percent of all claims. These data are in keeping with all earlier reports, Even so, we do not know exactly how common gallstones are.

For a number of years highly accurate contrast radiography has been performed to substantiate the diagnosis, but abdominal ultrasonography has recently become the diagnostic standard because it carries no risk of radiographic exposure but is as accurate as radiography. Consequently, more people are being screened for gallstones, and more positive diagnoses are made. The first effective oral medications for treatment are now available. Although these agents will benefit only approximately 13–20 percent of gallstone victims, these patients, whose gallstones are detected early and many of whom are younger, will presumably be spared the suffering and expense of major surgery.

As is true of colorectal cancer, the etiology of gallstones is now much better understood; unfortunately, the basic epidemiology has been poorly documented. The best data on prevalence are only now being collected by the Health and Nutritional Examination Survey (HANES) study of approximately 4,000 Hispanic patients. The study of this population should also provide the answer to the most pressing question in managing patients who have gallstones: how can we best treat the asymptomatic patient in whom gallstones are discovered?

Cirrhosis of the Liver

Cirrhosis, the eighth leading cause of mortality in the United States, accounted for 31,380 deaths in 1980. Men are affected about twice as often as women, and a disproportionate number of deaths from cirrhosis occur in the middle years.

The first concrete data on incidence and prevalence of cirrhosis were reported more than three decades ago.[12] The magnitude of the problem has not changed appreciably since, nor has the widespread use of what is overwhelmingly the most common cause—alcohol. The most conservative estimates are that 60 percent of cirrhosis in the United States is caused by alcohol,[11] but most liver experts place the figure closer to 90 percent.

During the last year of life, patients who have cirrhosis require an average of five hospitalizations.[13] Because of the complex care and often extensive transfusions required during these hospital stays, the cost of treating this illness is usually extremely high.

Because alcoholics are a difficult population to follow, data on the cumulative risk from alcohol use/abuse have been difficult to obtain. According to the best study of the subject, an average intake of 100 g (3.5 oz) per day over a period of five years is the minimal cirrhotogenic dosage for men.[14] However, according to another study, a markedly reduced dose, perhaps as low as 60 g (2 oz) per day, could cause cirrhosis in women.[14] Whether nutritional status contributes to the disease is uncertain. According to animal studies, nutrition does not seem to be an important factor,[15] but data on humans are lacking.

When liver transplantation becomes routine clinical practice, treatment of the cirrhotic patient will become more expensive and so will have an additional economic impact.

Peptic Ulcer Disease

Peptic ulcer disease is one of the oldest gastrointestinal illnesses mentioned in medical literature, having been first described by Jean Cruveilhier in about 1830.[16] The disease is responsible for five times more hospitalizations than either colorectal cancer or cirrhosis. Despite its being so widespread, peptic ulcer disease is not a leading cause of mortality. Death rates for colorectal cancer and cirrhosis are 15 and seven times higher, respectively. Furthermore, the death rate for peptic ulcer disease has been falling steadily since the 1950s because of improved diagnosis and treatment.[17]

The epidemiology of peptic ulcer disease has become clouded by the shifting demography of the illness, the change in classification of the International Classification of Diseases and Causes of Death (ICD codes), and the routine use of endoscopy for accurate diagnosis. Not only is the disease now diagnosed earlier, it can be treated much more effectively with newly developed oral medications. Federal Drug Administration approval of the H_2 receptor antagonists in 1979 dramatically changed the clinical approach to treatment. In fact, cimetidine was the largest-selling pharmaceutical agent in

1983: total sales were more than $1 billion (unpublished data from Smith Kline & French Laboratories).

Genetic influence and smoking appear to be the leading risks associated with peptic ulcer disease. Although smoking has not yet been shown to increase the incidence, it has been demonstrated to adversely affect the morbidity and mortality of peptic ulcer disease. At this time smoking appears to be the most clearly defined controllable risk factor for the disease.

The role of stress as a risk factor is still being debated. The marked increase of hospital admissions for peptic ulcers in London during the World War II bombings has been the classic "proof" cited for the role of stress.[18] However, recent work on the frequency of the disease in various socioeconomic groups has raised several questions concerning the role of stress and health. It seems that peptic ulcer disease is at least as common, if not more so, in lower as in higher economic groups.[19]

Despite the commonly held view that diet may influence the development of peptic ulcer disease, no risks have been shown for any foods, including alcohol. The use of some drugs (e.g., corticosteroids) does promote ulcers, but this accounts for a small percentage of patients.

Inflammatory Bowel Disease

The epidemiology of inflammatory bowel disease can be traced only for the past 25 years because the distinction between ulcerative colitis and Crohn's disease was not made until the 1960s. Although the disease is not a leading cause of mortality, it is an important cause of morbidity, as is shown by hospitalization rates.

Many gastroenterologists consider inflammatory bowel disease the most difficult to treat. Despite intensive research, we still lack a clear understanding of the cause or the risk factors, nor are there any guaranteed therapeutic approaches.

Patients who have had chronic ulcerative colitis for more than 20 years have a 32-fold increased risk of cancer.[20] There is a pathologic marker, epithelial dysplasia, which indicates a higher risk of cancer development in patients with this finding; the cancer that develops is not typical of colorectal cancer and is generally more severe. Careful surveillence of this population should reduce the cancer rate significantly.

Diverticular Disease

Diverticula are small saccular outpouchings of the colon that develop near nutrient arteries. It is thought that these arteries are located at naturally occurring weak spots in the bowel wall and that high colonic pressures over a lifetime lead to bulgings of the colon wall that develop into diverticula. Diet low in fiber has been associated with a high level of intracolonic pressure in the large bowel.[21]

No strong correlation exists between the presence of diverticula and the development of cancer. Diverticula do not cause symptoms in most patients. They are present at autopsy in as many as 60 percent of subjects over the age of 60,[22] but it is believed that in only approximately 1 percent of such patients do serious consequences of diverticular disease develop.[23] The poor classification system now in use poses some difficult methodologic problems in studying this illness. Again, the Loma Linda population provides an ideal group in which to explore the influence of dietary manipulation of diverticular disease.

We need to elucidate the link between fiber in the diet and diverticular disease in the elderly and irritable colon syndrome in the young. Irritable colon syndrome accounts for a large number of outpatient visits to gastroenterologists. The work-up of these patients is expensive, as the diagnosis is largely one of exclusion. At least four medical centers are currently developing positive diagnostic methods for this syndrome. Therapy is now directed at increasing the bulk of the fecal mass, which may yield valuable insights into the link between fiber and irritable colon/diverticular disease.

Other Digestive Diseases

A great many digestive diseases that produce significant morbidity and mortality are not discussed in this report, not because these diseases lack importance but because risks and interventions are impossible to identify at this time. For example, carcinoma of the pancreas has steadily become more frequent during the past 25 years. This illness ranks among the leading causes of cancer deaths, accounting for 20,000–23,000 deaths a year. Despite important advances in the direct assessment of the organ's anatomy and function, nothing has produced any real hope of changing the pattern of the disease, nor have clear risk factors emerged. Earlier recognition of pancreatic cancer has not been translated into an improved survival rate, and the outcome for the patient remains dismal. Most of these statements can also be made about cancer of the esophagus.

Hemorrhoids remain common, but very little research has been done in this field in the past few years. The Digestive Diseases Division of the National Institutes of Health has developed a study group under the direction of Dr. Donald Murphy to assess the magnitude and implication of anorectal disease.

One illness for which intervention may soon exist is heartburn, or esophageal reflux. New approaches are being developed to recognize and treat this illness, including H_2 receptor antagonists combined with metaclopramide.

INTERVENTIONS

Increased surveillance of all people over the age of 45 has the potential to yield an 85 percent reduction in mortality from colorectal cancer. Annual testing for fecal occult blood and fiber optic endoscopy every five years is strongly recommended. However, maximum compliance can be achieved only if the cost of endoscopy is reduced by approximately one third. In addition, the reliability of the FOBT should be improved so that the false-positive rate is under 5 percent.

Gallbladder disease can now be treated with oral medication, but only if it is detected early. Medication could benefit as many as 20 percent of gallstone victims. Because of the growing use of ultrasonography, we can now improve surveillance and make earlier diagnoses without radiography and without surgery.

Alcohol has been estimated as the cause of 60–90 percent of all cases of cirrhosis. Prevention of alcoholic cirrhosis lies in the early recognition and treatment of alcoholism and in preventing the development of alcoholism (see the accompanying papers "Alcohol Dependence and Abuse" and "Unintentional Injuries").

It has been well established that tobacco smoking exacerbates the morbidity and mortality of peptic ulcer disease; patients who have this disease should be encouraged to enroll in smoking cessation programs.

Because patients who have had chronic ulcerative colitis for 20 years are at increased risk for developing colorectal cancer, an annual FOBT and fiber otpic endoscopy every five years are recommended for these patients.

A diet high in fiber to increase the bulk of fecal mass is strongly recommended for all patients who have diverticular disease. Moreover, as a primary intervention, everyone should be encouraged to include adequate fiber in the diet.

SUMMARY

Digestive diseases are costly, though just how costly cannot be determined until more detailed statistics are available. The facts in one state suggest the extent of the social and economic burden of these disorders nationally.[11] Cancer and cirrhosis are clearly the most deadly of these diseases, but peptic ulcer is costly in hospital days, and the insidious drain on our health resources represented by less threatening disorders such as gallbladder disease and diverticular disease should not be overlooked (Table 3). Given the fact that the leading risk factors for these disorders overwhelmingly point to lifestyle choices—the kinds and amounts of food eaten and the use of alcohol and tobacco—it is clear that these costs need not remain at their current levels.

The full extent of the epidemiology of the more common gastrointestinal illnesses, however, cannot be easily measured because some elementary epidemiologic data are not available. The system of reporting digestive diseases, the lack of organization and support within the specialty (as opposed to disease-oriented disciplines such as cardiology and oncology), and the classification system itself have contributed to the lack of available information.

The ICD codes for digestive diseases extend from ICD 520 to ICD 579. The National Digestive Diseases Advisory Board showed that only 66 of the

Table 3. Estimated morbidity and mortality from digestive diseases for persons over the age of 64, United States, 1980

Disease	Risk factor	Deaths	Person-years lost before age 65	Hospital days (thousands)	Cost (millions of dollars)
Colon cancer	Polyps @ 75%	54,322	585,144	372.8	2,102
	Diet	7,243	78,019	50	280
Cirrhosis	Alcohol	26,631	589,120	48	303
Peptic ulcer	Smoking	1,897	14,926	132	69
Gallbladder	Obesity	311	3,074	46	14
Diverticula	Diet	280	2,805	20	13
Totals		90,684	1,273,088	668.8	2,768

Data from National Digestive Diseases Advisory Board.[21]

218 codes referable to digestive diseases actually fell within the ICD 520–579 series. For example, "Whipple's Disease" is listed under "Infectious Diseases," "Hemorrhoids" under "Cardiovascular Disease," and "Zollinger–Ellison Syndrome" under "Endocrine Disorders," to name but a few.[24] This lack of focus is the reason that the figures reported for digestive diseases are so disparate.

Unfortunately, the future may yield even less accurate figures. The Diagnosis Related Group (DRG) classification is placing high economic incentives on the pattern of disease reporting. The rewards for manipulating disease reporting may degrade the accuracy of the reports at a time when the value of accurate data is just beginning to be fully appreciated.

Despite this lack of crucial data, we know that digestive diseases constitute a significant health problem for our society. Much of the problem is currently solvable, however. Through improved preventive measures and more thorough patient education, we can stem the morbidity and mortality from these diseases.

REFERENCES

1. Current estimates from the National Health Interview Survey: United States, 1980. Hyattsville, Maryland: National Center for Health Statistics, 1981; DHHS publication no. (PHS) 82-1567. (Vital and health statistics; series 10; no. 139).

2. Prevalence of selected chronic digestive conditions: United States, 1975. Hyattsville, Maryland: National Center for Health Statistics, 1979; DHEW publication no. (PHS) 79-1558. (Vital and health statistics; series 11; no. 123).

3. Day DW, Morson BC. The adenoma–carcinoma sequence. In: Marson BC, ed. The pathogenesis of colorectal cancer. Philadelphia: Saunders, 1978;58–71.

4. Gilbertson VA. Proctosigmoidoscopy and polypectomy in reducing the incidence of rectal cancer. Cancer 1974;34:936.

5. Hardcastle JD, Armitage NC. Early detection of colorectal cancer: a review. J R Soc Med 1984;77:673–6.

6. Correa P, Strong JP, Ruif A, et al. The epidemiology of colorectal polyps. Cancer 1977;39:2258.

7. Brandeau ML, Eddy DM. The workup of the asymptomatic patient with a positive fecal occult blood test. Med Decision Making 1987;7:32–46.

8. Burkitt DP. Epidemiology of cancer of the colon and rectum. Cancer 1971;28:3–13.

9. Naraise Y, Kagamimori S, Watanabe M, et al. Mortality rates for farmers and fishermen in Japan compared with England and Wales. Soc Sci Med 1985;21:139–43.

10. Armstrong B, Doll R. Environmental factors and cancer incidence and mortality in different countries with special reference to dietary practices. Int J Cancer 1975;15:617–31.

11. Progress through action: second annual report of the national digestive diseases advisory board. Bethesda, Maryland: National Institutes of Health, 1983;1–8.

12. Lilienfeld AM, Korns RF. Some epidemiologic aspects of cirrhosis of the liver: a study of mortality statistics. Am J Hygiene 1950;52:65–81.

13. Garagliano CF, Lilienfield AM, Mandeloff AI. Incidence rates of liver cirrhosis and related diseases in Baltimore and selected areas of the United States. J Chron Dis 1979;32:543–54.

14. Selbach WK. Cirrhosis in the alcoholic and its relation to the volume of alcohol abuse. Ann NY Acad Sci 1975;252:85–105.

15. Seiber C. Alcohol and the liver: 1984 update. Hepatology 1984;4:1243–60.

16. Major RH. Classic descriptions of disease. Springfield, Illinois: Charles C. Thomas, 1945:628–32.

17. Kurata JH, Haile BM. Epidemiology of peptic ulcer disease. Clin Gastroenterol 1984;13:289–307.

18. Watkinson J. Epidemiological aspects. In: Topics in gastroenterology. 7th ed. Oxford: Blackwell, 1979:3–34.

19. Pulvertaft CN. Peptic ulcer in town and country. Br J Prev Soc Med 1959;13:131.

20. Lennard-Jones JE, Morson BC, Ritchie JK, et al. Cancer in colitis: assessment of the individual risk by clinical and histological criteria. Gastroenterology 1977;73:1280.

21. Painter NS. The etiology of diverticulosis of the colon with special reference to the action of certain drugs on behavior of the colon. Ann R Coll Surg Engl 1964:34:98.

22. Painter NS, Burkitt DP. Diverticular disease of the colon, a twentieth century problem. Clin Gastroenterol 1975;4:73.

23. Painter NS. Diverticular disease of the colon. In: Topics in gastroenterology. Oxford: Blackwell, 1973:295–307.

24. National Digestive Diseases Advisory Board. Third annual report. Bethesda, Maryland: National Institutes of Health, 1984; DHHS publication no. (NIH) 85-2482.

Drug Dependence and Abuse

Paul J. Goldstein, Ph.D., Dana Hunt, Ph.D.,
Don C. Des Jarlais, Ph.D., and Sherry Deren, Ph.D.

The impact of drug use on the health of the nation is enormous, complex, and stubbornly resistant to full and accurate documentation. No national health data bases specify the broad range of physical dysfunctions from drug use or enumerate their incidence and prevalence. No national criminal justice data bases specify the range of ciminally violent acts, enumerate resultant injuries, or link these acts to drug use of the victims or perpetrators. Yet, even without such data, evidence indicates that drug use is a major social and health problem in the United States.

- 2.5 million Americans are estimated to have serious drug problems.[1]
- In 1981, 443,000 (about 3 percent) of New York State residents experienced health problems related to drug use.[2]
- The societal costs of drug abuse have been estimated at $10 billion[1]–$47 billion[3] per year.
- The leading causes of death among teenagers and young adults—unintentional injuries, suicide, and homicide—are in many cases linked to drug abuse.
- Approximately 200,000 persons received publicly funded treatment for drug abuse in 1980.[4]
- Workers at all levels of industry report that drug use is a problem leading to increased absenteeism, theft, dissension, unintentional injuries, and decreased productivity.[5]

Drug use, a health problem in itself, also contributes to other problems. It can have a negative impact on family life, work and school performance, finances, and social life, and can result in hospitalization, incarceration, or death. The health consequences of drug use encompass a broad range of physical dysfunctions. Different types of drugs are associated with different lifestyles, means of ingestion, pharmacological properties, and consequently with different health problems.

A single drug can lead to specific health consequences, for example, amphetamine psychoses. Health consequences can also result from interactions between drugs or between drugs and alcohol. In many cases, it is difficult to attribute a specific dysfunction to a specific substance when many drugs are being ingested concurrently.

The consequences of drug abuse are far reaching, as varied as the substances available and the methods of ingestion. Because of the wide range of health consequences, we have selected just three areas for discussion: (1) infectious diseases, (2) unintentional poisoning/overdose, and (3) violence. Each contributes substantially to mortality and morbidity costs, yet each involves different drugs, modes of administration, and populations of users. Following these sections is a brief discussion of the health consequences parents' substance abuse has upon their children.

INFECTIOUS DISEASES

The majority of infectious diseases associated with drug use stem from bacterial infections caused by intravenous or intramuscular drug injection with nonsterile equipment. This practice may lead to localized infection problems, such as abscesses and cellulitis, or systemic problems, such as endocarditis, hepatitis, and acquired immune deficiency syndrome (AIDS).

The prevalence of infection is disproportionately high among the drug-using population. Needles are often shared or used repeatedly by the same person without sterilization. Microorganisms enter percutaneously and may cause a variety of local and systemic infections.

Hepatitis B

Although hepatitis B (serum hepatitis), may also originate from other sources of infection and in

From Narcotic and Drug Research, Inc., New York (Goldstein and Hunt) and New York State Division of Substance Abuse Services, Albany (Des Jarlais and Deren).

Points of view and opinions in this article do not necessarily represent the official positions or policies of Narcotic and Drug Research Inc. or of the New York State Division of Substance Abuse Services.

Address reprint requests to Dr. Goldstein, Narcotic and Drug Research, Inc., 55 West 125th Street, 8th Fl., New York, NY 10027.

other populations, it is particularly prevalent among intravenous drug users. Hepatitis B usually has a long incubation period, and persons may be actively infectious or longtime carriers of the virus. Although only 0.1–0.5 percent of the general population is estimated to carry hepatitis B surface antigen (HB$_s$Ag positive), clinical evidence suggests that as many as 30 percent of intravenous drug users may be HB$_s$Ag positive.[6] Approximately 10–12 percent of addicts entering methadone maintenance treatment are chronic carriers of hepatitis B antigens, 50 percent have hepatitis B core antibodies, and 96 percent show some evidence of prior hepatitis B infection.[7]

Hepatitis B carriers may be asymptomatic for many years; they may have low-grade, persistent hepatitis or chronic active episodes. The fatality rate from hepatitis B in the general population is low (0.1 percent), but because of its more frequent occurrence and the generally negligent health care associated with the lifestyle of intravenous drug users, fatalities in this group are ten times higher (1 percent).[8] In rare cases, hepatic necrosis ensues and rapidly progresses to coma. More typically, the drug user experiences recurrent episodes of jaundice, enlarged spleen, and fever, followed by progressive liver damage. In narcotics addicts, whose health care is notoriously sporadic and who may carry hepatitis B for many years, the incidence of hepatic complaints is as high as 81 percent.[8]

Included in Table 1 are the estimated incidence, prevalence, and mortality of hepatitis B attributable to drug use in the 1980 population, using an estimate of the number of intravenous narcotics users in the general population and a clinical estimate[7] of the proportion of heroin users with hepatitis B (10–12 percent).

Persons at greatest risk for hepatitis B are drug users 24–44 years of age who have been injecting for many years. Although users may be long-term carriers, symptoms may not surface for several years, and many problems are exacerbated by years of poor hygiene and sporadic health care. According to a study of narcotics users over 50 years old, the "survivors" of a lifetime of drug use were those who scrupulously cared for their needles and syringes and did not share their equipment with others.[9]

The costs associated with serum B hepatitis are shown in Table 2. This figure is an extremely low estimate of the costs of this illness, as visits to private physicians and many types of clinics are not included. Although these hospitalizations represent both major and minor complications of hepatitis B, many of the problems associated with systemic infections are ignored or handled through self-medications until they reach serious proportions and require extended treatment.

Acute Bacterial Infectious Endocarditis

Unlike other forms of endocarditis, acute infectious endocarditis among intravenous drug users is unique because it most often involves a normal heart; that is, a history of rheumatic heart disease or valvular abnormality is not necessarily present. According to a study of illnesses among drug users seeking hospital treatment, those who had acute infectious endocarditis were uniformly drug injectors, predominantly narcotics users.[8]

Although addicts who have no history of heart disease have a fairly good prognosis for management and survival of the disease, congestive heart failure from valvular destruction or progressive cardiac damage is not unknown. For example, 7 percent of IV drug users in the Blanck et al.[8] sample suffered congestive heart failure. This study reports the mortality associated with treated endocarditis in this population as 6.5 percent; mortality rates for untreated users, however, have been estimated to be as high as 85 percent.

The high mortality rates reflect the poor health

Table 1. Morbidity and mortality related to drug abuse, United States, 1980

	Annual prevalence		Incidence		Deaths[59]		Years lost
	n	Rate/ 100,000	n	Rate/ 100,000	n	Rate	before age 65[59]
Drug dependence	350,000	171	150,635	74.2	640	0.31	20,628
Poisoning/overdose	—	—	96,383	47.1	1,485	0.73	43,713
Serum B hepatitis	35,000	17	6,644	3.3	294	0.14	13,565
Bacterial endocarditis	42,000[a]	21	680	0.3	177	0.09	8,939
AIDS[b]	774	0.31			300	0.14	9,000
Assault/homicide	—	—	140,010[c]	78.2[d]	2,186	0.86	67,399

[a] The prevalence of bacterial endocarditis is calculated by taking 12 percent of the estimated number of serious drug users in the population, or the number of users estimated in clinical studies as having infective endocarditis.[8] The incidence is calculated by taking 12 percent, the number estimated by clinical studies for drug related endocarditis,[58] of the cases of infectious endocarditis reported in the HDS.
[b] Estimates are for 1984.
[c] Resulting in injuries.
[d] Based on population over 12 years of age.

Table 2. Hospitalizations, hospital days, and hospital costs related to drug abuse, United States, 1980

Health problem	No. of hospitalizations	No. of hospital days	Hospital costs
Drug dependence	30,635	435,767	$108,941,750
Poisoning/overdose	96,383	519,237	129,809,750
Serum B hepatitis	6,644	52,475	13,118,750
Bacterial endocarditis	869	20,520	5,130,000
Assault	5,667	45,774	11,443,500
Total	140,198	1,073,773	$268,443,750

Data from Hospital Discharge Survey (1980), and National Crime Survey, 1980.[43]

care of intravenous drug users, which allows advancing endocarditis to go undetected and become fatal. The morbidity associated with endocarditis stems from embolic complications, repeated acute episodes of infection, and progressive heart disease. Blanck et al.[8] indicated that approximately 12 percent of nonemergency hospital treatment of drug users in their sample is for complications of acute infectious endocarditis. The estimated incidence, prevalence, and mortality of this disease shown in Table 1 are based on this figure and the estimated number of narcotics users in the population. Estimates of both mortality and morbidity from drug-related endocarditis are invariably low, because many deaths from heart failure or embolism may not be recorded as complications of drug-related endocarditis but simply as heart failure or stroke.

The medical costs of infectious endocarditis include acute care and long-term management with antibiotics and are summarized in Table 2.

AIDS

The acquired immune deficiency syndrome (AIDS) is the most important new health problem to emerge in the United States during the past decade. The first cases were reported in the summer of 1981, and more than 10,000 cases were reported in the United States to the Centers for Disease Control through May 21, 1985. The number of cases has doubled approximately every ten months.

Intravenous (IV) drug users constitute the second largest group of persons who have developed AIDS. Seventeen percent of the AIDS cases in the United States have occurred in persons with IV drug use as their primary risk factor, and another 7 percent have occurred in persons with both IV drug use and male homosexual activity as risk factors.[10] Areas with large numbers of IV drug users are reporting rates as high as 40 percent among users.

IV drug users are also linked to two other groups at increased risk for AIDS. Over half of the children

who have developed AIDS have at least one parent who is an IV drug user, and over two thirds of the "heterosexual partners" (persons whose only known risk for AIDS is a heterosexual relationship with a member of the previously identified high-risk groups) are sexual partners of IV drug users.[10]

AIDS is a disorder of the immune system, particularly of the cell-mediated (T cell) subsystem.[11] The disease is thought to be caused by a virus, which has been variously named lymphadenopathy associated virus (LAV),[12] human T lymphotropic virus type III (HTLV-III),[13] and AIDS related virus (ARV).[14] We will refer to the virus as HIV.

According to the surveillance definition used by the Centers for Disease Control, patients are diagnosed as having AIDS if they have contracted Kaposi's sarcoma, *Pneumocystis carinii* pneumonia, or any of a long list of other "opportunistic infections" without any known reason for immunosuppression. The surveillance definition is clearly biased toward diagnosis of only the most severe cases of AIDS-related disease. This serves to limit the number of "false positive" cases that would require epidemiologic investigation but greatly underestimates the true prevalence of AIDS-related disease. It also inflates the fatality rate; for surveillance definition cases, approximately 80 percent have died within two years of diagnosis.

To date, AIDS cases among IV drug users have been heavily concentrated in the metropolitan New York City area. Approximately 80 percent of all U.S. cases in which IV drug use is the primary risk factor have been from the two states of New York and New Jersey.[10] Studies of the prevalence of antibody to HIV both confirm the concentration in New York and indicate a potential for major increases in other cities with large numbers of IV drug users. In serum samples collected from users in treatment in the middle of 1984, 59 percent of IV drug users in New York City had antibody to HIV, compared with 11 percent in Chicago and 9 percent in San Francisco.[15] Antibody prevalence among IV drug users in New Jersey ranged from 50 percent in the northern part of the state to only 2 percent in the southern part.[16]

The AIDS virus is apparently spread among IV drug users through the sharing of needles and syringes used for injecting drugs,[16,17] though it is possible that sharing of the "cookers" used for preparing the drugs may also be a means of viral spread. While more research is needed on viral transmission through sharing needles, it appears that the HIV virus is not as easily transmitted as the hepatitis B virus, to which it has often been compared epidemiologically. It is, however, also spread through sexual contact.

Estimating the incidence rates for AIDS among IV drug users is difficult because of the rapid changes in incidence during such an epidemic, the problem of estimating the population of IV drug users, and the overlap among IV drug use and homosexuality as risk factors. There were 1,007 cases of AIDS among male heterosexual and female IV drug users in New York City through May 20, 1985,[18] and the best estimate of the current number of IV drug users in New York City is 190,000.[19] (This latter figure includes persons who may not currently be injecting drugs because they are receiving treatment, incarcerated, or temporarily abstinent.) Our conservative estimate is that the incidence of AIDS among IV drug users in New York City is approximately 3 percent, including cases of homosexual male IV drug users.

The cost of treatment for AIDS among IV drug users is high. At present there is no known effective treatment for the underlying immune disorder in AIDS. Treatment for the various clinical manifestations—opportunistic infections and Kaposi's sarcoma—does not prevent repeated episodes of the same infection or the development of others. An IV drug user diagnosed with AIDS typically dies within one to two years. The AIDS IV patient usually spends one half to two thirds of this time in the hospital, at an average cost of approximately $500 per day. The cost per day is higher than for an "average" patient because much of the time is spent in intensive care or costly isolation units. This gives an approximate medical treatment cost of $160,000 per patient.

In addition to the direct cost, there is the considerable human suffering, both for the patient and for his or her family and friends, that occurs with any nontreatable fatal disease. Added to this normal suffering is the social stigma associated with drug use. This stigma greatly increases the difficulties in providing needed psychological and social services for AIDS patients. Providing housing for these patients, in particular, has been very difficult.

The AIDS epidemic is already a tragedy for IV drug users and a serious danger to their nonin-jecting sexual partners and children. The eventual magnitude of this problem will depend upon several factors, including whether successful treatment or vaccines can be developed. Until treatment and/or vaccines are developed, the size of the problem will be determined largely by the percentage of virally exposed IV drug users who develop the disease and by the effectiveness of risk reduction efforts among IV drug users. Estimates of the percentage of virally exposed persons who develop surveillance-definition AIDS now range between 4 and 19 percent.[20] Efforts to reduce the risk of viral exposure have already been noted among IV drug users in New York City,[21] but it is not yet possible to assess their effectiveness at this point.

We are not yet at a point where confident predictions can be made about the ultimate health and economic costs of AIDS among intravenous drug users. It is clear, however, that AIDS has emerged as one of the most important health problems associated with intravenous drug use.

POISONING/OVERDOSE

"Poisoning/overdose" refers to the ingestion of an unspecified amount of a drug such that physical or mental dysfunction is caused in the user. The amount ingested need not be large.

Opiates and Synthetic Analgesics

When a heroin addict dies without apparent cause, the death is usually attributed to too much heroin. In fact, death by overdose more often actually means death from unknown causes after injecting heroin and may be related to an adulterant or to an interaction with alcohol or some other drug.

A recent study of heroin-related deaths[22] reported a 1981 mortality rate (17.4 per 100,000) that appears to be the highest ever reported. Of the 266 documented heroin-related deaths in the District of Columbia between 1980 and 1982, 93 percent of the decedents were black, 82 percent were male, 48 percent were employed, and the average age was 31. Comparison with two control groups indicated that those who died from heroin overdose were more likely to have quinine in the lungs and positive blood ethanol levels and to have used heroin less chronically than did the controls. These findings suggest that sporadic or recreational heroin users who combine heroin with alcohol and whose heroin is "cut" (diluted) with a substantial amount of quinine are at high risk for heroin-related mortality.

National survey data[23] indicate a relatively low incidence and prevalence of use of opiates and synthetic analgesics (heroin, morphine, methadone, Demerol, Dilaudid, Percodan) in the general population. Only 1.2 percent of those 18–25 years of age and 5 percent of those 26 years of age or older reported that they have ever used heroin. However, the incidence of poisoning or overdose per user is high, making any use a serious risk.

Narcotic poisoning not resulting in death is frequently seen in hospital emergency rooms. Of all drug-related admissions mentioned by emergency rooms that reported to the Drug Abuse Warning Network (DAWN) in 1980, more than 20,000, or 10 percent, were the consequences of narcotics use.[4] Similar findings have been reported from the Hospital Discharge Survey.

Narcotic poisoning necessitates immediate medical attention and some aftercare. Acute poisoning occurs easily in children, in persons who have hepatic dysfunction or pneumonia, and in narcotic addicts who use drugs shortly after withdrawal. Addicts, not realizing that tolerance to narcotics declines quickly after withdrawal or detoxification, may take a formerly well-tolerated dose, which has serious or fatal consequences. In addition, poisoning results when narcotics users misjudge the purity of the drug or ingest too much of it. Clinical treatment includes resuscitation or revival of the respiratory response. Aftercare includes stabilization of the patient's general health, supportive psychological therapy, and referral to or initiation of treatment.

Barbiturates

Of the more than 50 different barbiturates marketed, only a handful are widely used: pentobarbital, secobarbital, amobarbital, aprobarbital, thiopental, barbital, secobarbital/amobarbital, and phenobarbital.

Acute intoxication can result from the intentional or unintentional ingestion of large quantities of barbiturates or from combining them with alcohol. Central nervous system depression or coma is induced at varying rates, depending on which barbiturate has been taken and whether other drugs are present.

Barbiturate dependency can occur from taking as little as 0.4 g daily for a few months. It develops more often and more rapidly among abusers who ingest larger quantities. Alcoholics may use barbiturates to reduce alcoholic tremors, and cross-tolerance results.[24] Withdrawal from barbiturate dependency may lead to seizures and convulsions, necessitating immediate medical intervention.

Approximately 20 percent of all hospital admissions for drug poisoning and 6 percent of all suicides involve barbiturates.[24] In a recent study, barbiturates were reported as the primary substance of abuse in 7 percent of drug-related hospital emergency room admissions.[25] DAWN reported that barbiturates constituted approximately 4 percent of all drug mentions in emergency room visits in 1980.

Sedative Hypnotics and Tranquilizers

Sedative hypnotics and tranquilizers—chlordiazepoxide, diazepam, meprobamate, and methaqualone—are widely prescribed for anxiety and depression and are popular on the illicit drug market. The combination of their widespread distribution, use as a method of suicide, and attractiveness as a euphoriant makes tranquilizers and sedatives the most common drugs in nonfatal poisoning and overdose.[26] They constitute approximately 50 percent of the acute drug cases seen in emergency rooms.[27] In 1980, 9 percent of all drugs mentioned to DAWN reports from emergency rooms were for this category of drugs.[4]

According to a study of sedative/tranquilizer users admitted to four large urban hospitals for overdose/poisoning,[28] 58 percent of the users had obtained the drugs from nonmedical sources and 33 percent of the users had obtained the drug from legal prescriptions and had been using it daily for more than a year before the overdose. Many (47 percent) had had at least one prior overdose; intentional harm was the motive of 34 percent of the users. Multiple abuse was common: of these users, 23 percent reported that they had taken heroin or methadone in the preceding year and 38 percent identified themselves as users of barbiturates, cocaine, or marijuana in addition to the sedatives or tranquilizers.

Acute poisoning with these drugs leads to somnolence, confusion, respiratory difficulties, and, in severe cases, coma. As is true of barbiturates, mortality from tranquilizers or sedatives is often associated with alcohol. Alcohol was involved in 47 percent of the overdoses reported by Shader et al.[28]

Not all victims require hospitalization. Shader et al.[28] reported that 23 percent of persons who overdosed on sedatives or tranquilizers were unconscious when brought to the hospital but that only 18 percent were admitted. A large number (40 percent) were treated and referred to other services—drug treatment, counseling, or another health facility. The time that medical services spend on the complications of tranquilizer/sedative abuse is not inconsequential, however. At the hospitals studied,[28] more than 8,000 emergency room hours and more than 4,000 inpatient hours over a one-year period were spent treating people poisoned by tranquilizers, sedatives, or barbiturates. More than 24,000 diagnoses for complications of poisoning by tranquilizers or sedatives were reported in the hospital discharge data for 1980.

Stimulants: Amphetamines and Cocaine

Cocaine and amphetamines, though of limited therapeutic use, are popular drugs of abuse. Amphetamines and dextroamphetamines are powerful analeptics whose hypertensive and respiratory stimulant action are prescribed primarily for narcolepsy, fatigue, and weight control. Cocaine is occasionally used as a local anesthetic in some surgical procedures.

The prevalence of experience with cocaine sometime in their life among people 18–25 years of age rose from 13 percent in 1976 to 28 percent in 1979.[23] Use during preceding month, which had been relatively rare in the mid-1970s, tripled in 1979 and dropped only slightly in 1982. The greatest increases were among young adults, whites, and middle-income users.

Cocaine deaths generally result from overdose due to two causes. First, the user overestimates his or her tolerance to the drug and consumes a large quantity, which produces convulsions, arrhythmia, or hypertension with fatal consequences. The second cause involves accidental poisoning during trafficking. The victim uses a body cavity (such as the rectum or vagina) or swallows sealed containers of cocaine, the containers open or leak, and massive respiratory arrest occurs.[29] At special risk of death are persons who have epilepsy or hypertension, or other cardiovascular diseases.

Cocaine-related morbidity stems from the properties of the drug or its mode of ingestion. Chronic use may lead to liver and respiratory problems. Nasal septal perforation, which requires surgical repair,[29] is a common outcome of snorting cocaine.

The chronic use of cocaine has also been clinically linked to a number of mental disturbances, varying from mild stimulation of the central nervous system to severe depression and psychotic behavior.[30] Acute cocaine psychosis can manifest itself in hallucinations, paranoia, and debilitating anxiety reactions that require extended hospitalization. Evidence indicates that even limited use of the drug can produce an abrupt onset of psychotic behavior, or a "kindling effect,"[31] in which small amounts set off a response normally expected from much larger doses.

The increasingly popular practice of freebasing cocaine presents new health problems: severe burns from accidents with the highly flammable materials used in the procedure, chronic bronchitis, and searing of the pulmonary tissues.[32] Recent evidence has suggested that freebasing significantly reduces the capacity to diffuse carbon monoxide and even produces some degree of pulmonary hypertension.[33]

According to hospital discharge data, 959 diagnoses were related to complications of cocaine use. Cocaine complications constituted 3 percent of all drug mentions in hospital emergency rooms in 1980.[4]

The population at greatest risk for problems associated with cocaine is young adults. The greatest percentage of current users is among those 20–30 years of age, and users increasingly come from all income levels.[23] Of all mentions of cocaine in hospital emergency rooms in 1980, 55 percent were from this age group.[4]

The popularity of amphetamines has decreased since the 1960s and 1970s. According to NIDA survey data for 1982,[23] only 2 percent of respondents were using amphetamines, though more than twice that number reported having taken these drugs in the preceding year. Amphetamine complications constituted 3 percent of all mentions of drugs in emergency rooms in 1980.[4]

Treatment of amphetamine abuse includes long-term hospitalization for severe amphetamine psychoses in psychiatric facilities and short-term treatment to stabilize the patient's nutrition and sleep, eliminate the drug, and refer the patient to drug treatment.

Marijuana

Since their rapid rise to popularity in the 1960s, cannabis and its derivatives have been the most frequently consumed illicit substances. Since that time a plethora of contradictory information about the drug has emerged both in the clinical and the popular literature. In contrast to the situation a decade ago, people now are more likely to try marijuana at an earlier age and, if they continue, to use it more frequently. The prevalence of its use, however, is declining. In the 1979 NIDA drug use survey, 35 percent of young adults reported using marijuana in the month prior to the survey, but by 1982 this figure had dropped to 27 percent.[35]

Health problems associated with marijuana are derived both from the method of ingestion (inhalation) and the properties of the drug itself. In most people, low to moderate intake produces few ill effects: mild impairment of memory and coordination. Even mild intoxication, however, produces problems in operating machinery or driving. In a small percentage of users, a single dose of marijuana can produce mild anxiety or panic.[36] These reactions, which may occur in naive users or when a particularly strong variety of the drug is encountered, are usually treated with psychiatric assistance for a few days.

Most of the health risks from marijuana are associated with the inhalation of the heavy tars and a number of carcinogens. Marijuana cigarettes produce 50 percent more tar than do equal quantities of strong tobacco. Marijuana, however, is typically smoked to a butt of 30 mm or less, yielding twice as much tar as an ordinary cigarette. Concentrations of carcinogens such as benzopyrene are 70 percent higher in marijuana than in the same amount of tobacco. Clinical evidence shows that regular marijuana smokers are subject to more rhinitis, sore throats, and bacterial infections of the lung and bronchi than nonusers.[37]

Tolerance to and mild dependence on the drug can occur. In heavy users, withdrawal of the drug can produce irritability, gastrointestinal disturbances, and sleep disorders. Heavy cannabis use over extended periods may produce psychological dependence, but there has been little indication of serious psychological problems among persons who were not already experiencing psychiatric difficulties.[37]

Deaths directly attributable to cannabis are rare, though marijuana intoxication has been increasingly implicated in automobile fatalities.[37]

VIOLENCE

Drugs and violence are related in three possible models: the psychopharmacologic, the economically compulsive, and the systemic. In the psychopharmacologic model some persons, as a result of short- or long-term ingestion of specific substances, may exhibit irrational or violent behavior. Substances commonly associated with this mode of violence include alcohol, stimulants, barbiturates, and PCP (phencyclidine).

According to the economically compulsive model, some drug users engage in economically oriented violent crime (e.g., mugging) in order to support costly drug use. Heroin and cocaine, because they are expensive drugs characterized by compulsive patterns of use, fit this model well. However, most users avoid violent acquisitive crime if they have nonviolent alternatives, partly because violent crime is more dangerous and carries an increased threat of prison. Such users more commonly obtain cash or drugs by working within the drug business or by engaging in petty theft, prostitution,[38] and a variety of miscellaneous "hustling" activities.[39]

In the systemic model, violence is intrinsic to involvement with any illicit substance. Systemic violence refers to traditionally aggressive patterns of interaction within the system of drug distribution and use. Substantial numbers of users (of any drug) become involved in distribution as their drug-using careers progress, and they therefore risk becoming a victim or a perpetrator of systemic violence. Examples of systemic violence include "wars" over territory between rival drug dealers, assaults and homicides committed within dealing hierarchies as a means of enforcing normative codes, robberies of drug dealers and the usually violent retaliation by the dealer or his bosses, elimination of informers, and punishment for selling adulterated or phony drugs or for failing to pay one's debts.

There are no definitive data on how much of the violence engaged in by drug users may be attributable to each of the three models. However, knowledgeable observers of the drug scene suggest that systemic violence accounts for most of the violence perpetrated by, or directed at, drug users. For example, Zahn[40] points to the scarcity of drugs, their inelastic demand, and the ready availability of guns among illicit drug users and traffickers, and concludes that homicide is likely to result. Zahn further showed that peaks in the homicide rate occurred during periods of establishing and maintaining markets for illegal goods (alcohol in the 1920s and early 1930s; heroin and cocaine in the late 1960s and early 1970s). This connection is explained by the need to control or reduce competition, solve disputes between suppliers, eliminate dissatisfied customers, and the constant fear of being caught by a rival or the police.

National data sets collected in the criminal justice and health care systems are not very useful for elaborating on the drugs/violence nexus, because they do not link acts of criminal violence and resultant injuries to antecedent drug activity of victims or perpetrators. Some local studies provide more insight. For example, a New York City Police Department analysis[41] showed that 24 percent of known homicides in 1981 were drug related. Drug-related homicides were the second most common form, following only the category "disputes." Handguns were used more often in drug-related homicides (84 percent) than in any other form. In robbery-related homicide, which ranked second, handguns were used 61 percent of the time. In approximately 40 percent of the drug-related homicides, the victim was a drug dealer who was robbed. Finally, in 94 percent of the drug-related homicides, the victim and perpetrator were friends or acquaintances.

A recent national report conservatively estimated that 10 percent of the homicides and assaults nationwide are the result of drug abuse.[3] The authors include the caveat that their estimate should be viewed as an approximation in the face of inadequate empirical data to support an estimate derived in a systematic fashion. Use of this conservative 10 percent national estimate produces a drug-related homicide rate of about 1 per 100,000 population. This rate is substantially higher in major drug distribution localities such as New York City (5 per 100,000).

In addition to homicide, health consequences of the drugs/violence nexus include wounds (gunshot, knife), concussions, abrasions, broken bones, amputations, cripplings, burnings, and lost teeth. Being the victim of such violence, or even just fearing it, may lead to anxiety, depression, or other mental disorders.

According to the Uniform Crime Reports (UCR) there were 618,548 aggravated assaults in 1980. However, this is a measure of crimes known to the police; many assaults go unreported. The National Crime Survey[42] projected a total of 4,626,000 assaults for the United States in 1980. Of these, 1,661,000, or nearly three times the number reported by the UCR, were aggravated assaults. From the previously cited national estimate, 10 percent (462,600) of these assaults were drug related. The drug-related assault rate is thus approximately 257 per 100,000 population.

Of the estimated 4,626,000 total assaults, 1,401,000 (30 percent) were reported to have involved injury. The injury rate in drug-related assaults is probably higher than that of other assaults because of the prevalence of weapons among drug users and traffickers. Thus the estimates shown in Table 3 may actually be much higher.

The persons most at risk for being victims of assault were men between the ages of 16 and 24 who had never married and who were unemployed and living below the poverty level. Hispanics were slightly more likely to be assault victims than were either blacks or whites. Blacks were more likely than whites to incur injury from aggravated assaults.[42] There is no reliable base from which to project the demographic characteristics of drug-related assault victims, though the literature suggests that poor, young, black, and Hispanic men make up an especially high risk group.

In nearly 8 percent of assaults, hospital care was required. In the majority of cases, only emergency room treatment was given (Table 3). Men between the ages of 35 and 64 were most likely to require hospital attention. Blacks were almost twice as

Table 3. Drug-related assaults, United States, 1980

Type of assault	Number
Total drug-related assaults	462,600
Assaults with injury	140,010
Any medical attention given	67,360
Hospital care	34,878
Emergency room only	29,211
Inpatient	5,667
Other medical care	29,136
Unknown/NA	3,346

These estimates were made by taking 10% of the total reported in the National Crime Survey.[43]

likely as whites to receive hospital care because of an assault.[42] See Table 2 for the costs and the numbers of hospitalization days resulting from assaults.

The National Center for Health Statistics (NCHS) reported that approximately 10 percent of all assault cases involved loss of time from work.[43] If this figure holds constant for drug-related assault cases, approximately 46,000 drug-related assault cases resulted in victims' loss of time from work. Black assault victims were somewhat more likely to report loss of time from work than were white victims.

This discussion of drug-related violence has focused only on homicide and assault. Other areas—robbery, rape, and arson—also merit attention but, because of space limitations, are not included in this report.

CHILDREN OF DRUG ABUSERS

The effects of drug abuse on the abusers' children may begin during the prenatal phase, extend to neonatal withdrawal symptoms, and continue as the child is raised in a drug-abusing environment. In 1977 an estimated 5,000 infants were born to addicted mothers.[44] Further, it has been estimated that more than 234,000 children in the United States have heroin-addicted mothers.[45] The number of children whose mothers abuse nonnarcotic drugs is difficult to determine. However, based on a recent estimate of 800,000 such children in New York City,[46] a conservative projection for the nation is between 1.5 million and 2 million.

Addicted mothers usually receive little or no prenatal care. They are also likely to suffer complications during pregnancy—abruptio placenta, intrauterine growth retardation, preeclampsia, and eclampsia.

Newborns of addicted mothers are more likely to be born prematurely, and about 50 percent are low-birth-weight infants.[47] Up to 90 percent of infants born to heroin-addicted or methadone-maintained mothes experience withdrawal symptoms, including irritability, tremors, hyperactivity, and sleep and feeding problems, which can persist for several months. Many of these children require extended hospital stays.[48] Infants born to methadone-maintained mothers, as compared with heroin-addicted mothers, have improved outcomes on some of these measures (e.g., lower mortality and higher birth weight).[48]

In New York City, between 1979 and 1981, infants born to heroin-addicted mothers had a mortality rate almost three times that of the general population. Of infants who died in their first year, sudden infant death syndrome was diagnosed in 25 percent of the infants of addicted mothers, compared with 10 percent in the general population.[49] Though their numbers are small as yet, recent evidence indicates that the number of children of addicted mothers being born with AIDS is increasing.

Substance abuse in parents has been associated with higher rates of substance use in children.[50] Drug-abusing parents may be prone to greater impulsivity, unresponsiveness to infants' needs, and other parenting difficulties.[51,52] An association between child abuse and substance abuse is believed to exist, but this association has not been systematically examined. Some evidence indicates that children of substance abusers are at greater risk for learning problems and juvenile delinquency.[53]

INTERVENTIONS

Environments characterized by poverty, unemployment, racism, and boredom are breeding grounds for substance abuse. Many of the health problems discussed in preceding sections, such as inadequate medical care and poor hygiene, are common to persons who live in poverty, regardless of whether they are substance abusers or not. Although many ways to ameliorate specific problems associated with substance abuse are available, we have chosen the following because they are reasonable and humane and can be achieved in a short time.

Get more people into treatment. If the estimate of persons reported to be in drug treatment programs is reliable (181,500), only about 7 percent of the people who are estimated to have serious drug problems (2.5 million) are in treatment programs. Many of the remaining 93 percent are undergoing progressive and chronic physical deterioration, as well as committing crimes and being involved in accidents that lead to injuries to themselves and others. Such persons are also candidates for acute drug-related health crises.

Entering treatment programs often leads to a decrease in drug users' criminal activity and illict drug use. These decreases in turn may reduce the incidence of overdose, unintentional poisoning, homicide, vehicular injury, assault, abscesses, and infectious diseases. A recent study documented reductions of 45 percent in medical hospitalizations, 66 percent in psychiatric admissions, 54 percent in physician office visits for injuries, and 25 percent in office visits for illness (Blue Cross–Blue Shield, unpublished report, April 1982). These reductions mean reduced expenditures for these patients' medical care.[54] As indicated in Table 4, the average yearly cost per client in methadone-maintenance treatment programs and ambulatory drug-free programs is less than the costs of just ten days of hospitalization at $250 per day.

Even without more rigorous empirical research, it appears likely that getting more substance abusers into treatment would reduce or eliminate many of the health problems that affect this population. In the following sections we propose specific strategies for getting more drug abusers into treatment.

Identify users early. From an epidemiologic perspective, new drug users may be considered infectious agents. Most drug users have a honeymoon with a new drug; during the honeymoon the drug is perceived as wonderful, and the new user may spread the word about the "discovery," thus recruiting other new users. The duration of this euphoric phase varies for different persons. Users rarely volunteer for treatment during this period. By the time the honeymoon is over, other new users have been recruited.

It is important to identify new users as early as possible in the honeymoon phase, provide them with information about the potentially deleterious effects of the drugs they are using, and care for any physical problems that may already be occurring. Such early identification should not have as its goal a punitive response. Rather, early identification should be undertaken in an epidemiologic spirit, that is, to identify the affected person so that the condition is not transmitted to others. The potential ramifications of drug use and the treatment available can be explained to the user, who can then make an informed choice about personal health care.

Young people who begin to abuse drugs are likely to come into contact with certain social agents: law enforcement personnel, family court officers, social service workers, shelters for runaway youth, teachers, school guidance counselors, physicians and other medical personnel, recreation workers, and the clergy. These "gatekeepers" can

Table 4. Costs of long-term drug treatment, United States, 1982

Type of treatment	No. of patients[a]	Cost per person ($)[b]	Total cost ($)
Drug-free: outpatient and residential	95,874	$5,520	$529,224,480
Detoxification	5,146	3,000	15,438,000
Methadone maintenance	72,010	2,200	158,422,000
Other	449	—	—
Total	173,479		$703,084,480

[a] Total number of persons in each treatment modality in federally funded treatment programs. (From personal communication from George Beschner, Treatment Research Division, National Institute on Drug Abuse.)
[b] Costs per treatment type are based on treatment costs in New York State. Although higher than in many other states, the costs are comparable to those in states that have large populations of drug users.

function as frontline fighters in the struggle for a healthier society. They should be trained to detect signs of drug abuse, should have the best possible training in counseling abusers, and should be part of a referral network geared toward providing the highest quality drug treatment, counseling, and medical care to those in need.

The phrase "those in need" is critical. Not all users are abusers. While all users deserve attention, not all users need treatment. Many young people go through relatively brief periods of experimental and recreational drug use before moving on to full, healthy, and productive lives. Heavy-handed intervention with such persons would be ill considered and counterproductive.

Early intervention should seek those in need of intervention, i.e., those young people who are manifesting marked behavioral changes. These changes may be identified, for example, by teachers who observe that a good student is beginning to cut classes, fail exams, sleep in class, or speak in a slurred fashion.

Improve and expand drug treatment services. Four recommendations to improve the quality of drug treatment have been selected for their potential to affect the health consequences of substance use immediately: (1) increase medical services, (2) make methadone available to those not formally enrolled in treatment programs, (3) increase focus on polydrug abuse, (4) implement a medical maintenance model.

Medical services in many drug treatment programs are scanty. Having physicians available at least half time would increase the potential services that drug treatment programs can offer. Treatment programs could be used as medical way stations where users of all ages could be offered medical services. Early treatment of infections and other drug-

related illnesses could begin before the user seeks treatment, perhaps forestalling later health problems. Prenatal care could be offered to drug-abusing or addicted mothers, both to those already in treatment and to those not yet in treatment. Medical services could also be offered to the infants and children of these mothers. These programs could be valuable sources of information about drugs, hygiene, and treatment options.

If methadone clinics offered short-term doses of methadone to addicts who are not immediately interested in treatment, not only might the addicts' criminal activity be reduced, if even for one day, but the dispensing of methadone could also be an opportunity to provide medical care and information to an addict population not currently in treatment. Other services, e.g., education and counseling, which are often sought by drug users, could also be provided. The provision of these services might attract opiate users into treatment.

Higher treatment enrollment could be achieved through greater financial commitment to drug treatment and through reorganization of existing programs to direct minimal services to a specific population of users. We recommend pharmacy-style pickup of methadone for those who need limited services. This change would allow expanded service for those in need and would permit a larger number to be treated.

Persons whose primary drug of abuse is marijuana, cocaine, or barbiturates have difficulty finding treatment facilities for their problem. In addition, many persons who enter treatment for heroin use are using three or more nonopiate substances. Estimates of heavy alcohol consumption in methadone treatment populations range from 20 to 50 percent.[51,55,56] Understanding drug use as a multifaceted problem will open treatment facilities to a wider range of users and enable these facilities to better serve their current patients.

Certain drugs, such as barbiturates, necessitate hospitalization for detoxification. Access to such treatment is often available only as a follow-up to emergencies. Improved access to treatment programs is essential to reducing mortalities from barbiturate withdrawal. Currently, because they have little choice but self-medication, many barbiturate users, particularly the young, try to detoxify themselves from these drugs, often with fatal consequences.

Improve and expand employee assistance programs. Many drug abusers are employed, and their work sites provide an excellent opportunity for intervention. Employers or other supervisory personnel are usually in a good position to identify drug abuse at an early stage. For example, good workers may begin to arrive late and leave early, fail to adhere to established standards of productivity, fall asleep on the job, become unusually argumentative, or injure themselves unintentionally. Because most of them wish to remain employed, they have a special motivation to enter and succeed in treatment.

The well-designed employee assistance program (EAP) includes a clear statement of policy about drug abuse, a referral system that ensures that employees get the kind of treatment they need, and support for the employee's rehabilitative efforts. Such programs should maintain appropriate standards of confidentiality, provide health insurance coverage for substance abuse treatment, and publicize these benefits. Every effort should be made to allow the employee to continue work while in treatment. Certain employees (e.g., single working mothers) may find it exceptionally difficult to attend treatment on their own time. Everything possible should be done to allow such employees to obtain treatment on company time.

Expanded EAPs could also provide information and counseling to employees who fear that their children might have a developing drug problem. Finally, because children of substance abusers are at high risk for becoming abusers, expanded programs should encourage family therapy for drug-abusing employees.

Decriminalize possession of paraphernalia and allow needles and syringes to be sold without prescription. Current laws promote needle sharing and continued use of the same needle by making the possession of equipment a crime and by prohibiting the sale of needles and syringes without a prescription. These laws increase the likelihood of infection and contribute to higher health care costs.

Intravenous drug users share needles essentially for three reasons. First, needle sharing is a social activity that bonds members of a drug-using group. Second, in those locations where needles and syringes are not legally available, they are frequently obtained from friends, from other drug users who make money by "renting out" their "works," from a drug dealer, or from the "proprietor" of a "shooting gallery." Finally, IV drug users may be deterred from carrying paraphernalia by fear of arrest. Even though they may have clean needles at home, when they are out users may share the same needle.

We recommend decriminalizing possession of needles and syringes and allowing over-the-counter sales. Such items, sold legally, should cost less than street addicts are now paying to "rent" or purchase them illicitly. Enactment of this recommendation would remove much of the legal and economic compulsion to share needles and could significantly reduce the spread of infectious disease in the future.

Increase funding for youth programs. Participation in groups and activities that are incompatible with drug use decreases the likelihood that a person will move from experimental to heavy drug use. For example, participation in theater, dance, or religious activities may increase the person's "stake in conformity"[57] and diminish the attraction of groups in which drug use is the norm.

The recent financial cuts in extracurricular programs in sports and the arts are costly errors. Youths who might otherwise be involved in such activities may choose drug taking as an alternative, particularly in urban areas where access to drugs is easy and organized alternatives are few. Funds for extracurricular activities for youths in these areas are a valid prevention strategy and will be cost effective in the long run.

Improve and expand existing data bases. To obtain better-quality information about the health impact of substance abuse, we recommend the following:

1. Modify criminal justice reporting systems to better measure the impact that drugs have on criminal violence.

2. Modify health care reporting systems to better measure the impact that drugs have on physical dysfunction.

Better understanding of the relationships between substance use, criminal violence, and health problems will allow more informed prevention and treatment policies to be implemented.

The authors are grateful to the many individuals who shared their time, data, and expertise with us. Special thanks are due to

Douglas S. Lipton, New York State Division of Substance Abuse Services; Craig White, Centers for Disease Control; Edgar Adams, Mike Backenheimer, Barry Brown, and Sue Becker of the National Institute on Drug Abuse; Victoria Paukstys, Blue Cross and Blue Shield Association; Michael R. Rand, Bureau of Justice Statistics; John French, New Jersey Department of Health; and Barry Spunt, Narcotic and Drug Research, Inc.

REFERENCES

1. Promoting Health/Preventing Disease: Objectives for the Nation. Atlanta: Centers for Disease Control, 1980.

2. Drug use among New York State's household population. Albany: New York State Division of Substance Abuse Services, 1981.

3. Harwood H, Napolitano DS, Kristiansen P, et al. Economic costs to society of alcohol and drug abuse and mental illness. Rockville, Maryland: National Institute on Drug Abuse, 1984.

4. Annual data report, data from the drug abuse warning network. Rockville, Maryland: National Institute on Drug Abuse, statistical series 1.

5. Drug use in industry. Services research report. Rockville, Maryland: National Institute on Drug Abuse, 1980.

6. Dienstag J, Wands J, Koff R. Acute hepatitis. In: Petersdorf R, Adams R, Braunwald E, et al., eds. Principles of internal medicine. 10th ed., New York: McGraw-Hill, 1983:1789–1801.

7. Kreek M, Hartman N. Chronic use of opiates and anti-psychotic drugs: side effects, effects on endogenous opioids and toxicity. Ann NY Acad Sci 1982;642:20.

8. Blanck R, Ream N, Deleese J. Infectious complications of illicit drug use. Int J Addict 1984;19:221–32.

9. Des Jarlais D, Joseph H, Courtwright D. Old age and addiction: the study of elderly patients in methadone maintenance treatment. In: Gottheil E, Druley KA, Skoloda TE, Waxman HM, et al., eds. Combined problems of alcoholism, drug addiction, and aging. Springfield, Illinois: Charles C. Thomas, 1985:201–9.

10. Weekly surveillance report. In: United States AIDS Activity Center for Infectious Diseases. Atlanta: Centers for Disease Control, 1985 May 20.

11. Update on acquired immunodeficiency syndrome (AIDS). Morbid Mortal Weekly Rep 1982;13:507–8.

12. Barre-Sinouss F, Cherman JC, Rey F. Isolation of a T-lymphotrophic retrovirus from a patient at risk for acquired immune deficiency syndrome (AIDS). Science 1983;220:868–71.

13. Popovic M, Sarngadharam MD, Read E, Gallo RC. Detection, isolation and continuous production of cytopathic retroviruses (HTLV-III) from patients with AIDS and pre-AIDS. Science 1984;224:497–500.

14. Levy JA, Hoffman AD, Kramer SM, et al. Isolation of lymphocytopathic retroviruses from San Francisco patients with AIDS. Science 1984;225:840–2.

15. Spira TJ, Des Jarlais D, Bokos D. HTLV-III/LAV antibodies in intravenous drug abusers: comparison of high and low risk areas for AIDS. Presented at the International Conference on AIDS, Atlanta, 1985.

16. Weiss SH, Ginzburg HM, Goedert JJ. Risk for HTLV-III exposure and AIDS among parental drug abusers in New Jersey. Presented at the International Conference on AIDS, Atlanta, 1985.

17. Cohen HW, Marmor M, Des Jarlais D. Behavioral risk factors for HTLV-III/LAV seropositivity among intravenous drug abusers. Presented at the International Conference on AIDS, Atlanta, 1985.

18. AIDS surveillance report. New York: City Department of Health, May 1985.

19. New York State Plan Update. Albany: New York State Division of Substance Abuse Services, 1983.

20. Goeddert JJ, Weiss SH, Biggar RJ. Natural history of HTLV-III seropositive persons from AIDS risk groups. Presented at the International Conference on AIDS, Atlanta, 1985.

21. Des Jarlais D, Friedman S, Hopkins W. Risk reduction for the acquired immunodeficiency syndrome among intravenous drug users. Ann Intern Med 1985;103:755–9.

22. Ruttenber A, Luke J. Heroin related deaths in the District of Columbia, 1979–1982: new insights into the dynamics of an epidemic.

23. Miller J, Cisin I, Gardner-Keaton H, et al. National Survey on Drug Abuse: main findings 1982. Rockville, Maryland: National Institute on Drug Abuse, 1982.

24. Victor M, Adams R. Opiates and synthetic analgesics. In: Petersdorf R, Adams R, Braunwald E, et al., eds. Principles of internal medicine. 10th ed., New York: McGraw-Hill, 1983:1278–82.

25. Inciardi J, Russe B, Pottieger A, et al. Acute reactions in a hospital emergency room. Services research report. Rockville, Maryland: National Institute on Drug Abuse, 1979.

26. Greenblatt D, Allen M, Harmatz J, et al. Acute overdose with benzodiazepine derivatives. Clin Pharmacol Ther 1977;21:497–514.

27. Brandwin M. Drug overdose emergency room admissions. Am J Drug Alcohol Abuse, 1976;3:605–19.

28. Shader R, Anglin C, Greenblatt D, et al. Emergency room study of sedative–hypnotic overdosage: a study of the issues. Treatment research monograph series, Rockville, Maryland: National Institute on Drug Abuse, 1982.

29. Wetli C. Death from recreational cocaine use. In: Proceedings of symposium on cocaine. Albany: New York State Division of Substance Abuse Services, 1982:39–48.

30. Sokolov S, Motzer E. Drug abuse detection, guidelines and policies. Hospitals 1972;14:37–9.

31. Post R. Cocaine, kindling and reverse tolerance. Lancet 1975:409–10.

32. Smith D. Diagnosis and treatment of cocaine abuse. In: Proceedings of symposium on cocaine. Albany: New York State Division of Substance Abuse Services, 1982:88–102.

33. Schnoll S. Pulmonary dysfunction in cocaine freebase smokers. Rockville, Maryland: Alcohol, Drug Abuse and Mental Health Administration, 1984.

34. Trend report January 1978–September 1981. Rockville, Maryland: National Institute on Drug Abuse, 1982; statistical series 24.

35. Annual data report. Rockville, Maryland: National Institute on Drug Abuse, 1983.

36. Fehr K, Kalant O, Single E. Cannabis: adverse effects on health. Toronto: Addiction Research Foundation of Ontario, 1981.

37. Peterson R. Marijuana research findings: 1980. Rockville, Maryland: National Institute on Drug Abuse, 1980; research monograph 31.

38. Goldstein P. Prostitution and drugs. Lexington, Massachusetts: Lexington Books, 1979.

39. Goldstein P. Getting over: economic alternatives to predatory crime among drug users. In: Inciardi J, ed. The drugs/crime connection. Beverly Hills, California: Sage Press, 1981:67–84.

40. Zahn M. Homicide in the twentieth century United States. In: Inciardi JA, Faupel CE, eds. History and crime. Beverly Hills, California: Sage Press, 1980.

41. Homicide Analysis 1981. New York: New York City Police Department, 1983.

42. Criminal victimization in the United States, 1980. Washington, D.C.: US Department of Justice, 1982.

43. Statistical abstract. Washington, D.C.: National Center for Health Statistics, 1980.

44. Estimate of opiate addicted births. Services research branch notes. Rockville, Maryland: National Institute on Drug Abuse, 1979.

45. Cuskey W, Watney B. Female addiction. Lexington, Massachusetts: Lexington Books, 1982.

46. Carr J. Drug patterns among drug-addicted mothers: incidence, variance in use, and effects on children. Pediatr Ann 1975:66–77.

47. Householder J, Hatcher R, Burns W, et al. Infants born to narcotic-addicted mothers. Psychol Bull 1982;92:453–68.

48. Stimmel B, Goldberg J, Reiman A, et al. Fetal outcome in narcotic-dependent women: the importance of maternal narcotic use. Am J Drug Alcohol Abuse 1982;9:383–95.

49. Mortality in infants of addicted mothers. New York: City Health Department, 1983.

50. Fawzy F, Coombs R, Gerber B. Generational continuity in the use of substances: the impact of parental substance use on adolescent substance use. Addict Behav 1983;8:109–14.

51. Coppolillo H. Drug impediments to mothering behavior. Addict Dis 1975;2:201–8.

52. Bauman P, Dougherty F. Drug addicted mothers' parenting and their children's development. Int J Addict 1983;18:291–302.

53. Sowder B, Burt M. Children of heroin addicts. New York: Praeger, 1980.

54. Jones K, Vischi T. Impact of alcohol, drug abuse and mental health treatment on medical care utilization. Med Care 1979;17(suppl):1–82.

55. Hunt D, Strug D, Goldsmith D, et al. Alcohol use and abuse: heavy drinking among methadone clients. Am J Drug Alcohol Abuse (in press).

56. Belenko S. Alcohol abuse by heroin addicts: a review of research findings and issues. Int J Addict 1979;14:965–75.

57. Briar S, Piliavin I. Delinquency, situational inducements and commitment to conformity. Soc Prob 1966;18:35–6.

58. Kaplan E, Rich H, Gersony W, et al. A collaborative study of infectious endocarditis in the 1970s. J Circulation 1979;59:327–35.

59. Vital statistics of the United States, 1980. Washington, D.C.: US Government Printing Office, 1981.

Infectious and Parasitic Diseases

John V. Bennett, M.D., Scott D. Holmberg, M.D.,
Martha F. Rogers, M.D., and Steven L. Solomon, M.D.

Most of the health problems identified in *Closing the Gap* relate directly or indirectly to infectious diseases. Infections and infection-related deaths are important contributors to circulatory, respiratory, and gastrointestinal diseases, to infant morbidity and mortality, and to arthritis. Infections also play an important role in morbidity and mortality that may complicate unintentional injuries, malignancies, attempted homicides or suicides, and diabetes mellitus. Microbial agents probably play a crucial role in dental caries and periodontal disease. Further, in the past few years viruses have been found to cause malignancies in humans, and other oncogenic viruses will no doubt be identified. Because of these interrelationships, the information in this report overlaps with and complements information in other position papers of the Carter Center Health Policy Project.

The effective control of each health problem will reduce the morbidity and mortality associated with infectious disease. Conversely, improvements in infection prevention and treatment will reduce the morbidity and mortality associated with other health problems.

DATA SELECTION

Infectious and parasitic diseases occupy the International Code of Diseases (ICD) codes 1–113, but at least 125 additional specific ICD codes reflect infections. Indeed, only 17 percent of all deaths from infections can be identified within ICD codes 1–113. Some ICD codes represent entities that are not always caused by infectious agents (for example, bronchitis), and some codes encompass situations in which infections may be either primary events or secondary to other inciting episodes (for example, peritonitis). These deficiencies in classification make it difficult to obtain a clear picture of the true magnitude of infections from data systems based on ICD codes. For this reason, we relied on other data to establish the burden of illness caused by infections.

To estimate the negative impact of infectious diseases in the United States, we first divided all infectious diseases into mutually exclusive groupings, then used published material and survey data from the National Center for Health Statistics to derive morbidity and mortality estimates for each grouping. The groupings were then combined to give totals for all infectious diseases. We refer to this information as the consultants' data. (The details of this data set are presented in a 361-page appendix which is on file with the Carter Center.)

The second group of data, referred to as CDC Survey Data, was collected from experts in the various divisions of the Center for Infectious Diseases and the Center for Prevention Services, Centers for Disease Control (CDC). Data were provided in 1985 on the current incidence of symptomatic infections, current and estimated future case–fatality ratios attributable to these infections, and current and estimated future overall efficiency in preventing infections caused by 117 specific microbial agents or agent groupings (Table 1, first five columns). Estimates included the morbidity and mortality averted by use of all applicable intervention strategies in both the public and private sectors. Estimates are given of current effectiveness as well as likely future effectiveness deriving from known or likely upcoming improvements in the effectiveness of various intervention strategies. Estimates of the effectiveness of prevention efforts vary in reliability. In some instances, such as nosocomial infections, these estimates are well established. In other instances, such as rotaviruses, they are based on the assumed efficacy of a yet-to-be-fully-devel-

From the Center for Infectious Diseases, Centers for Disease Control, Atlanta.

Address reprint requests to Dr. Bennett, Center for Infectious Diseases, Centers for Disease Control, 1600 Clifton Road, Atlanta, GA 30333.

oped vaccine. Some estimates represent solely the cautious guesses of experts.

The data provided in the CDC survey were then used to derive additional parameters by which prevention could be assessed as described in Table 2. The resulting estimates of the numbers of cases and deaths prevented now and in the future and other derivative data appear in the last nine columns of Table 1.

The 117 specific infections or infection groupings were assigned subsequently to appropriate, mutually exclusive etiologic groups and to one or more of 13 additional infection categories that were not necessarily mutually exclusive (Table 3). In some instances, such as the category "zoonotic," all infections potentially transmissible from animals to humans were included. In other instances, such as the category "foodborne," the proportion of each specific infection acquired in that fashion was estimated as indicated in Table 3, and only that proportion of overall morbidity and mortality attributable to foodborne acquisition was included under the "foodborne" heading. "Vaccine-preventable" infection data could not be apportioned reliably in this fashion, although it is recognized that the vaccine itself may sometimes not be responsible for all prevented cases (e.g., anthrax).

In general, the CID survey data underestimated the overall magnitude of infections compared with the consultants' data, since not all known specific infectious agents were included in the survey results, and clinically diagnosed infections of known and unknown causes were encompassed in the consultants' data. Thus, we have relied primarily on the consultants' data for estimates of negative impact and on the CDC survey data for prevention estimates.

SCOPE OF THE PROBLEM

The consultants' data indicate that more than 740 million infectious disease events and nearly 200,000 attributable deaths occur annually in the United States (Table 4). Included in the total incidence are infections that, although not life threatening for persons who have normal host defenses, may result in days lost from work (or other major activities) or that incur a direct financial burden. The total number of deaths attributed to infectious diseases includes those cases for which either prevention or successful treatment would have prolonged the life of the affected person.

We estimate that each year infectious diseases result in more than 2 million years of life lost before the age of 65, more than 52 million hospital days, and nearly 2 billion days lost from work, school, and other major activities. The total direct cost of infectious diseases—not including the cost of deaths, lost wages and productivity, reactions to treatment, or other indirect costs—exceeds $17 billion annually.

The leading contributors to these negative impacts, as assessed from the CDC survey data, are listed by nonexclusive category in Table 5. The five most important contributors to mortality from infections, in decreasing order of magnitude, are: bacterial infections, lower respiratory infections (pneumonia and influenza), nosocomial infections, vaccine-preventable infections, and viral infections. The five major causes of symptomatic infections, in decreasing order of magnitude of cases, are: viral, upper respiratory, cutaneous, vaccine-preventable, and bacterial infections.

The annual monetary costs of infectious diseases derive largely from the cost of hospital care. Nosocomial infections themselves account for the greatest direct costs; they complicate the course of recovery among hospitalized patients, increase the severity of illness, increase mortality, or prolong hospital stay, thus adding substantially to the consumption of expensive hospital services.

The consultants' data indicate that nosocomial infections account for almost 12 million excess hospital days annually and pose direct costs of close to $3.5 billion. Enteric and lower respiratory infections account for 9 million and 7.5 million hospital days, respectively, and are estimated to involve direct costs of $3 billion and more than $2 billion, respectively. Genitourinary tract infections, soft-tissue infections, and upper respiratory infections are not major causes of death. However, they result in appreciable costs for outpatient care. Approximately $5 billion was spent on genitourinary tract and upper respiratory infections, and $2 billion on soft-tissue infections.

ESTIMATES OF PREVENTION GAPS

We can prevent many additional infections every year simply by expanding our current efforts in prevention and utilizing recent technological advances. Specific infections or infection groupings where more than a million additional future cases may be preventable each year include infections caused by rotaviruses, enteroviruses, Norwalk and other 27-nanometer particles, campylobacter, salmonella, and toxoplasma (Table 1, column 12 minus

Table 1. Domestic infections, United States, 1985

Disease or agent	Current incidence[a]	Case/fatality ratio (%)[b] Now	Future	Effectiveness[c] Now	Future	Deaths now
Bacterial						
Chlamydia neonatal	50,000	0.0001	0.0001	0	35	0
Psittacosis	700	1.0	0.5	40	50	7
Trachoma	100	0.0	0.0	50	50	0
Mycoplasma pneumonia	1,000,000	0.01	0.01	0	1	100
Anthrax	1	5.0	5.0	99	99	0
Bacillus cereus	5,000	0.0	0.0	80	84	0
Botulism incl. infants	200	4.0	2.0	99	99.3	8
Brucellosis	400	0.5	0.5	97	99	2
Campylobacteriosis	2,100,000	0.1	0.02	75	95	2,100
Chancroid	4,000	0.0005	0.0001	50	80	0
Chlamydia trach. gen. inf.	2,200,000	0.05	0.02	5	50	1,100
Cholera	25	1.0	0.0	95	98	3
Clost. perfringens	10,000	1.0	0.0	80	85	100
Dial. pyrogen, py. reac., sep.	5,000	0.1	0.08	10	15	5
Diphtheria	10	10.0	3.0	>99.9	>99.9	1
E. coli–enteric.	200,000	0.2	0.1	90	98	400
End. bact.–aer. and anaer.	10,000	0.05	0.05	10	10	5
Gardnerella vaginale inf.	6,000,000	0.0	0.0	1	10	0
Gonococcal infection	2,000,000	0.05	0.02	40	65	1,000
H. influ. incl. menin.	20,000	5.0	5.0	3	75	1,000
Legionellosis	75,000	15.0	15.0	3	12	11,250
Leprosy	400	1.5	1.0	4	4	6
Leptospirosis	1,100	3.0	1.0	55	60	33
Listeriosis	220	12.5	12.5	1	35	28
Meningococcal inv.	6,000	10.0	10.0	4	50	600
Misc. unclass.	1,000	0.05	0.05	0	1	1
Miscellaneous enteric	200,000	1.0	0.5	50	80	2,000
Miscellaneous zoonotic	2,000	1.0	0.5	5	10	20
Mycobacteria nontb.	10,000	0.5	0.4	1	2	50
Mycoplasma hom. genital	100,000	0.002	0.001	1	25	2
Mycoplasma/ureaplasma	250,000	0.001	0.001	1	7.5	3
Pasteurella multocida	14,000	0.25	0.2	20	25	35
Pertussis	34,000	0.2	0.2	80	85	68
Plague	50	15.0	10.0	50	75	8
Pneumococcal invasive	400,000	8.0	6.0	4	55	32,000
Relapsing FVR.–tick/louse	264	0.5	0.5	5	5	1
Rickettsioses	2,000	5.6	5.0	5	10	112
S. aureus–TSS	4,500	3.0	1.5	75	90	135
S. aureus excl. TSS	8,900,000	0.08	0.05	3	5	7,120
Salmonellosis, nontyphi.	2,000,000	0.1	0.05	80	95	2,000
Shigella	300,000	0.2	0.2	55	75	600
Strep. Group A	10,000,000	0.03	0.02	1	1.5	3,000
Strep. Group B neonatal	7,000	20.0	15.0	5	25	1,400
Syphilis	70,000	0.08	0.01	75	85	56
Tetanus	150	30.0	30.0	98	99	45
Tuberculosis	27,000	5.0	4.0	40	40	1,350
Tularemia	402	1.0	0.8	15	17	4
Typhoid	600	6.0	5.5	95	99	36
Vibrio inf. excl. cholera	10,000	4.0	2.0	80	95	400
Yersiniosis excl. plague	5,000	0.05	0.04	0.5	2	3
Fungal						
Actinomycotic diseases	1,400	5.0	4.0	10	10	70
Aspergillosis	2,300	7.0	4.0	5	5	161
Blastomycosis	100	7.0	4.0	5	5	7
Candidiasis	4,000	10.0	2.0	5	5	400
Chromoblastomycosis	50	0.0	0.0	5	5	0
Coccidioidomycosis	8,000	4.0	2.0	10	10	320
Cryptococcosis	1,000	10.0	10.0	4	4	100
Dermatophytoses	18,000,000	0.0	0.0	1	1	0
Histoplasmosis	10,000	1.0	1.0	5	7	100
Mycetomas	25	0.0	0.0	0	0	0

	Without prevention		With prevention		Preventable annually[d]		Future incidence[e]	
	Cases	Deaths	Cases	Deaths	Cases	Deaths	Cases	Deaths
Bacterial								
Chla. neon.	50,000	0	0	0	17,500	0	32,500	0
Psittacosis	1,167	12	467	45	583	9	584	3
Trachoma	200	0	100	0	100	0	100	0
Mycopl. pneu.	1,000,000	100	0	0	10,000	1	990,000	99
Anthrax	100	5	99	5	99	5	1	0
B. cereus	25,000	0	20,000	0	21,000	0	4,000	0
Bot. in infant	20,000	800	19,800	792	19,860	797	140	3
Brucellosis	13,333	67	12,933	65	13,200	66	133	1
Campylobact.	8,400,000	8,400	6,300,000	6,300	7,980,000	8,316	420,000	84
Chancroid	8,000	0	4,000	0	6,400	0	1,600	0
Chla. tra. gen.	2,315,789	1,158	115,789	58	1,157,894	926	1,157,895	232
Cholera	500	5	475	2	490	5	10	0
C. perfring.	50,000	500	40,000	400	42,500	500	7,500	0
Dial. pyro.–sep.	5,556	6	556	1	833	2	4,723	4
Diphtheria	15,000	1,500	14,990	1,499	14,990	1,500	10	0
E. coli.–ent.	2,000,000	4,000	1,800,000	3,600	1,960,000	3,960	40,000	40
End. bac.–Ae&An	11,111	6	1,111	1	1,111	1	10,000	5
Gardner. vag.	6,060,606	0	60,606	0	606,060	0	5,454,546	0
Gonococcus	3,333,333	1,667	1,333,333	667	2,166,666	1,434	1,166,667	233
H. inf. in men	20,619	1,031	619	31	15,464	773	5,155	258
Legionellosis	77,320	11,598	2,320	348	9,278	1,392	68,042	10,206
Leprosy	417	6	17	0	16	2	401	4
Leptospirosis	2,444	73	1,344	40	1,467	63	977	10
Listeriosis	222	28	2	0	78	10	144	18
Meningo. inv.	6,250	625	250	25	3,125	312	3,125	313
Misc. unclass.	1,000	1	0	0	10	1	990	0
Misc. ent.	400,000	4,000	200,000	2,000	320,000	3,600	80,000	400
Misc. zoo.	2,105	21	105	1	211	12	1,894	9
Mycobac. nontb.	10,101	51	101	1	202	11	9,899	40
Mycop. hom. gen.	101,010	2	1,010	0	25,252	1	75,758	1
Mycop./ureapla.	252,525	3	2,525	0	18,939	1	233,586	2
Pasteur. multoc.	17,500	44	3,500	9	4,375	18	13,125	26
Pertussis	170,000	340	136,000	272	144,500	289	25,500	51
Plague	100	15	50	7	75	12	25	3
Pneumo. inv.	416,667	33,333	16,667	1,333	229,167	22,083	187,500	11,250
Relap. fever	278	1	14	0	14	0	264	1
Rickettsioses	2,105	118	105	6	210	23	1,895	95
S. aur.—TSS	18,000	540	13,500	405	16,200	513	1,800	27
S. aur. ex TSS	9,175,258	7,340	275,258	220	458,763	2,982	8,716,495	4,358
Salm.–nontyphi.	10,000,000	10,000	8,000,000	8,000	9,500,000	9,750	500,000	250
Shigellosis	666,667	1,333	366,667	733	500,000	1,000	166,667	333
Strep. gp. A	10,101,010	3,030	101,010	30	151,515	1,040	9,949,495	1,990
Strep. gp. B neo	7,638	1,528	638	128	1,974	678	5,664	850
Syphilis	280,000	224	210,000	168	238,000	220	42,000	4
Tetanus	7,500	2,250	7,350	2,205	7,425	2,227	75	23
Tuberculosis	45,000	2,250	18,000	900	18,000	1,170	27,000	1,080
Tularemia	473	5	71	1	80	2	393	3
Typhoid	12,000	720	11,400	684	11,880	713	120	7
Vibrio ex. chol.	50,000	2,000	40,000	1,600	47,500	1,950	2,500	50
Yersinio ex. pl.	5,025	3	25	0	100	1	4,925	2
Fungal								
Actinomycosis	1,556	78	156	8	156	22	1,400	56
Aspergillosis	2,421	169	121	8	121	77	2,300	92
Blastomycosis	105	7	5	0	5	3	100	4
Candidiasis	4,211	421	211	21	211	341	4,000	80
Chromoblastomy.	53	0	3	0	3	0	50	0
Coccidioidomyc.	8,889	356	889	36	889	196	8,000	160
Cryptococcosis	1,042	104	42	4	42	4	1,000	100
Dermatophytos.	18,181,818	0	181,818	0	181,818	0	18,000,000	0
Histoplasmosis	10,526	105	526	5	737	7	9,789	98
Mycetomas	25	0	0	0	0	0	25	0

Table 1. Continued

Disease or agent	Current incidence[a]	Case/fatality ratio (%)[b]		Effectiveness[c]		Deaths now
		Now	Future	Now	Future	
Paracoccidioidomycosis	2	0.0	0.0	0	3	0
Sporotrichosis	200	6.0	4.0	3	4	12
Zygomycosis	100	15.0	15.0	0	5	15
Nosocomial						
Acute care	2,200,000	1.2	1.2	6	32	26,400
Chron. care	1,900,000	1.3	1.3	1	16	24,700
Parasitic						
Amebiasis	12,000	0.3	0.01	50	50	36
Ascariasis	50,000	0.1	0.01	20	50	50
Babesiosis	20	10.0	10.0	10	10	2
Cryptosporidiosis	50	50.0	50.0	20	50	25
Echinococcosis	200	1.5	0.75	50	60	3
Filariasis	300	0.001	0.001	0	0	0
Flukes	9,000	0.001	0.0001	0	0	0
Giardiasis	120,000	0.0001	0.0001	50	90	0
Hookworm	200	0.0001	0.0001	90	95	0
Leishmaniasis	35	0.1	0.1	0	0	0
Malaria	2,500	1.0	1.0	75	98	25
Meningoencephal., amoebic	4	99.99999	50.0	0	10	4
Pediculosis	9,000,000	0.0	0.0	10	10	0
Pneumocystis	600	20.0	1.0	90	90	120
Scabies	10,000,000	0.0	0.0	1	1	0
Schistosomiasis	1,000	0.001	0.0001	75	90	0
Strongyloidiasis	10,000	1.0	1.0	1	20	100
Taeniesis/cysticercosis	1,000	1.0	0.2	50	80	10
Toxocariasis VLM	10,000	0.0001	0.0001	1	80	0
Toxoplasma congenital	3,000	15.0	2.0	5	50	450
Toxoplasmosis excl. cong.	2,300,000	0.0001	0.0001	5	50	2
Trichinosis	100,000	1.0	0.001	10	90	1,000
Trichomoniasis	5,000,000	0.0	0.0	5	10	0
Trypanosomiasis, African	2	10.0	5.0	0	0	0
Trypanosomiasis, Amer.	1	10.0	5.0	0	0	0
Viral						
Adenovirus	10,000,000	0.01	0.01	10	15	1,000
CMV congenital	1,900	15.0	10.0	30	60	285
Colorado tick fever	2,500	0.01	0.01	1	20	0
Coronavirus	18,080,000	0.0	0.0	0	0	0
Dengue–classical	46	0.0	0.0	25	60	0
Encephalitides, N.A.	5,000	12.0	1.0	20	75	600
Enteroviral dis.–nonpolio	6,000,000	0.001	0.0001	50	80	60
Hepatitis A	48,000	0.3	0.3	40	50	144
Hepatitis B	128,000	3.0	3.0	15	80	3,840
Hepatitis non-A non-B	50,000	0.4	0.4	0	15	200
Herpes simplex (gen.)	400,000	0.00001	0.00001	5	30	0
HIV	80,000	10.0	10.0	20	50	8,000
HSV neonatal	1,000	50.0	20.0	30	80	500
Influenza	20,000,000	0.005	0.005	5	7.5	1,000
Lymphocytic choriormenin.	200	1.0	0.01	10	10	2
Measles	2,500	0.01	0.01	>99.9	>99.9	0
Mumps	10,000	0.004	0.004	99.6	99.9	0
Norwalk/other 27 nmpar.	6,000,000	0.0001	0.0001	30	50	6
Papilloma virus	3,000,000	0.001	0.001	0	0	30
Poliomyelitis	7	10.0	10.0	99.9	99.9	1
Rabies	10	99.0	99.0	99	99	10
Rhinovirus	125,000,000	0.00001	0.00001	10	10	13
Rotavirus	8,000,000	0.01	0.01	0	50	800
Rubella congenital	70	50.0	50.0	99	100	35
Rubella excl. congenital	20,000	0.0001	0.0001	98.6	99.9	0
Varicella	3,500,000	0.003	0.0002	0	2	105
Virus, respiratory sync.	7,000,000	0.005	0.005	0	30	350

	Without prevention		With current prevention		Preventable annually[d]		Future incidence[e]	
	Cases	Deaths	Cases	Deaths	Cases	Deaths	Cases	Deaths
Paracoccidioid.	2	0	0	0	0	0	2	0
Sporotrichosis	206	12	6	0	8	4	198	8
Zygomycosis	100	15	0	0	5	1	95	14
Nosocomial								
Acute care	2,340,426	28,085	140,426	1,685	748,936	8,987	1,591,490	19,098
Chron. care	1,919,192	24,950	19,192	250	307,070	3,992	1,612,122	20,958
Parasitic								
Amebiasis	24,000	72	12,000	36	12,000	71	12,000	1
Ascariasis	62,500	63	12,500	13	31,250	60	31,250	3
Babesiosis	22	2	2	0	2	0	20	2
Cryptosporidio.	63	32	13	7	31	16	32	16
Echinococcosis	400	6	200	3	240	5	160	1
Filariasis	300	0	0	0	0	0	300	0
Flukes	9,000	0	0	0	0	0	9,000	0
Giardiasis	240,000	0	120,000	0	216,000	0	24,000	0
Hookworm	2,000	0	1,800	0	1,900	0	100	0
Leishmaniasis	35	0	0	0	0	0	35	0
Malaria	10,000	100	7,500	75	9,800	98	200	2
Meningoenc.–amo.	4	4	0	0	0	2	4	2
Pediculosis	10,000,000	0	1,000,000	0	1,000,000	0	9,000,000	0
Pneumocystis	6,000	1,200	5,400	1,080	5,400	1,194	600	6
Scabies	10,101,010	0	101,010	0	101,010	0	10,000,000	0
Schistosomiasis	4,000	0	3,000	0	3,600	0	400	0
Strongyloidiasis	10,101	101	101	1	2,020	20	8,081	81
Taeniasis/cys.	2,000	20	1,000	10	1,600	19	400	1
Toxocara vlm.	10,101	0	101	0	8,081	0	2,020	0
Toxoplas. cong.	3,158	474	158	24	1,579	442	1,579	32
Toxopla. ex. con.	2,421,053	2	121,053	0	1,210,526	1	1,210,527	1
Trichinosis	111,111	1,111	11,111	111	100,000	1,111	11,111	0
Trichomoniasis	5,263,157	0	263,157	0	526,316	0	4,736,841	0
Trypanosom.–Af	2	0	0	0	0	0	2	0
Trypanosom.–Am	1	0	0	0	0	0	1	0
Viral								
Adenovirus	11,111,111	1,111	1,111,111	111	1,666,667	167	9,444,444	944
CMV congenital	2,714	407	814	122	1,629	298	1,085	109
Colorado tk. fv.	2,525	0	25	0	505	0	2,020	0
Coronavirus	18,080,000	0	0	0	0	0	18,080,000	0
Dengue–classic	61	0	15	0	37	0	24	0
Encephaliti.–NA	6,250	750	1,250	150	4,688	734	1,562	16
Enterov. non-po.	12,000,000	120	6,000,000	60	9,600,000	118	2,400,000	2
Hepatitis A	80,000	240	32,000	96	40,000	120	40,000	120
Hepatitis B	150,588	4,518	22,588	678	120,471	3,614	30,117	904
Hepa. non-A non-B	50,000	200	0	0	7,500	30	42,500	170
Herpes sim.–gen.	421,053	0	21,053	0	126,316	0	294,737	0
HIV	100,000	10,000	20,000	2,000	50,000	5,000	50,000	5,000
HSV neonatal	1,429	714	429	214	1,142	657	287	57
Influenza	21,052,632	1,053	1,052,632	53	1,578,947	79	19,473,685	974
Lymph. choriom.	222	2	22	0	22	2	200	0
Measles	3,500,000	350	3,497,500	350	3,497,500	350	2,500	0
Mumps	2,500,000	100	2,490,000	100	2,497,500	100	2,500	0
Nor./oth. 27 nmp.	8,571,429	9	2,571,429	3	4,285,714	5	4,285,715	4
Papillomavirus	3,000,000	30	0	0	0	0	3,000,000	30
Poliomyelitis	7,000	700	6,993	699	6,993	699	7	1
Rabies	1,000	990	990	980	990	980	10	10
Rhinovirus	138,888,889	14	13,888,889	1	13,888,889	2	125,000,000	12
Rotavirus	8,000,000	800	0	0	4,000,000	400	4,000,000	400
Rubella congen.	7,000	3,500	6,930	3,465	7,000	3,500	0	0
Rubella ex. con.	1,428,571	1	1,408,571	1	1,427,142	1	1,429	0
Varicella	3,500,000	105	0	0	70,000	98	3,430,000	7
Virus–resp. syn.	7,000,000	350	0	0	2,100,000	105	4,900,000	245

Data from CDC survey
[a] Estimated true annual number of clinically significant infections.
[b] Attributable to the infection.
[c] Total effectiveness, in percent, of all public and private interventions in preventing cases.
[d] Assuming future effectiveness and case-fatality ratios.
[e] Unprevented morbidity and mortality.

column 10). Similarly, more than a thousand additional deaths might be preventable each year by improved prevention of infections caused by pneumococci, HIV-1 (human immunodeficiency virus–type 1), hepatitis B, *Staphylococcus aureus*, campylobacter, salmonella, and miscellaneous bacterial enteric pathogens (Table 1, column 13 versus column 11).

Similar analyses can be applied to categories of infection (Figure 1). Substantial increments are possible in the number of prevented cases of enteric (13 million), viral (12.9 million), bacterial (6.6 million), vaccine-preventable (5.4 million), zoonotic (4.3 million), foodborne (3.5 million), lower respiratory (3.0 million), and sexually transmitted infectious diseases (2.9 million). Marked increases in the proportion of infections prevented (cases prevented in the future divided by cases prevented now) are envisioned for nosocomial infections (6.9-fold), meningitis (5.1-fold), perinatal infections (3.4-fold but not shown in Figure 1 because numbers are too small for the scale used), lower respiratory infections (3.3-fold), sexually transmitted infections (2.5-fold), and day-care-center-related infections (2.4-fold).

Impressive gains in the numbers of deaths prevented (in decreasing order) can be achieved (Figure 2) with bacterial diseases (35,900), vaccine-preventable infections (25,300), lower respiratory infections (23,300), and nosocomial infections (11,100). The largest proportional gains in deaths prevented are envisioned with meningitis (10.5-fold), fungal infections (7.0-fold), nosocomial infections (6.8-fold), lower respiratory infections (6.7-fold), cutaneous infections (5.9-fold), day-care-center-related infections (4.2-fold), and vaccine-preventable infections (3.1-fold).

Prevention of infection translates readily into economic savings. The results of applying current and achievable effectiveness in preventing cases (from CDC survey data) to negative impacts (from the consultants' data) are depicted in Figure 3. Despite impressive accomplishments in prevention, substantial gaps between what we are achieving and what we could achieve in preventing infection remain. For example, we estimate that an additional $1.3 billion in direct costs, 56 million cases of infection, 3.2 million hospital days, and 144 million disability days could be saved merely by broader application of available or soon-to-be-available interventions.

The estimated gaps between current and future achievements in preventing deaths and reducing the number of years of life lost are shown in Figure 4. An additional 80,000 deaths and nearly 1 million years of life lost may be saved annually. Indeed, more than twice as many deaths as are annually prevented now are likely to be prevented in the future. These gains result both from improved primary prevention of cases and from improved diagnosis and treatment of cases that do occur. However, such gains could occur simultaneously with and be offset by increases in unprecedented deaths from any expanding lethal infection problem. Only HIV infections are foreseen to pose such a threat.

Table 2. Derivations of additional parameters from CDC survey data

Deaths now	= (current cases) (current case-fatality ratio[a,b])
Cases in absence of prevention	= (current cases) ÷ (1 − current effectiveness[a])
Deaths in absence of prevention	= (cases in absence of prevention) (current case-fatality-ratio[a])
Cases prevented now	= (cases in absence of prevention) (current effectiveness[a])
Deaths prevented now	= (deaths in absence of prevention) − (deaths now)
Cases prevented in the future	= (cases in absence of prevention) (future effectiveness[a])
Future annual cases	= (cases in absence of prevention) − (cases prevented in the future)
Future annual deaths	= (future annual cases) (future case-fatality-ratio[a])
Deaths prevented in the future	= (deaths in absence of prevention) − (future annual deaths)

[a] Expressed as a decimal.
[b] Italics: data provided by CDC survey.

NARROWING THE GAPS

Each prevention estimate in the foregoing material depends on the composite efficacy of applicable interventions. Thus, a detailed scrutiny of each intervention capable of preventing morbidity or mortality from infection seems appropriate.

Intervention strategies for preventing infectious diseases can be divided into two basic groups: (1) strategies that are generically applicable to all infectious diseases (indeed, to all diseases), such as disease surveillance, epidemiologic investigations, diagnosis, and treatment; and (2) strategies that are applicable to subsets of infectious diseases, such as immunization, chemo- or immunoprophylaxis, screening, contact tracing, control of environmental sources and vehicles (food, water, air, medical devices), control of insect and animal reservoirs and vectors, isolation precautions and quarantine, and behavior modification. These 12 strategies interact synergistically with each other.

Rapid and accurate identification, both of individual cases and of clusters of disease, is important in preventing new cases as well as in initiating early and appropriate treatment of those who are already ill. The potential for the rapid identification of specific infectious diseases has been greatly enhanced in recent years by developments in the microbiology laboratory and by the revolution in data pro-

Table 3. Domestic infections, United States, 1985: percentage attributed to various infection categories

Disease or agent	Pneumonia and lower respiratory	Upper respiratory	Perinatal	Zoonotic	Cutaneous	Food-borne	Enteric	Water-borne	STD	Meningitis	Vector-borne	Day care	Vaccine preventable
Bacterial													
Chlamydia neonatal	100	100											
Psittacosis	100			100									
Trachoma					100								
Mycoplasma pneumonia	100												
Anthrax				100									100
Bacillus cereus						100	100						
Botulism incl. infants						90	100						
Brucellosis				100		5							
Campylobacteriosis				100		100	100	15					
Chancroid									100				
Chlamydia trach. gen. inf.									100				
Cholera						100	100						
Clost. perfringens						100	100						
Dial. pyrogen, py. reac., sep.													
Diphtheria		100											100
E. coli–enteric.						25	100	75				5	
End. bact.–aer. and anaer.	50									5			
Gardnerella vaginale inf.									100				
Gonococcal infection									100				
H. influ. incl. menin.	12									50		30	100
Legionellosis	98												
Leprosy					100								
Leptospirosis				100									
Listeriosis				100						60			
Meningococcal inv.										80		5	100
Misc. unclass.	1									1			
Miscellaneous enteric						95	100	5					
Miscellaneous zoonotic				100									
Mycobacteria nontb.	20									1			
Mycoplasma hom. genital									100				
Mycoplasma/ureaplasma									100				
Pasteurella multocida				100									
Pertussis	100											0.5	100
Plague	20			100						10	100		
Pneumococcal invasive	95									5		5	100
Relapsing FVR.–tick/louse				100							100		
Rickettsioses											100		
S. aureus–TSS													
S. aureus excl. TSS	1				75	17				1		2	
Salmonellosis, nontyphi.				100		96	100	3				1	
Shigella						30	100	10				25	
Strep. Group A	1	75			25	5				1		2	
Strep. Group B neonatal	20		100							50			
Syphilis									100				
Tetanus													100
Tuberculosis	85									0.6			
Tularemia				100							100		
Typhoid						80	100	10					
Vibrio inf. excl. cholera						90	100	10					
Yersiniosis excl. plague				100		65		35					
Fungal													
Actinomycotic diseases													
Aspergillosis	100												
Blastomycosis	95												
Candidiasis												5	
Chromoblastomycosis					100								

Table 3. Continued

Disease or agent	Pneumonia and lower respiratory	Upper respiratory	Perinatal	Zoonotic	Cutaneous	Food-borne	Enteric	Water-borne	STD	Meningitis	Vector-borne	Day care	Vaccine preventable
Coccidioidomycosis	100												
Cryptococcosis										60			
Dermatophytoses					100							5	
Histoplasmosis	100												
Mycetomas					100								
Paracoccidioidomycosis	100												
Sporotrichosis					100								
Zygomycosis					100								
Nosocomial													
Acute care	15				6								
Chron. care	11				16		8						
Parasitic													
Amebiasis							100					0.5	
Ascariasis							100					5	
Babesiosis											100		
Cryptosporidiosis							100					2	
Echinococcosis				100									
Filariasis											100		
Flukes							100						
Giardiasis							100	60				15	
Hookworm							100						
Leishmaniasis					90						100		
Malaria											100		100
Meningoencephal., amoebic										100			
Pediculosis					100							0.5	
Pneumocystis	100												
Scabies					100							0.5	
Schistosomiasis													
Strongyloidiasis							100						
Taeniesis/cysticercosis				100									
Toxocariasis VLM				100									
Toxoplasma congenital			100										
Toxoplasmosis excl. cong.				100									
Trichinosis				100		100							
Trichomoniasis									100				
Trypanosomiasis, African											100		
Trypanosomiasis, Amer.											100		
Viral													
Adenovirus		100										2	100
CMV congenital			100										
Colorado tick fever											100		
Coronavirus		100										1	
Dengue–classical											100		
Encephalitides, N.A.											100		
Enteroviral dis.–nonpolio							100					2	
Hepatitis A						10	100					15	
Hepatitis B			1										100
Hepatitis non-A non-B													
Herpes simplex (gen.)					100					100			
HIV			1						75				
HSV neonatal			100										
Influenza	100											1	100
Lymphocytic choriormenin.				100						95			
Measles					100								100
Mumps		100											100
Norwalk/other 27 nmpar.							100	5				0.5	
Papilloma virus					100				5				
Poliomyelitis							100						100
Rabies				100									100
Rhinovirus		100											
Rotavirus							100					10	100
Rubella congenital			100										100
Rubella excl. congenital					100								100
Varicella					100								
Virus, respiratory sync.	100											5	

Table 4. The annual negative impact of infections, United States: consultants' data

Cases	742,248,261
Deaths	194,704
Years lost before the age of 65	2,192,370
Hospital days	42,029,624
Disability days[a]	1,901,847,705
Cost[b]	$17,191,400,000

[a] Days lost from work, school, preschool, or housekeeping.
[b] Excludes costs of death, sequelae of infections, home care, and reactions to treatment.

cessing. Advances in molecular biology and microbial genetics have led to the development of rapid, sensitive, and specific diagnostic tests, and additional discoveries are imminent.

Surveillance and epidemiologic investigations establish risk factors for disease by defining the sources of infection, the means by which the causative agent is spread, and the host factors that make people susceptible to infection. Surveillance identifies new problems, focuses control efforts, and provides a means to monitor the effectiveness of control efforts.

Our ability to perform surveillance has been greatly enhanced by advances in data processing, which permit rapid transmission of data among public health agencies and health care providers and allow for immediate analysis of large amounts

Table 5. Current annual impacts by infection category, United States: CDC survey data

Infection group	Deaths[a]	Incidence[b]
Bacterial	68,200	36,026,000
Cutaneous	11,800	53,534,000
Day-care-related	2,600	3,713,000
Enteric	10,800	25,227,000
Food-borne	9,100	6,496,000
Fungi	1,200	18,027,000
Meningitis	3,500	229,000
Nosocomial	51,100	4,100,000
Parasitic	1,800	26,620,000
Perinatal	2,800	65,000
Pneumonia and lower respiratory	52,000	29,321,000
Sexually transmitted	8,200	16,234,000
Upper respiratory	3,300	160,590,000
Vaccine-preventable	40,400	38,623,000
Vector-borne	800	13,000
Viral	17,000	207,329,000
Water-borne	900	940,000
Zoonotic	5,300	6,536,000

[a] Rounded to the nearest 100.
[b] Rounded to the nearest 1,000.

of data as they are gathered. Disease surveillance and investigation, combined with new diagnostic techniques, permit the other interventions discussed to be performed efficiently and effectively for specific infections. Potentially communicable persons and reservoirs within the environment can be identified, treatment or decontamination can be

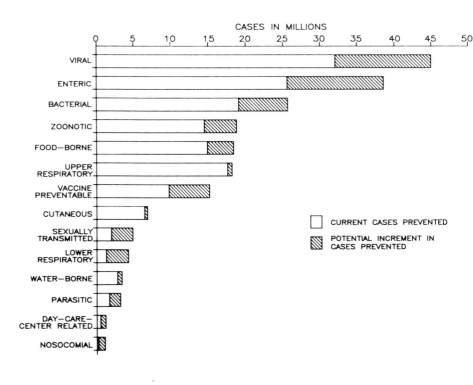

Figure 1. *The prevention of infectious diseases in the United States, current and potential: number of cases prevented annually, by infection categories, based on CDC survey data.*

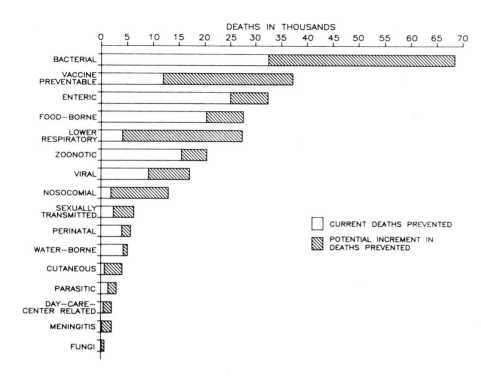

Figure 2. The prevention of infectious diseases in the United States, current and potential: number of deaths prevented annually, by infection categories, based on CDC survey data.

initiated, and, when necessary, chemoprophylaxis and immunoprophylaxis can be offered to exposed and potentially exposed persons. Disease investigations continue to identify new sources of transmission for well-known agents.

Advances in molecular biology offer great opportunities to improve the immunogenicity, safety, and quantity of older vaccines and to develop highly effective and safe new ones. The production of more effective vaccines with a longer duration of protection in large quantities at low cost may ulti-

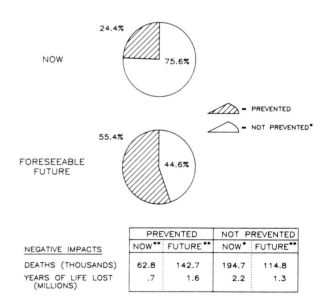

NEGATIVE IMPACTS	PREVENTED		NOT PREVENTED	
	NOW**	FUTURE**	NOW*	FUTURE**
COSTS (BILLIONS)	3.1	4.4	17.2	15.9
CASES (MILLIONS)	135.1	191.3	742.2	686.0
HOSPITAL DAYS (MILLIONS)	7.6	10.8	42.0	38.8
DISABILITY DAYS (MILLIONS)	346.2	490.1	1901.8	1757.9

Figure 3. Annual morbidity from infections, United States. *Unprevented morbidity is equivalent to the current negative morbidity impacts shown in Table 4. **Derived from above prevention estimates and current negative morbidity impacts.

NEGATIVE IMPACTS	PREVENTED		NOT PREVENTED	
	NOW**	FUTURE**	NOW*	FUTURE**
DEATHS (THOUSANDS)	62.8	142.7	194.7	114.8
YEARS OF LIFE LOST (MILLIONS)	.7	1.6	2.2	1.3

Figure 4. Annual mortality from infections, United States. *Unprevented mortality is equivalent to current negative mortality impacts in Table 4. **Derived from above prevention estimates and current negative mortality impacts.

mately make routine immunization of the entire population with a variety of vaccines (e.g., hepatitis B, meningococcal vaccine) economically feasible. Improved vaccines might also play major roles in management of persons known or likely to be exposed to particular infectious agents, and make it possible to develop highly effective immunoprophylactic agents.

Ongoing research has led to new antimicrobial agents, especially antiviral and antifungal drugs, that are available or undergoing experimental trials. These drugs offer the promise of successful therapy for persons who have infections that until now have been untreatable. Such therapy will lessen the burden of illness and reduce the likelihood that the diseases will be communicated to others. Surveillance of microbial resistance of infectious agents improves the appropriateness and thus the effectiveness of both treatment and prophylaxis.

Contact tracing is often associated with finding persons exposed to sexually transmitted diseases. This method may also be used to identify people who are at risk for other infections, such as infections caused by eating contaminated food, by contact with persons who have communicable diseases in day care centers or institutions, or by exposure to contaminated pharmaceutical products and medical devices. The rapid institution of effective therapy in persons already infected, at times before the onset of symptoms, may be critical to the prevention of disability, mortality, and spread of infection.

Screening, the systematic and routine use of tests to detect infection, is especially useful when a large percentage of infected persons are without clinical symptoms, and the progress or spread of the infection can be influenced if its presence is known. Infections detected through screening contribute to surveillance and contact tracing and may lead to chemo- or immunoprophylaxis, immunization, or counseling to influence changes in behavior.

Environmental control is the process of ensuring that food, water, and air do not become a source of infectious diseases. Examples of areas where further progress can be made include finding ways to reduce antibiotic-resistant salmonella in meat products and developing new approaches to reduce the hazard of legionella in cooling towers and potable water.

The control of insects and animals involved in arthropod-borne and zoonotic infections continues to be of great importance. Expanded efforts at prevention will further reduce the impact of illnesses as diverse as campylobacteriosis, plague, rabies, and infectious encephalitis.

Quarantine, the detection and total physical isolation of infected persons, has some applicability in preventing the introduction of certain hazardous communicable infections from other parts of the world into the United States. However, it plays little part in the prevention of domestic infections. Isolation, the implementation of precautions appropriate for the known ways in which infections are spread, is effective in preventing spread from patients to other patients, hospital staff, and visitors.

The final intervention strategy is behavior modification. Convincing people to alter aspects of their lifestyles that predispose them to infectious diseases or that enable them to spread infections to others is difficult. Personal hygiene, sexual behavior, and the use of tobacco products, alcoholic beverages, and licit and ilicit drugs, as well as a person's willingness to make appropriate use of health care providers and public health services, profoundly affect one's risk of becoming a victim of an infectious disease.

We believe that the interventions likely to have the most impact on closing the demonstrated gap between current achievements and future attainments in preventing cases and deaths from infections include improved epidemiologic services, improved diagnosis and treatment, more widespread immunization, more effective environmental control, and more effective behavior modification. The risks for infectious disease are multifactorial, and a broad-based approach to prevention that uses many intervention strategies will yield the best results.

SUMMARY

More than 740 million symptomatic infections occur annually in the United States, resulting in 200,000 deaths a year. Such infections result in more than $17 billion annually in direct costs, not including cost of deaths, lost wages and productivity, reactions to treatment, and other indirect costs. About 135 million infections, 63,000 deaths, and $3.1 billion in direct costs are now prevented annually, but an additional 56 million cases, 80,000 deaths, and $1.3 billion in direct costs could be prevented by using currently and soon-to-be-available interventions.

The advances made in preventing infectious diseases during this century have been among the most dramatic developments in medicine. However, it is likely that we will be able in the future to prevent nearly one and a half times more infections and more than twice as many deaths as can be prevented now. Indeed, it is conceivable that we will be able during the next decade to match the entire accumulated progress to date in preventing morbidity and mortality from infections. Unfortunately, the presently expanding mortality from HIV infection will lessen the net effects of these remarkable advances in prevention.

The authors express appreciation to many persons at the Centers for Disease Control who provided information and estimates on the morbidity and mortality of specific infections. Special thanks are extended to the following reviewers: Drs. Miriam J. Alter, Libero Ajello, Larry J. Anderson, Paul A. Blake, Joel G. Breman, Claire V. Broome, Walter R. Dowdle, John C. Feeley, Steven C. Hadler, Ann M. Hardy, George R. Healy, Kenneth Herrmann, Alan R. Hinman, James M. Hughes, Dennis D. Juranek, Robert L. Kaiser, Arnold F. Kaufmann, and William G. Winkler.

Respiratory Diseases

Laurence S. Farer, M.D., M.P.H., and Carl W. Schieffelbein

Respiratory diseases constitute a tremendous health problem, as measured by the number of persons affected, the number of days of productive activity and years of productive life lost, and the direct costs of caring for persons suffering from them. This report provides an overview mainly of chronic lung diseases, which, because of their chronicity, are more significant in the huge costs incurred for care than in years of life lost prematurely. Other lung diseases, especially acute respiratory infections and lung cancer, contribute enormously to the overall problem of respiratory diseases.

According to the National Institutes of Health (NIH), lung diseases are a leading cause of death and disability in the United States. Nearly 240,000 deaths each year are directly attributable to lung diseases, and these diseases are a contributing cause to perhaps as many additional deaths. Thus, lung diseases may cause one out of every eight deaths and play a role in one out of every four. Almost 17 million Americans have chronic bronchitis, emphysema, or asthma, and more than 100 million cases of influenza, pneumonia, and acute bronchitis occur annually. Respiratory diseases account for approximately 2.5 million hospital discharges, 21 million days of hospital care, and 25 million physician visits. In 1979 the costs of these services were estimated at $29 billion. According to the American Lung Association, lung diseases account for more workdays lost (more than 31 million annually) than any other category of illness.

To this economic impact must be added the social costs and human suffering associated with these diseases. The devastating psychosocial and personal economic effects of a chronic, incurable lung disease are obvious. Progressive pulmonary impairment results in a decreasing ability to carry on the usual activities of daily living. The impairment may eventually lead to severe limitation of function, with loss of earning capacity and dependence on public assistance. Worry and anxiety may produce

From the Division of Tuberculosis Control, Center for Prevention Services, Centers for Disease Control, Atlanta.

Address reprint requests to Dr. Farer, Division of Tuberculosis Control, Center for Prevention Services, Centers for Disease Control, Atlanta, GA 30333.

intense stress for both the patient and the family. They may have to deal with a usually nonfatal but incurable disease such as asthma, face the possibility of fatal cancer as a complication of asbestos exposure, or cope with the inevitability of death in a disease such as cystic fibrosis.

Smoking is unquestionably the main cause of chronic lung disease. Other exogenous causes are hazardous substances found in the workplace, allergens, and infectious agents such as tuberculosis bacteria. Some lung diseases, notably cystic fibrosis, are hereditary. Many acquired lung diseases are of known cause. Acute viral respiratory infections in children may contribute to chronic lung disease later in life. Although probably not a cause, air pollution clearly can exacerbate chronic lung disease.

Information is presented in this paper on chronic obstructive pulmonary disease (COPD), asthma, occupational lung diseases, tuberculosis, and a group of other lung diseases. For most of the conditions described, complete and reliable data could not be found, and data from different sources were often found to conflict. Interpretation of the data was made difficult by the sometimes obscure lines dividing diagnostic categories, the variation among data sources in the diagnostic categories used, and the different years for which information on various aspects of a particular condition were available. The data provided here are more likely to understate than exaggerate the problems. Particular note should be taken of the effects of inflation on current costs wherever dollar figures are given. Despite these shortcomings, the estimates in this report give enough information to delineate the relative magnitude of the disease problems presented (Figures 1, 2).

RESPIRATORY PROBLEMS

Chronic Obstructive Pulmonary Disease

Chronic obstructive pulmonary disease (COPD) is a common health problem most prevalent in white males. However, its frequency among women is increasing. The spectrum of disease under the COPD

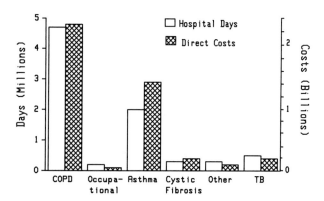

Figure 1. Respiratory diseases: hospital days and direct costs, United States, 1980. Source: Ten-year review and five-year plan, National Heart, Lung, and Blood Institute, vol. 3. Tables 2, 7.

rubric includes emphysema, chronic bronchitis, bronchiectasis, and a variety of other conditions. Such conditions frequently coexist, and the contribution of each to the obstruction of airflow varies from individual to individual. COPD strikes people in middle age, disables them with unremitting shortness of breath, destroys their ability to earn a living, results in their frequent use of the health care system, and disrupts the lives of their family members for one to two decades before death eventually occurs.

Cigarette smoking is the most important exogenous etiologic factor in COPD. Death rates from COPD have been reported to be 20 times higher for smokers than for nonsmokers. In the development and progression of COPD, cigarette smoking interacts additively, and sometimes synergistically,

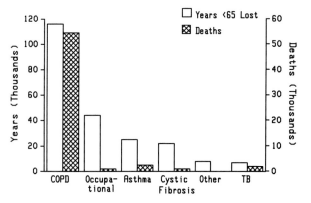

Figure 2. Respiratory diseases: potential years of life lost before the age of 65 and deaths, United States, 1980. Sources: Ten-year review and five-year plan, National Heart, Lung, and Blood Institute, vol. 3. Tables 2, 4, and 7; " 'Closing the Gap' Consultant's Guide," tables 3, 6; National Center for Health Statistics, Advance report on final mortality statistics, 1980, 1983.

with other inhaled toxic agents such as dust and fumes in the workplace and air pollutants. Most patients who have severe COPD are smokers, but only 10–15 percent of all smokers develop severe COPD. Genetic factors may be associated with COPD; the best known of these is severe alpha$_1$-antitrypsin (AAT) deficiency. Recurrent antecedent respiratory infections, usually beginning in childhood, are also associated with COPD.

Typically, COPD begins when a young person starts smoking cigarettes. Several years may elapse without recognized symptoms, although measurable abnormalities of pulmonary function may be present. Later, a chronic, productive cough develops. After about the age of 40, shortness of breath begins to occur. Advanced, incapacitating disease typically appears after age 55 but may occur earlier.

In 1980 more than 50,000 deaths ranked COPD and allied conditions as the fifth most common cause of death, having risen from tenth place in 1970. The seasonable pattern of COPD mortality is related to the frequency and severity of influenza and pneumonia in COPD patients during the winter. Because deaths of COPD patients are often attributed to pneumonia, the number of deaths related to COPD is probably underestimated.

The prevalence of COPD is approximately 10 million persons, and more than 1.5 million new cases are diagnosed annually in the United States. Its chronic, progressive nature makes COPD a major cause of functional impairment and suffering, producing a disability that inevitably affects a person's ability to earn a living and lead a productive life. In 1979 the estimated direct costs for hospital care, continuing care, physician visits, and medication were $2.3 billion; indirect costs of lost earnings due to disability were estimated to be $2 billion; and lost earnings due to mortality were estimated to be $2.2 billion. Thus, the total economic cost of COPD may now have reached $6.5 billion.

Asthma

Asthma is a disease characterized by hyperresponsiveness of the airways to a variety of different stimuli, including infectious agents, allergens, drugs, industrial and occupational chemicals, air pollutants, and exercise. These stimuli can trigger paroxysmal attacks of severe airway narrowing associated with coughing, wheezing, and difficulty in breathing. The dimensions of the public health problem posed by asthma are large. It is estimated that the number of Americans affected will soon reach 10 million. The most common chronic disease of childhood, asthma affects approximately 3 million children under 15 years of age, or about 5 percent of all children in this age group; it accounts for approximately 3 percent of pediatric hospitalizations and 6.5 percent of pediatric outpatient visits.

The number of deaths from asthma is in the range of 2,000–3,000 annually. However, because asthma is a common chronic disease that has a low fatality rate, the direct costs of health care and the indirect costs of absenteeism from school and work are high. In 1979 asthma cost the nation an estimated total of almost $2.4 billion. The direct cost for physician visits (almost 6.8 million visits annually), hospital care, and drugs (bronchodilators, corticosteroids, and over-the-counter remedies) amounted to approximately $1.4 billion; indirect costs related to morbidity and mortality amounted to almost another $1 billion.

Asthma accounts for more than 100 million days of restricted activity, and asthmatic children lose more than 6 million school days annually. The asthmatic child is thus likely to fall behind in school and be handicapped in learning. Asthma disrupts family life; managing the asthmatic child can be a stressful and time-consuming process, particularly during acute attacks.

Occupational Lung Disease

Occupational lung disease is caused by the inhalation of toxic substances present in the work environment. It is a man-made problem and is thus, in principle, completely preventable. However, the association between lung disease and occupational exposure may not always be apparent or simple. Industrial processes change and evolve; new hazards may emerge even as known hazards are controlled. It is not clear in all cases whether there is a safe threshold for exposure; what is clear is that as exposure to a known hazardous substance increases, so does the risk of lung disease.

Only infrequently are responses to lung injury distinctive for a specific agent. Recognizing occupational respiratory illness may be hampered by the nonspecificity not only of symptoms and of lung function impairment but of radiographic and pathologic findings as well. Workplace exposures can cause disease or exacerbate existing disease, and work-related lung disease may be synergistically complicated by the effects that cigarette smoking has on the lung. There is often a long delay between exposure and the appearance of clinical symptoms. Moreover, the manifestations of occupational lung diseases are many. They range from reversible airway disease (asthma) to permanent airway damage (chronic bronchitis) to lung tissue damage (allergic alveolitis, pneumoconiosis) to cancer. Illness may be acute, subacute, or chronic. If exposure ceases in time, it may be possible to interrupt the progression of disease; later, cessation of exposure will not necessarily halt the disease.

We have virtually no data on the incidence of occupational lung diseases, but in 1977 the NIH estimated that each year approximately 400,000 workers manifest occupational diseases. An unknown number of these people have diseases that involve the respiratory system. The NIH further estimated that approximately 100,000 persons die from occupational diseases each year; about half of them have diseases of the lung, including lung cancer. According to the NIH, estimated losses of work output and costs of treatment for pneumoconioses (all cases are considered occupational in origin) in 1972 were $85 million ($6 million for loss of work output, $9 million for medical treatment, and $70 million for loss of productivity due to premature death).

This discussion will focus on four occupational lung disease problems, in two of which (byssinosis and coal worker's pneumoconiosis) substantial progress in control has been made and in two of which (silicosis and asbestos-related disease) a large gap between problem and progress remains. There are others, including "occupational asthma" and work-related hypersensitivity pneumonitis.

Byssinosis. Caused by the inhalation of cotton dust (or certain other organic dusts), byssinosis is generally characterized by acute respiratory symptoms, including chest tightness, cough, and shortness of breath, most noticeable on return to work after a period without dust exposure. Symptoms are more severe in smokers. Chest films show no changes, and no specific pathologic changes are detected in the lung. The term byssinosis is also used to describe a chronic, irreversible airway disease that may occur in workers who have had long-term exposure to cotton, flax, or hemp dust.

The National Institute for Occupational Safety and Health (NIOSH) has estimated that more than 500,000 U.S. workers are exposed to cotton dust. Epidemiologic and clinical studies have demonstrated a widely variable risk of byssinosis for these workers. Those in the cotton knitting industry appear to be at very low risk. In contrast, those in cotton yarn manufacturing are at much higher risk; among these, cardroom workers have a reported prevalence rate as high as 50 percent, compared with approximately 10 percent among spinning workers. Byssinosis is becoming a less common problem because major improvements in dust control have been made in much of the U.S. cotton textile industry.

Coal worker's pneumoconiosis (CWP). This type of pneumoconiosis is caused by the inhalation and deposition in the lung of carbonaceous dust. It is primarily a disorder of coal miners, although graphite workers and carbon black workers are also at risk. CWP is commonly divided into a simple, nondisabling form and a more advanced, complicated form (progressive massive fibrosis, or PMF). The disease usually takes ten or more years to develop to the point that it can be detected by radiography. PMF, which may develop and progress after exposure ends, can lead to substantial functional impairment and premature death. There is no effective therapy for CWP. Numerous studies showing a clear dose–response relationship between carbonaceous dust exposure and the development of CWP indicate that the disease can be prevented if dust exposure is sufficiently reduced.

The economic impact of CWP has been huge. Since 1969 almost $10 billion has been paid in federal "black lung" benefits (not entirely related to CWP, as smoking was a confounding factor in the lung disease of many of the miners who received benefits). This figure does not include the millions of dollars spent for direct medical care costs. Progress to date in CWP prevention is another example of what can be done to close a gap and the potential benefits of doing so. Data from the third round of the National Coal Study (1981–1982) showed radiologic changes compatible with CWP in 5 percent of miners, compared with 30 percent in the first study (1969–1970). These data suggest that CWP is declining, largely because of enforcement of dust standards in mines.

Silicosis. A form of nodular pulmonary fibrosis, silicosis is caused by inhalation and pulmonary deposition of free silica ("quartz dust"). Silica dust is commonly encountered in mining, quarrying, and tunnel drilling, especially when power tools and blasting are used. Some other industrial activities in which the risk of silica exposure is high are foundry work, grinding and polishing with sandstone abrasives, sandblasting, boiler scaling, manufacturing refractory brick, working with fillers that contain finely ground quartz (in paint, rubber, plastic, and paper manufacturing industries), vitreous enameling and enamel spraying, and stonemasonry. Abrasive blasting is especially hazardous because finely divided silica can be scattered through the air in poorly ventilated, restricted spaces.

Chronic silicosis takes 15–20 years or longer to develop; acute silicosis can occur within months.

The fibrotic lung damage caused by silica is presumed to be irreversible, and treatment can be only palliative. In a minority of silicosis cases PMF does develop; it is more common than in coal worker's pneumoconiosis. It can progress after exposure ends and may be associated with substantial cardiopulmonary impairment and premature death. There is an increased risk of tuberculosis and other mycobacterial diseases in persons who have silicosis.

The quantity of crystalline silica and the duration of exposure are the most important factors influencing the development of silicosis. In 1979 the NIOSH estimated that some degree of silicosis might develop in nearly 60,000 workers then being exposed in mines and foundries, abrasive blasting operations, and in stone, clay, and glass manufacturing. In addition, the NIOSH issued a special warning in 1981 concerning the silica flour industry after investigations revealed PMF in several workers who had been exposed for six years or less to silica flour dust.

Estimating the cost of care for a silicosis patient is difficult; the amounts reported vary from state to state. An estimate of the cost to the North Carolina worker's compensation system for 1981 was $20,000 for a case of uncomplicated silicosis. Given the estimate of 60,000 projected new cases and the North Carolina cost estimate, the cost of care could eventually reach $1.2 billion for the workers already exposed.

Asbestos-related disease. Lung disease that results from the inhalation of asbestos fibers presents a spectrum of clinical manifestations, including diffuse interstitial pulmonary fibrosis (asbestosis); cancer of the lung, pleura, and peritoneum; and cancer of other organ systems, particularly the gastrointestinal tract. "Asbestos" is a generic term used to describe a certain group of silicate minerals. Since the turn of the century millions of tons of asbestos have been used in the construction industry and in manufactured products. Between 1940 and 1979, 27.5 million Americans, of whom 21 million were still alive in 1980, had possibly been exposed at a level now known to be associated with a significant risk of asbestos-related disease.

Asbestosis was recognized in asbestos factory workers as early as 1906. It is associated with abnormalities of the pulmonary function and characterized radiographically by the presence of small, irregular opacities with a predilection for lower and midlung fields. Its prevalence in workers correlates directly with increasing dose and increasing time from first exposure. Although exposure differences have resulted in varying estimates of mortality, in one study involving 17,800 insulation workers, asbestosis was identified as the cause of death in 7 percent of those who died.

Bronchogenic carcinoma is the most common malignancy associated with exposure to asbestos, and malignant mesothelioma, a rapidly fatal tumor that is extremely rare in the general population, has accounted for up to 10 percent of deaths in several asbestos-exposed cohorts. The relation of lung cancer to asbestos dose has been shown to be linear. Smoking interacts synergistically with asbestos exposure as a risk factor in lung cancer. In a study of lung cancer death rates in asbestos workers and a reference population, nonsmoking asbestos workers demonstrated a fivefold and smoking asbestos workers a 50-fold increase in lung cancer death rates, compared with similarly aged, nonsmoking, nonexposed men. There are now approximately 8,200 asbestos-related cancer deaths every year. This number is expected to rise to approximately 9,700 by the year 2000 but should then start decreasing. It will remain substantial, however, for another three decades.

Because it is a useful substance with many applications, asbestos has become ubiquitous, and exposure to it is not limited to workers. Household contacts of workers as well as persons living in the neighborhood of industrial facilities may show radiographic abnormalities consistent with asbestos exposure. Presumably, family members inhale asbestos fibers carried home by the worker on the person or on clothing, and people in the neighborhood are exposed to ambient asbestos levels. The public may also be subject to asbestos exposure, as in the indoor environment of schools constructed with materials containing asbestos.

The complex natural history and pathogenesis of asbestos-associated disease pose formidable obstacles to effective surveillance and control. In view of the long latency periods associated with asbestosis (15 or more years) and asbestos-related cancer (two to four decades), disease observed today and during the next several decades must reflect past exposure. It will take decades to assess the efficacy of recent, current, and future interventions. The handling and disposition of the more than 1 million tons of asbestos currently in buildings, ships, and assorted products will determine the additional impact of present and future environmental exposure.

Tuberculosis

Tuberculosis was once a chronic, relapsing, incurable disease that necessitated years of isolation in the hospital and was responsible for enormous suffering, disability, and mortality. Now, with appropriate drug treatment, it is a curable and preventable disease. Nevertheless, tuberculosis has not been eliminated from the United States and is not likely to disappear in this century. Over 22,000 new cases of tuberculosis disease are reported each year, and an estimated 10 million Americans are infected with tuberculosis.

Tuberculosis is an infectious disease caused by the *Mycobacterium tuberculosis* bacillus. Once a disease striking mainly young adults, in this country it is becoming more and more a geriatric disease. However, the nearly 1,400 cases in children reported during 1982 indicate that tuberculosis continues to be transmitted. Tuberculosis is a systemic disease that can involve any part of the body, but the lung is by far the most common site. This is of particular public health significance because transmission is usually through the air: a symptomatic person with pulmonary tuberculosis coughs the bacteria into the air, and the organisms are inhaled by susceptible persons who share the environment. Not all infected persons develop the disease. Only approximately 10 percent of them have clinical manifestations, some shortly after becoming infected but others years or even decades later. In the rest, the infection heals spontaneously, with no further problems. In those who do develop tuberculosis, the disease process can, without treatment, remit spontaneously, become chronic, or lead to death. Chronic cases remain infectious and in the past were the main reason for the perpetuation of the disease.

Because modern drug treatment rapidly relieves symptoms and reduces infectivity, most persons with tuberculosis today can quickly resume the usual activities of daily life. High-risk infected persons can be treated prophylactically to prevent the later development of overt disease. Nevertheless, tuberculosis is still responsible for millions of days of restricted activity (3.7 million days in 1979), especially during the early period of clinical illness, diagnostic evaluation, and initiation of treatment. Diagnostic procedures may take weeks, and cure requires that uninterrupted drug treatment continue for nine months or longer. In 1979 the direct costs of medical care for tuberculosis were more than $142 million for hospitalization, more than $16 million for physician visits, and more than $6 million for pharmaceuticals. Achieving patient adherence to the treatment regimen for the prescribed duration is probably the greatest challenge in tuberculosis control.

Although no longer the major killer it once was, tuberculosis is still an important cause of death from communicable disease. For example, in 1979 it was the leading cause of death among 38 specific, reportable communicable diseases (not including the pneumonias). In 1982 a provisional total of almost 2,000 tuberculosis deaths (more than 1,600 pulmonary) was reported, and almost 5 percent of new cases each year are discovered and reported at the time of death. Tuberculosis mortality showed essentially no decline for the period 1979–1982. In 1983 more than 23,000 cases of tuberculosis were reported in the United States, the case rate being about 10 per 100,000 population. The morbidity trend has been downward for decades, though some fluctuation has occurred, such as the leveling off from 1979 to 1981, largely due to the influx of Indochinese refugees. The decline has been steady but slow, at an average pace of approximately 5–6 percent annually.

A group of diseases similar to tuberculosis in many respects is caused by related mycobacteria. These diseases are not communicable, their epidemiology is poorly understood, and they are often difficult to manage clinically. The magnitude of the nontuberculous mycobacterial disease problem is unknown.

Other Respiratory Diseases

Other respiratory diseases that are not now amenable to specific or primary intervention include cystic fibrosis and acute infectious bronchiolitis, both of which are predominantly pediatric problems, and a heterogeneous group of interstitial lung diseases, the most prominent of which is sarcoidosis. However, secondary interventions can reduce the morbidity and, in some instances, the mortality of these diseases.

Cystic fibrosis. Cystic fibrosis is an inherited, progressive, incurable disease of childhood. It is the most common fatal genetic disease of white children, occurring in approximately 1 per 2,000 live births; it also accounts for most cases of chronic progressive pulmonary disease in the first three decades of life. The prevalence is estimated to be more than 30,000 cases. The mechanism of the hereditary defect is unknown. Cystic fibrosis presents a wide spectrum of clinical manifestations, but it is uniformly fatal. Typically, large quantities of thick secretions are produced, obstructing airways, impairing pulmonary function, and predisposing to respiratory infections that damage lung tissue. Patients with mild or early disease can function well and lead productive lives for a time if properly treated.

Before 1960 the median survival rate was less than five years, but with good supportive therapy (e.g., physical therapy, postural drainage, treatment of infections), approximately 50 percent now survive to 18–20 years of age. Cystic fibrosis is associated with impaired growth and development, chronic disability, and limited endurance, and imposes a predictably heavy psychosocial burden on the patient and the family. As the disease progresses, frequent hospitalizations are usually necessary. The estimated annual costs amount to more than $6,000 per patient, a large part of which has to be provided from governmental sources such as Medicaid and state Crippled Children Services, because many private insurers will not cover cystic fibrosis.

Acute viral bronchiolitis. Acute viral bronchiolitis is the most common lower respiratory tract infectious disease of infants. Respiratory syncytial virus (RSV) is by far the most important cause of bronchiolitis; however, there are other viral etiologic agents. There is no specific treatment for viral bronchiolitis.

Annually, approximately 200,000 children below the age of 2 years (approximately 6.5 percent of all children in this age group) have bronchiolitis. Of these, fewer than 1 percent require intensive care in the hospital. The illness does not last long, and hospitalization, if required, is usually brief. However, 1.5 percent of those hospitalized die, most deaths occurring in children who have some underlying defect such as congenital heart disease.

Bronchiolitis may be associated with impaired lung function and is of particular importance in its potential contribution to obstructive airway disease (asthma, COPD) in adult life. Until an antiviral vaccine or treatment agent, particularly against RSV, is developed, aggressive clinical management through quality health services and education remains the only intervention.

Interstitial lung disease. More than 100 agents are known to cause interstitial disease, but in two thirds of all cases no cause can be identified. Palliative corticosteroid treatment is usually given for interstitial lung disease of unknown cause. Avoiding exposure to the causative agent is the obvious intervention when the cause is known. Most cases develop insidiously over months or years, but there are reports of cases that have developed within days or weeks. Early symptoms are fatigue and breathlessness on exertion. As it progresses, the disease interferes with pulmonary gas exchange, leading to poor oxygenation and decreased capacity for physical activity and work. Annually, there may be as many as 5 to 10 cases of interstitial lung disease per 100,000 population; these cases account for more than 10,000 hospital admissions.

INTERVENTIONS

The single most important thing that can be done to reduce morbidity and mortality from lung disease is to eliminate cigarette smoking. Both COPD and lung cancer are directly related to smoking; asthma and other chronic lung diseases are exacerbated by smoking; and smoking may interact synergistically with occupational exposures, particularly to asbestos, to greatly increase the risks for workers.

Physicians' attitudes and the advice they give patients about smoking can influence patient behavior, as can counteradvertising, the promotion of smoke-free workplaces, and such financial incentives as lower premiums for health, life, and fire insurance for nonsmokers. Behavior modification programs to help people stop smoking are important, but most effective of all is behavior modification that discourages smoking in the first place.

Since the majority of smokers start during adolescence, the antismoking effort must focus on children. Comprehensive health education should begin in kindergarten and continue through grade 12. Health curricula that emphasize physiology and broad principles of health maintenance have been developed even for young children; older children are taught about decision making and how to understand and resist peer pressure and advertising. Such school health programs, combined with efforts to eliminate cigarette advertising and to use local and national leaders as role models to "advertise" good health as a symbol of maturity and status, can decrease the number of adolescents who start smoking. The long-term payoff will be the prevention of morbidity and premature mortality in young people. Such an approach is undoubtedly more cost effective than postponing, through treatment, the deaths of chronically ill older persons.

Other interventions to ameliorate the chronic lung disease problem include reducing occupational exposures to hazardous substances; enforcing established clean air standards; providing information to the public and to health professionals on ways to prevent lung disease; educating patients and health care providers about clinical management and treatment of chronic lung diseases, including self-help skills; and ensuring access to health care, including home health care, for patients with chronic lung disease. These interventions can enhance the functional ability of most patients and help them to cope with chronic illness, but once the manifestations of disease are present, the course of the disease usually cannot be substantially altered. Major advances in the control of many of these diseases will depend on new insights into therapy and prevention, which can be acquired only through continued research.

Chronic Obstructive Pulmonary Disease

Because cigarette smoking is the major cause of COPD, long-term control of the disease depends upon the elimination of smoking. Although the mechanisms are not fully understood, there is really no controversy about the epidemiologic association between smoking and lung disease. Several surgeons general of the Public Health Service have issued reports to the public on the hazards of smoking. Smoking cessation benefits the individual smoker and can reduce the frequency of lung disease in the population. Because at least 80 percent of the cases of COPD can be attributed to smoking, elimination of smoking could theoretically reduce the mortality, morbidity, disability, direct costs, and indirect costs associated with COPD by up to 80 percent while improving the quality of life for both ex-smokers and those who never start to smoke.

Other ways to intervene include the elimination of pollutants from the workplace, the home, and the outdoor environment; the prevention and treatment of pulmonary infections, which in childhood may predispose to later COPD and which in patients with COPD may produce additional morbidity and mortality; education and support for all COPD patients to promote self-help at home, reduce morbidity, and decrease reliance on medical care facilities; and supportive and palliative medical care, such as bronchial drainage, physical therapy, and oxygen provision (preferably at home), for chronically disabled COPD patients.

Asthma

Little can be done to prevent the inception of asthma until its cause is understood. Intervention must therefore be directed toward preventing asthma attacks. Of greatest importance is removal or avoidance of asthma-provoking stimuli in both the home and the workplace. Cessation of smoking and avoidance of secondhand smoke may be of significant benefit. Hyposensitization may have a role if specific allergens can be established as the cause of asthma. Information on the causal association between asthma and aspirin, other drugs, and food additives should be made available to asthmatic patients and their physicians, and product labels should list all contents. Patients, parents, and health care providers need to know about self-help programs and to be familiar with the clinical management of asthma and the appropriate use of medications such as bronchodilators.

Because the etiologic factors and the individual responses to them vary so much, it is difficult to measure the effect interventions might have. It is likely that intense, organized application of known interventions can substantially reduce the frequency of acute asthmatic attacks, thus reducing the number of emergency room visits and hospitalizations and the rate of absenteeism, with all their social and economic consequences.

Occupational Diseases

Occupational lung disease is almost entirely preventable. Largely a legacy of the past, it need not be a bequest to the future. Responsibility for its prevention is shared by government and industry and, within industry, by workers and management. Management has a stake in actively contributing to the health of the worker, and labor has a stake in promoting its own health interests. The control of these work-related diseases provides an opportunity to put the principles of health maintenance and health promotion into practice. The success of this approach is demonstrated by the reduction in the incidence (and presumably eventual elimination) of byssinosis and coal worker's pneumoconiosis.

The most obvious strategy is to avoid exposure to hazardous substances. Exposures to substances such as cotton or coal dust in mills or mines are easily recognized and more readily controlled than exposures to ubiquitous substances such as asbestos and silica. Avoiding exposure can be accomplished many ways, including the installation of engineering controls, the use of personal protection devices, and the substitution of new substances or processes. Nonessential uses of asbestos and silica could be eliminated as, for instance, in Britain, where silica has been banned as an abrasive blasting material for more than 30 years, with salubrious results. One risk in substitution, however, is that a new substance or process may present problems of its own.

Because useful, albeit potentially hazardous, substances cannot and will not be entirely eliminated or avoided, standards must be set for their use and for controlling exposure to them. Government has the responsibility for setting and enforcing such standards, monitoring the workplace, and providing consultation on exposure control, especially for small industrial operations and for new or emerging technologies. Better definition of the problem of occupational lung disease requires the establishment of surveillance systems to provide information on mortality and morbidity that is presently unavailable. Because of the long latency period that often exists between exposure and disease, and the chronicity of some of the manifestations of disease, registries may be needed for tracking workers at risk, even as they change jobs, so that hazardous exposures and disease occurrence can be recognized and counted.

Education can be important at several levels. Managers need to be aware of the financial and human costs of occupational lung diseases. This information should be part of the curriculum for business and engineering students. Management has an obligation to employees and consumers to disclose potential hazards connected with the manufacture or use of its products. Employers should develop and distribute materials that alert workers to the occupational hazards to which they are exposed and the protective measures they can take. Such employee education should be part of new employee orientation in industries using hazardous substances and is particularly important for young people who are just entering the workplace. On the other hand, workers have a responsibility to use the information provided to protect their health, and it is within management's prerogative to use such measures as preemployment spirometry to assess the employee's risk at the time of employment.

Because smoking and occupational exposures interact to increase a person's risk of having COPD and cancer, programs focused on the alteration of personal habits must be an integral part of the prevention of work-related lung diseases. Education about the hazards of smoking and programs that discourage smoking are vitally important, especially for persons who may be exposed to asbestos. Having documented the synergistic effect between cigarette smoking and asbestos exposure in regard to lung cancer, we now know that persons exposed to asbestos should not smoke and smokers should not work with asbestos. Though controversial, one way of dealing with this problem is for management to refuse to hire smokers.

Continuing research in health and industry is needed to establish safer standards, develop better control methods, and identify substitute materials and processes. As an example, the ultimate strategy for preventing byssinosis would be to develop, through genetic manipulation or otherwise, cotton and other organic fibers with low "byssinogenic" activity.

Tuberculosis

With current interventions, tuberculosis can be controlled and reduced but not eliminated in the foreseeable future. A common misconception about tuberculosis is that it is a problem of the past, one that has been solved; this misconception has increased the difficulty of maintaining local resources for tuberculosis control so that existing diagnostic, therapeutic, and preventive tools can be used to maximum advantage. Another misconception is that although tuberculosis is a problem not yet solved, good enough tools for its solution are at hand; this misconception has inhibited crucial research to identify the control techniques that will be necessary if tuberculosis is to be eliminated.

The current level of control activity will reduce morbidity to 8 cases per 100,000 by 1990. A more rapid decline could be achieved with intensified application of existing methods, which can ensure cure, interrupt transmission, and avert future cases. Noncompliance with drug regimens is the major problem; failure to ensure compliance can lead to treatment failures and relapses, return of infectivity, and drug resistance. Expensive inpatient care, solely to ensure the taking of medication, has been a traditional approach to this problem. A less expensive alternative is to use community outreach workers to monitor the patients' taking of medication directly. This approach is now being used by many health departments.

To control tuberculosis we must provide adequate health department resources, which means financing and organizing health services for delivery not only to tuberculosis patients but also to their contacts and other high-risk persons in the population. It should be possible to save hundreds of millions of dollars in direct and indirect costs by intensified application of existing methods. However, the eventual elimination of tuberculosis will require new diagnostic, treatment, or prevention techniques, which can be developed only if research is funded.

Other Respiratory Diseases

Although these diseases are not currently amenable to specific or primary interventions and although research is needed to elucidate causes and develop more effective treatment and prevention strategies, it is important to recognize and provide appropriate care for persons who have these conditions. Health services must be available and accessible to the patient, health care providers must be knowledgeable in the management of these problems, and patients and their families must be taught self-help measures. Such secondary interventions can decrease morbidity and mortality.

SUMMARY

The high cost of respiratory disease in America is masked in two ways: first, respiratory problems are often secondary to other health problems; and second, the data we now collect cannot alert us to the longer-range trends for individual diseases nor to the interactive or accumulative effects of all lung disorders considered together.

One barrier to more precise data collection is the fact that respiratory diseases typically present a blurred picture to the diagnostician. Treating the symptoms pragmatically perhaps offers relief but leaves an enormous amount of disease imprecisely diagnosed and unreported. As a result, we know very little about the overall costs of lung disorders.

Respiratory diseases extract a high price from American society, in terms of both the direct costs of the health care they require and the indirect costs that result from the disruption of normal activities that they cause. Much of the respiratory disease problem is preventable, particularly that which is related to smoking and occupational exposure. Other aspects of the problem are amenable to amelioration; health care costs can be reduced and the quality of life improved.

This paper was prepared in consultation with the American Thoracic Society.

SELECTED READINGS

Entries preceded by an asterisk are of primary importance.

Acute Conditions—Disability, 1978. Hyattsville, Maryland: National Center for Health Statistics. (Vital and health statistics; series 10; no. 132).

Acute conditions: incidence and associated disability—US July 1977–June 1978. Hyattsville, Maryland: Centers for Disease Control. (Vital and health statistics; series 10; no. 132).

Advance report on final mortality statistics, 1980. Hyattsville, Maryland: National Center for Health Statistics, 1983. (Vital and Health Statistics; series 32; no. 4).

*Adult lung diseases and allied conditions: data reference manual, 1984 (unpublished data). New York: American Lung Association, Division of Medical Affairs, Epidemiology and Statistics Unit.

Anderson HA, Lisis R, Daum SM, Selikoff IJ. Asbestos among household contacts of asbestos factory workers. Ann NY Acad Sci 1979;330:387.

Asthma and the other allergic diseases. Bethesda, Maryland: National Institutes of Health, 1979; DHEW publication no. 79-387.

Centers for Disease Control. Table V. Estimated number of physician contacts. Morbid Mortal Weekly Rev 1984;33:75.

Centers for Disease Control. Premature mortality, U.S., 1982. Table V. Years of potential life lost, deaths, and death rates, by cause of death, and estimated number of physician contacts, by principal diagnosis, United States. Morbid Mortal Weekly Rev 1984;33:2.

Chretien J, Holland W, Macklem P, et al. Acute respiratory infections in children. N Engl J Med 1984;340:982–4.

Cropp GJA. The problems of lung disease in children and adolescents. Bull Am Lung Assoc 1976 Dec.

Crystal RG, Bitterman PB, Rennard SI, et al. Interstitial lung diseases of unknown cause. N Engl J Med 1984;310:154–66, 235–44.

Cystic fibrosis facts and figures, 1983. Rockville, Maryland: Cystic Fibrosis Foundation, 1983.

Days of restricted activity per 100 persons per year, 1979. (Data from National Health Interview Survey.)

Deaths and death rates for 72 selected causes, United States, 1981 and 1982. Hyattsville, Maryland: National Center for Health Statistics. (Vital and health statistics; series 31; no. 13).

Epidemiology of respiratory diseases—Task force report. Bethesda, Maryland: National Institutes of Health, 1980; DHEW publication no. 81-2019.

Health consequences of smoking—the changing cigarette. A Report of the Surgeon General. U.S. Public Health Service, 1981; Rockville, Maryland: DHHS publication no. (PHS)81-05156.

Health consequences of smoking for women, A Report of the Surgeon General. Rockville, Maryland: U.S. Public Health Service, 1980.

Higgins M. Epidemiology of COPD: state of the art. Chest 1984;85(suppl):3S–8S.

IMS America: National disease and therapeutic index (NDTI) monthly report 1982 Dec.

McConnochie KM, Roghmann KJ. Bronchiolitis as a possible cause of wheezing in childhood: new evidence. Am J Pediatr (in press).

National Institute of Occupational Safety and Health. Control of occupational lung diseases. 1983. (DHHS Draft 15—internal document for review and possible revision).

Number of office visits for bronchitis, acute, 1980. Hyattsville, Maryland: National Center for Health Statistics. (Vital and health statistics; series 13; no. 71).

Patients' reasons for visiting physicians, 1977–1978. Hyattsville, Maryland: National Center for Health Statistics. (Vital and health statistics; series 13; no. 76).

Pattern of ambulatory care in pediatrics, January 1980–December 1981. Hyattsville, Maryland: National Center for Health Statistics. (Vital and health statistics; series 13; no. 75).

Personal Health Care Expenditures According to the Condition, Sex and Age: United States, 1980. Rockville, Maryland: National Center for Health Statistics, 1983.

Physician visits, 1980. Hyattsville, Maryland: National Center for Health Statistics. (Vital and health statistics; series 10; no. 144).

Prevalence of selected chronic respiratory conditions, United States—1970. Hyattsville, Maryland: National Center for Health Statistics. (Vital and health statistics; series 10; no. 84).

Respiratory diseases—task force report on prevention, control, and education. Bethesda, Maryland: National Institutes of Health, 1977; DHEW publication no. (DLD) 77-1248.

*Ten-year review and five-year plan, National Heart, Lung, and Blood Institute, vol. 3. Bethesda, Maryland: National Institutes of Health, 1984; DHEW publication no. (DLD) 84-2358.

Socioeconomic Status and Health

George A. Kaplan, Ph.D., Mary N. Haan, Dr.P.H.,
S. Leonard Syme, Ph.D., Meredith Minkler, Ph.D.,
and Marilyn Winkleby, Ph.D.

As early as the twelfth century, it was recognized that people at the lowest socioeconomic levels in the community have higher death and illness rates. This pattern has been observed throughout the world, regardless of whether the major causes of death and disability were from infectious or noninfectious diseases and regardless of how socioeconomic position was measured.[1-16] Certainly the overwhelming majority of diseases addressed by *Closing the Gap* fit this pattern.

A study we conducted in Alameda County, California,[17] demonstrated a difference in survival over an 18-year period for people with various levels of family income.[18] As shown in Figure 1, improved survival was associated with higher socioeconomic position. Those who had higher incomes at the beginning of the study survived better. At the end of the 18-year period, the death rate for persons with inadequate income was twice that for those with adequate income. Data for the United States show similar results. For example, in one analysis of a sample of 340,000 deaths in 1960,[16] it was found that in every age group white men with incomes below $2,000 had mortality rates approximately 50 percent higher than all other men.

The prevalence of specific diseases among lower socioeconomic groups is also higher.[19] For example, in 1972 people with incomes less than $3,000 had three times the rate of heart disease as those with incomes greater than $15,000. The burden of diabetes was almost 3.5 times greater in the poorest group. Similarly, rates of anemia and arthritis were 2.5 times higher for the poor.

Table 1 lists other health problems that are more severe in the lower socioeconomic levels. The most obvious explanations are inadequate medical care,

low income, poor nutrition, unemployment, race, and hazardous living circumstances. However, these possible explanations are inadequate for two reasons. First, although it is true that higher rates of morbidity and mortality occur among those in the lowest socioeconomic group, high rates are not exclusive to that group. Instead, a gradation of rates is often seen, increasing from the highest socioeconomic level to the lowest. It is difficult to argue that those at level 2 or 3 have inadequate medical care or nutrition or that they live in hazardous circumstances, and yet those at levels 2 and 3 have higher rates of disease than those at levels 1 and 2, respectively. The issue posed by the observation of higher disease rates relative to socioeconomic position is not simply that of position based on the subject's amount of money or of poverty compared with near-poverty or affluence, but of other factors as well.

From the Human Population Laboratory, State of California Department of Health Services (Kaplan) and California Public Health Foundation (Haan), the Program in Epidemiology (Syme and Winkleby), and the Department of Social and Administrative Health Services, University of California, Berkeley (Minkler).

Address reprint requests to Dr. Kaplan, Human Population Laboratory, State of California, Department of Health Services, 2151 Berkeley Way, Berkeley, CA 94704.

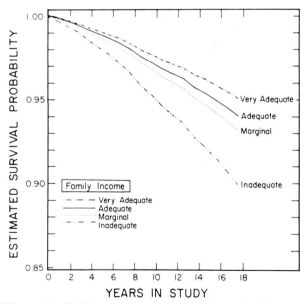

Figure 1. Eighteen-year survival of Alameda County, California, residents by family income.[17] Family income was adjusted for family size compared with federal standards.[18]

Table 1. Health problems that are more frequent at lower socioeconomic levels in the United States

Total mortality
Heart disease
Arthritis
Diabetes
Hypertension
Angina
Epilepsy
Rheumatic fever
Respiratory infections
Anemia
Lung cancer
Esophageal cancer
Sino-nasal cancer
Infant and child mortality
Neural tube defects
Tuberculosis
Unintentional injury
Low birth weight
Decreased survival from cancer
Decreased survival from heart attack
Restricted activity and bed days
Days in short-term hospitals
Number of hospital discharges

The second reason for doubting the most obvious explanations for the observed gradient is that so many organ systems are affected. Although one could understand how poor nutrition, inadequate medical care, or a hazardous environment might explain higher rates of one or even several diseases and conditions, the gradients by socioeconomic position involve virtually every disease of almost every organ system and also include such causes of death as accidents, suicide, and murder.

Furthermore, even within specific organ systems, the gradients of disease are not easily explained. In one study of cardiovascular disease among 18,000 British civil servants, it was possible to examine the contribution of serum cholesterol, smoking, and blood pressure to this gradient of cardiovascular disease.[20] Those in administrative classifications had the lowest death rates from coronary heart disease, followed by those in professional/executive positions, clerical, and other occupations. However, even when an adjustment for the major cardiovascular risk factors was made, the gradient of disease associated with socioeconomic position persisted. Other investigators of cardiovascular disease[6,21] have arrived at similar conclusions. Similarly, the differences in survival of breast cancer associated with socioeconomic position remain even when the stage of disease at diagnosis is taken into account.[22]

Because socioeconomic position and race are re-

lated, racial differences in risk factors or medical care are often proposed as explanations for gradients of disease associated with socioeconomic position.[23] However, socioeconomic gradients are found within racial and ethnic groups,[24,25] and, in some cases, socioeconomic position may actually account for what appear to be racial differences in health.[26]

A recent study[27] that we carried out in Oakland, California, further illustrates our difficulty in providing a simple explanation for the observed differentials in mortality from all causes among different socioeconomic groups. The mortality rates of people who resided in a federally designated poverty area of Oakland were compared with those who resided in other areas of Oakland. The poverty area was defined on the basis of census data on unemployment, income, and other markers of disadvantage. This area is a ten-mile-long strip on the western side of Oakland that is divided from the remainder of the city by an interstate highway and composed of residences alongside warehouses, manufacturing industries, and railways. During the years 1965–1974 the mortality rates in this population were considerably higher than for persons living in nonpoverty areas. Many factors that might have explained this difference in mortality were examined, but none could account for it. After adjustment for interarea differences in income, baseline health status, lack of medical care, unemployment, race, smoking, alcohol consumption, relative weight, physical activity, and several psychological factors, mortality rates in the poverty area were still 47 percent higher than in the nonpoverty area. Given these findings and others, it seems important to identify other risk factors that might account for a generalized vulnerability to many diseases among persons in lower socioeconomic positions.

The consistent evidence for socioeconomic position as a generic risk factor is overwhelming, and it is surprising that so little attention has been given to this factor in health promotion and disease prevention efforts. Perhaps one reason is the presumed impossibility of altering socioeconomic position. Socioeconomic position is often conceptualized as an amalgam of financial, educational, and occupational influences, but this does not necessarily help us understand why it exerts an influence on health. However, there is an underlying framework that can both help us understand socioeconomic position and develop interventions to reduce the associated health risks.

We believe that the important underlying characteristics of socioeconomic position relate to demands and resources. Specifically, those at low socioeconomic levels face greater environmental demands, both physical and social, and have fewer resources to deal with these demands. By resources, we include system resources such as money and access to medical care, interpersonal resources such as social support, and personal resources such as coping styles.

This conceptualization, which combines demands and resources, may help to explain why not all persons of low socioeconomic position become ill. For example, a person living in a high crime area on a fixed income may have better health if she or he has friends and neighbors on whom to rely for help than another person who lives in the same circumstances but has fewer social connections.

Furthermore, the balance between demands and resources changes as one moves up the socioeconomic ladder. Although demands may increase, resources increase even faster. Such a view of socioeconomic position is important because it suggests that changes in demands and resources may help to alleviate the burden of illness associated with lower socioeconomic status.

There are examples of interventions that help overcome socioeconomic risks. It has been shown in several studies that high physical and psychological demands and factors such as monotonous and repetitive work lead to higher rates of cardiovascular disease, especially in workers who have little control over the pace and timing of work or contact with coworkers.[28-30] Job design interventions such as those related to flextime or autonomous work units change the balance of demands and resources, and the evidence suggests a resultant lowering of rates of disease.[31-33] High demands and low resources in the work environment have also been shown to be associated with higher rates of risk behaviors such as smoking. Because of this, workplace smoking cessation programs are unlikely to be effective unless they also direct attention to reduction of demands and increase of resources.

Changes in the balance of demands and resources are also possible in maternal and child health. Educational interventions provide children with additional resources in the form of cognitive and social skills, which counteract some of their environmental demands. Interestingly, a recent 22-year follow-up study of Head Start enrollees reported significant gains in health for those enrolled compared with others not enrolled.[34] Prenatal programs have demonstrated lowered rates of low-birth-weight infants and perinatal mortality in association with increases in medical, behavioral, and social resources, which favorably affect the balance of demands and resources.[35,36]

Finally, in poor neighborhoods, intervention efforts that have focused on demands and resources appear to be associated with improved health among residents. A program now under way in the Tenderloin area of San Francisco[37] is aimed at increasing social ties among isolated, elderly, and poor residents of this area. Reductions in neighborhood crime and improved food access have already been accomplished, and there are some indications of improved health. Bringing residents of these areas together to work on common problems has allowed them to develop social resources that have reduced some of the environmental demands in these locations. These heightened social resources in combination with system resources such as Meals on Wheels, home health aides, and other services show real promise in improving the health of residents in these areas.

It is possible to estimate the impact on health of changes in socioeconomic position. For example, the nationwide indirect and direct costs associated with cardiovascular diseases were over $25 billion in 1977.[38] If the bottom 25 percent of the socioeconomic distribution had had the same disease rates as the median income category, there would have been a quarter of a million fewer cases of heart disease in 1972. This would have resulted in a savings of $3.3 billion annually. Of course, these figures do not include the costs of pain, suffering, and family disruption associated with cardiovascular disease.

Similar estimates for lung cancer lead us to equally striking conclusions. If white men and women with 1970 incomes less than $6,000 had had the same rates of lung cancer as those with incomes of $8,000–$13,000, there would have been approximately 12,000 fewer cases of lung cancer, a reduction of approximately 13 percent.[26] This decrease in the incidence of lung cancer would have resulted in a savings of $661 million in 1977 dollars.[39]

In 1980, those in the lowest 20 percent of the income distribution had more than twice the number of disability days per person than those at the median income level.[40] If this lowest group had had the same number of disability days as the average group, there would have been a net savings of over 194 million disability days. Looking only at savings for those who were working full time or keeping house, and using conventional cost-of-illness techniques, we translate this to an annual savings of $5.75 billion.[41]

In summary, we believe that socioeconomic position represents a true generic risk factor worthy of consideration in *Closing the Gap*. A substantial burden of illness is associated with lower socioeconomic position in the United States. Socioeconomic position also exerts an influence on the acquisition and maintenance of other generic risk factors. Interventions that focus on demands and resources can reduce the substantial toll of socioeconomic position on medical costs, lost productivity, and human suffering.

REFERENCES

1. Syme SL, Berkman LF. Social class, susceptibility and sickness. Am J Epidemiol 1976;104:1–8.

2. Antonovsky A. Social class, life expectancy, and overall mortality. Milbank Mem Fund Q 1967;45:31–73.

3. Black D, Morris JN, Smith C, Townsend P. Inequalities in health: the Black report. Middlesex, UK: Penguin, 1982.

4. Nayha S. Social group and mortality in Finland. Br J Prev Soc Med 1977;31:231–7.

5. Derrienic F, Ducimetière P, Kritsikis S. La mortalité cardiaque des Français actif d'âge moyen selon leur catégorie socio-professionelle et leur région de domicile. Rev Epidemiol Med Soc Sante Publique 1977;25:131.

6. Holme I, Helgeland A, Hermann I, et al. Four-year mortality by some socioeconomic indicators: the Oslo study. J Epidemiol Community Health 1980;34:48–52.

7. Hollingsworth JR. Inequality in levels of health in England and Wales, 1891–1971. J Health Soc Behav 1981;22:268–83.

8. Fisher S. Relationship of mortality to socioeconomic status and some other factors in Sydney in 1971. J Epidemiol Community Health 1978;32:41–6.

9. Pearce NE, Davis PB, Smith AH, Foster FH. Mortality and social class in New Zealand. II. Male mortality by major disease groupings. NZ Med J 1983;96:711–6.

10. Behm H. Socioeconomic determinants of mortality in Latin America. In: Proceedings of the Meeting on Socioeconomic Determinants and Consequences of Mortality. Geneva: WHO, 1980.

11. Caldwell JC. Education as a factor in mortality decline: an examination of Nigerian data. In: Proceedings of the Meeting on Socioeconomic Determinants and Consequences of Mortality. Geneva: WHO, 1980.

12. Tyroler HA, Knowles MG, Wing SB, et al. Ischemic heart disease risk factors and twenty-year mortality in middle-aged Evans County black males. Am Heart J 1984;108:738–46.

13. Frey RS. The socioeconomic distribution of mortality rates in Des Moines, Iowa. Public Health Rep 1982;97:545–9.

14. Simpson SP. Causal analysis of infant deaths in Hawaii. Am J Epidemiol 1984;119:1024–9.

15. Keil JE, Loadholt CB, Weinrich MC, Sandifer SH, Boyle E. Incidence of coronary heart disease in blacks in Charleston, South Carolina. Am Heart J 1984;108:779–86.

16. Kitagawa EM, Hauser PM. Differential mortality in the United States: a study in socioeconomic epidemiology. Cambridge, Massachusetts: Harvard University Press, 1973.

17. Berkman LF, Breslow L. Health and ways of living: the Alameda County study. New York: Oxford University Press, 1983.

18. Hochstim JR. Health and ways of living—the Alameda County, California, population laboratory. In: Kessler II, Levine ML, eds. The community as an epidemiologic laboratory. Baltimore: Johns Hopkins University Press, 1970:149–76.

19. US Department of Commerce: Social indicators III. Selected data on social conditions and trends in the United States. Washington, D.C.: US Government Printing Office, 1980.

20. Marmot MG, Rose G, Shipley M, Hamilton PJS. Employment grade and coronary heart disease in British civil servants. J Epidemiol Community Health 1978;32:244–9.

21. Salonen JT. Socioeconomic status and risk of cancer, cerebral stroke, and death due to coronary heart disease and any disease: a longitudinal study in eastern Finland. J Epidemiol Community Health 1982;36:294–7.

22. Dayal HH, Power RN, Chiu C. Race and socioeconomic status in survival from breast cancer. J Chron Dis 1982;35:675–83.

23. Health Indicators for Hispanic, black and white Americans. Hyattsville, Maryland: National Center for Health Statistics, 1984; DHHS publication no. (PHS) 84-1576. (Vital and Health Statistics; series 10, no. 148).

24. Health characteristics of minority groups, United States 1976. Washington, D.C.: US Government Printing Office, 1978; DHEW publication no. (PHS) 78-1250.

25. Differentials in health characteristics by color, United States—July 1965–June 1967. Hyattsville, Maryland: National Center for Health Statistics, 1969; DHEW publication no. 1000. (Vital and health statistics; series 10, no. 56).

26. DeVesa SA, Diamond EL. Socioeconomic and racial differences in lung cancer incidence. Am J Epidemiol 1983;118:818–31.

27. Haan M, Kaplan GA, Camacho T. Poverty and health: prospective evidence from the Alameda County Study. Am J Epidemiol 1987;125:989–98.

28. Karasek RA, Baker D, Marxer F, Ahlbom A, Theorell T. Job decision latitude, job demands and cardiovascular disease: a prospective study of Swedish men. Am J Public Health 1981;71:694–705.

29. Karasek R, Theorell T, Tores GT, et al. Job characteristics and coronary heart disease. Adv Cardiol 1981;29:62–7.

30. Alfredsson L, Karasek R, Theorell T. Myocardial infarction risk and psychosocial work environment—an analysis of the male Swedish working force. Soc Sci Med 1982;16:463–8.

31. Wright I, Wallin L. Psychosocial aspects of working environment among blue and white collar workers. Stockholm: Volvo, 1984.

32. Pierce JL, Newstrom JW. The design of flexible work schedules and employee responses: relationships and process. J Occup Behav 1983;4:247–62.

33. Wall TD, Clegg CW. A longitudinal field study of group work redesign. J Occup Behav 1981;2:31–49.

34. Weikart D. Perry Preschool Project. Ypsilanti, Michigan: High Scope Educational Research Foundation, 1984.

35. Minden S. A review of the literature regarding evaluation of programs for multi-disciplinary prenatal care. Sacramento, California: California Department of Health Services, Maternal and Child Health Branch, 1983.

36. Final Evaluation of the Obstetrical Access Pilot Project. Sacramento, California: California Department of Health Services, Maternal and Child Health Branch, 1984.

37. Minkler M, Frantz S, Wechsler R. Social support and social action organizing in a "grey ghetto": the Tenderloin experience. Int Q Comm Health Educ 1982–3;3:3–15.

38. Arteriosclerosis 1981: report of the Working Group on Arteriosclerosis of the National Heart, Lung, and Blood Institute. Bethesda, Maryland: National Institutes of Health, 1981.

39. Social and economic implications of cancer in the United States. Hyattsville, Maryland: National Center for Health Statistics, 1981; DHEW publication no. (PHS) 81-1404. (Vital and health statistics, series 3, no. 20).

40. Disability days: United States, 1980. Hyattsville, Maryland: National Center for Health Statistics, 1981; DHEW publication no. (PHS) 83-1571. (Vital and health statistics, series 10, no. 143).

41. Cost of illness and disease, fiscal year 1975. Washington, D.C.: Georgetown University, 1977.

Unintended Pregnancy and Infant Mortality/Morbidity

World Health Organization Collaborating Center in Perinatal Care and Health Service Research in Maternal and Child Care

In the United States, a large and unacceptable gap still exists between what is and what could be with respect to unintended pregnancy, infant mortality, and infant morbidity. The problem can be summarized in four simple phrases: each year we have (1) too many unintended pregnancies, (2) too many deaths of normal-birth-weight infants, (3) too many infants whose birth weights are low, (4) too many infants who have developmental disabilities.

This long-standing gap indicates that our society has yet to deal effectively with what should be one of our greatest concerns: our reproductive health and the raising of healthy children. Although the rates of unintended pregnancy, infant mortality, and infant morbidity are excessive in all segments of society, the highest rates are found among adolescent, black, and educationally disadvantaged people. This suggests that current knowledge, skill, and resources are not uniformly available, accessible, acceptable, or affordable to all citizens.

DEFINITIONS

Certain terms used in this paper have specific meanings. The following definitions will clarify these terms for the reader.

Birth-weight–specific mortality rate (BWSMR): the death rate among infants in a specific birth weight category. BWSMR depends on gestational age, race, and sex, and intrapartum, neonatal, and postneonatal care.

Educationally disadvantaged: having completed fewer than 13 years of education.

From the Collaborating Center composed of the Emory University Regional Perinatal Center, Woodruff Health Sciences Center; the Division of Public Health, Georgia Department of Human Resources; and the Centers for Disease Control, U.S. Department of Health and Human Services. Contributors: Brian J. McCarthy, M.D., M. J. Adams, Jr., M.D., Susan Zaro, M.P.H., Lynn S. Wilcox, M.D., Deborah C. Abels, M.B.A., Cathy L. Holt, B.S.N., James W. Buehler, M.D., Michael R. LaVoie, M.A., Alfred W. Brann, M.D., Godfrey P. Oakley, Jr., M.D., and James Alley, M.D.

Address reprint requests to Dr. McCarthy, Centers for Disease Control, 1600 Clifton Road, Bldg. 1, Rm. 4054, Atlanta, GA 30333.

Infant: birth through 12 months of age.

Low birth weight (LBW): weight at birth of less than 2,500 g (5 lb 8½ oz).

Neonatal period: birth through 27 days of age.

Poor woman: one whose family income is less than $10,000 per year.

Postneonatal period: 28 days to 1 year of age.

Unintended pregnancy: a pregnancy that was not planned.

Very low birth weight (VLBW): a weight at birth of less than 1,500 g (3.3 lb).

UNINTENDED PREGNANCY

The Problem

Of about 6 million reported pregnancies in the United States in 1980, 3.6 million (62 percent) were live births, 1.5 million (22 percent) were induced abortions, and 900,000 (16 percent) included early fetal losses, late fetal deaths, and ectopic pregnancies.[1,2]

Unintended pregnancy is an important reproductive public health problem. Fifty-five percent (3.3 million) of the 6 million pregnancies in 1980 were unintended, either unwanted or mistimed. Of these, 900,000 pregnancies occurred in women who did not want another pregnancy, and 2.4 million pregnancies occurred in women before they wanted to be pregnant. More than 376,000 infants, 1 in 10 of all live births, were born to women who did not want another child.[2]

In 1978 there were an estimated 4 million sexually active women who did not intend to become pregnant but who were using no or inadequate contraceptive methods. The Census Bureau projects that there will be one third more women of childbearing age at the end of the 1980s than there were at the beginning of the 1970s.[3] The increasing number of women of reproductive age, the widening interval between the onset of sexual activity and marriage, and the reliance on traditional, safe, but less effective contraception indicate that the magnitude of the problem will continue to increase.

Unintended pregnancy affects the mother, father, child, family, and community. When an unintended pregnancy occurs, the decisions to abort or maintain the pregnancy, to marry if the mother is single, or to keep the child or place it for adoption have far-reaching consequences. These decisions vary with the age, race, and social class of the mother. The likelihood that a teenager will choose abortion, for example, decreases as her age increases. More black women between 18 and 19 years of age seek abortion than do white women of these ages. White teenagers are more likely to marry than are black teenagers. But people who marry as teenagers are twice as likely to divorce as those who marry in their 20s.[4]

The social impact that giving birth has on teenage lives continues to plague our society. Out of every ten women, four become pregnant in their teens, 80 percent of them unintentionally.[5] Women bearing children during teenage years cut short their education and decrease their employment opportunities. In 1978 only 1.6 percent of women who bore children during high school had completed college by the age of 29, compared with 22.4 percent of women who had delayed childbearing past the age of 24.[4]

Thus, it appears that teenage women, a group at high risk for inadequate contraception and unintended pregnancy, tend to move into another group at high risk—low-income women—as the teenagers experience the consequences of unintended births. Teenage mothers are particularly likely to find themselves in the low-income group if there is no male partner in the household. In 1979, white families headed by women had only 40 percent of the median income of white husband–wife families. For blacks and Hispanics the percentages were even lower.[4]

Intuitively, we link unintended pregnancy and infant mortality. The sociodemographic characteristics of women most likely to give birth after an unintended pregnancy are similar to those of women with infants at high risk of dying. Many of these women smoke, drink alcohol, do not begin early prenatal care, and do not practice good nutrition. In addition, they may have fewer of the parenting skills needed to provide care essential to infant health.

The Cost

Estimating the cost of unintended pregnancy is difficult because data are sparse. Because 80 percent of teenage pregnancies are unintended (JG Dryfoos, Z Stein, unpublished observations, 1976), data concerning teenage mothers in the Aid to Families with Dependent Children (AFDC) program give some insights into the price paid for unintended pregnancies.

Women who bore their first child as teenagers are significantly overrepresented in the AFDC population. In 1975 approximately 56 percent of AFDC recipients were women whose first child was born while they were teenagers. In 1975, 265,144 teenagers were receiving benefits. An additional 870,600 AFDC recipients in their 20s had been teenagers when they first gave birth.[4] These women and their children accounted for $8.55 billion in annual public expenditures for food stamps, AFDC payments, and Medicaid benefits. The expenditure amounts to $18,000 for each birth to a teenager.

Public asistance expenditures, most of which may be avoidable, can be contrasted with the public cost of providing family planning services—approximately $63 per year per woman. Federal appropriations for family planning services now amount to approximately $285 million per year[4]—0.3 percent of the cost of public expenditures.

High-Risk Groups

Although unintended pregnancies are costly at all social levels, the burden weighs most heavily on three groups least able to bear the cost: black women, women in lower socioeconomic groups, and teenage women.

Black women are 2.5 times more likely to have an unintended pregnancy than are white women. Among black women, one pregnancy in four is unintended, compared with one in ten among white women.[2]

Poor women are twice as likely to have an unintended pregnancy than are other women. People with low incomes also use contraception less effectively, showing higher rates of unintended pregnancy whether using condoms, the rhythm method, the pill, an IUD, spermicides, or a diaphragm.[2]

Teenage women are at least twice as likely to have an unintended pregnancy as are older women, and they are 3.5 times more likely to use no contraception when sexually active and not intending to become pregnant.[2]

INFANT MORTALITY

The Problem

For 1980 the National Center for Health Statistics (NCHS) reported that 45,526 infants died in the first year of life, 67 percent (30,701) in the neonatal period, and 33 percent (14,813) in the postneonatal period.[1] Although the NCHS provides causes of infant deaths, birth weight and maternal data related to infant deaths have not been reported since 1960.

Birth weight and maternal data are crucial to understanding the infant mortality problem. The low-birth-weight rate (LBWR) is assumed to reflect primarily socioeconomic and maternal or fetal biological factors. Because the birth-weight-specific mortality rate (BWSMR) is associated with gestational age, race, sex, and intrapartum, neonatal, and postneonatal care,[6] it can be used to indicate the quality of medical care received by the mother and baby during these periods. Maternal characteristics, such as age, race, and level of education, can be used to describe high-risk populations of women and infants.

To obtain birth weight and maternal data on infant deaths, we aggregated data from nine states that have linked birth and death certificates. These states are California, Georgia, Massachusetts, Michigan, Missouri, New York, North Carolina, South Carolina, and Tennessee. We obtained infant mortality rates by birth weight and maternal characteristics from this aggregated data base and applied these rates to 1980 natality data for the entire United States from NCHS. Using these calculations, we estimated that there were 40,553 infant deaths in the United States in 1980—67 percent in the neonatal period and 33 percent in the postneonatal period. Seventy percent (28,467) occurred in white infants and 30 percent (12,086) in black infants. Of the infants who died, 45 percent weighed less than 1,500 g, 17 percent weighed 1,500–2,499 g, and 38 percent weighed more than 2,500 g. The causes of death were respiratory complications and immaturity, 27 percent; congenital anomalies, 21 percent; other perinatal conditions, 18 percent; sudden infant death syndrome (SIDS), 13 percent; birth trauma, 6 percent; infection, 5 percent; injuries, 3 percent; and all other causes, 7 percent.

Analysis of age at death, birth weight, and cause of death indicates that the main problems of infant mortality can be grouped into four categories:

1. Conditions (excluding congenital anomalies) occurring in low-birth-weight babies. These conditions resulted in 17,843 infant deaths.

2. Postneonatal disease other than congenital anomalies. These conditions accounted for almost 11,000 infant deaths.

3. Congenital anomalies, which accounted for over 8,000 deaths.

4. Perinatal complications of normal-birth-weight infants. These resulted in about 3,700 deaths.

Very low birth weight has long been regarded as a major contributor to infant mortality, and data from the aggregated data base support this conclusion. For example, 45 percent of the total estimated deaths were VLBW infants, even though these babies represented only 1.2 percent of all births. Unfortunately, current knowledge of how to reduce mortality in this group is approaching its limit. Further research is needed to identify specific causes of VLBW and design effective interventions to prevent these causes from leading to VLBW.

Our recommendations, which focus on implementing known interventions, are influenced by the fact that 38 percent of infant deaths occurred in normal-birth-weight babies. These are newborns who, because of their satisfactory size, need not be at increased risk and should survive the first year of life.

The Cost

The Office of Technology Assessment of the U.S. Congress estimated that 6 percent of all births in 1978 required neonatal intensive care at a cost of $1.5 billion (0.8 percent of the $189 billion in national health expenditures).[7] Most of this care is provided to VLBW infants. In general, the lower the birth weight, the higher the cost. Estimates vary, but the average cost per stay for VLBW infants is $15,000.[8] Hospital charges for a single infant's intensive care have been as high as $500,000. Survivors generally cost more than nonsurvivors because of longer hospitalizations and long-term morbidities. We have not attempted to estimate the indirect costs associated with infant death; a major cost would be the productivity loss of the child, but the productivity losses of the parents would also be important. Interventions that would prolong pregnancy for premature infants would save millions of dollars just in neonatal intensive care costs.

High-Risk Groups: Defining the Gap

Birth weight is a key factor in determining the gap between what is and what could be in infant mortality. Although total infant mortality in the United States has been declining since 1900, the difference between the LBW rates of blacks and whites has been increasing. But birth weight is not the only factor to be considered. The unacceptably high rate of infant mortality in this country is also the result of an excess of deaths among infants of normal birth weight.

A marked gap exists between what we know to be the best conditions for childbearing and what is actually happening in the United States. Only 29 percent of all births are to the lowest-risk women—those women 20 years of age or older with 13 or more years of education. We label this group "the best standard population." Whites are more likely than blacks to be in this category.

The infant mortality rate is 7.5 deaths per 1,000 live births among infants born to white women in the best standard population. This infant mortality contrasts with rates of 10.8 and 23.8 per 1,000 found on average among white and black infants, respectively. The gap between the best standard and actual white and black rates exists because of differences in low-birth-weight distributions and differences in birth-weight-specific mortality rates.

There are important differences between the best standard and acutal white and black populations with regard to the proportions of infants born with low birth weights (Figure 1). Infants of black women are almost three to four times as likely to be of low birth weight than are those of women in the best standard population. In addition, teenage and educationally disadvantaged women, white and black, are more likely to have LBW infants than are women in the best standard population (Figure 2). Such differences clearly point to the socioeconomic

divisions that exist in health care in our society.

The differences in birth-weight-specific infant mortality are much greater among infants with birth weights of 2,500 g and above than among low-birth-weight infants (Figure 3). The differences in the 2,500 g and above birth-weight group are important because the vast majority of all infants are in this group.

The differences in infant mortality among infants weighing 2,500 g and above at birth show different patterns in the neonatal and postneonatal periods (Figure 4). In the neonatal period normal-birth-weight black infants have nearly twice the mortality of the best standard rate, although there is no difference among the three sociodemographic groups for black infants. For white infants, there is also no difference among the three sociodemographic groups.

The most obvious sociodemographic differences appear in the postneonatal mortality rates for white and black infants (Figure 4). Infants with birth weights of 2,500 g or more should have an equal chance of surviving the first year of life, regardless of the prenatal care of the mother and the antenatal environment. But infants born to mothers in different socioeconomic groups do not in fact survive

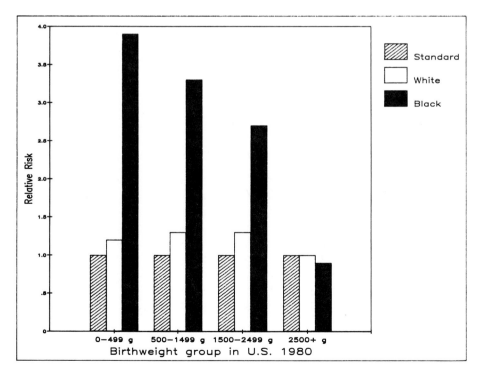

Figure 1. The relative risk of different birth weights by race, United States, 1980. Comparison of standard with race-specific data from NCHS natality data (computer tape). Relative risk: the ratio of the risk in one group to the risk in another. In Figures 1, 2, and 3, if the relative risk is 1, the risk is equal to that of the standard. If the relative risk is 2, the risk is twice that of the standard. The standard group consists of infants of white women 20 years of age or older who have 13 or more years of education and who sought prenatal care in the first trimester. The BWSMR of the group weighing at least 2,500 g at birth is further reduced by excluding deaths reportedly due to causes thought preventable (i.e., obstetrical, hypoxia, infection, and injury) and by using rates in white infants for black infants.

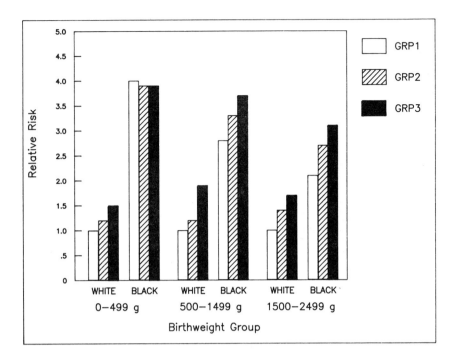

Figure 2. The relative risk of infant birth weight group by sociodemographic status and race of mother, United States, 1980. Comparison is with white group 1. Group 1: infants of women 20 years of age or older who have 13 or more years of education. Group 2: infants of women 20 years of age or older who have 12 or fewer years of education. Group 3: infants of women 19 years of age or younger.

at the same rate. The incidence of congenital anomalies does not explain the differences.

Furthermore, there is a striking difference between the survival of black and white infants, regardless of socioeconomic position (Figure 4). Although the greatest difference occurs in teenage mothers, black infants born to educationally advantaged mothers over age 19 also have a higher mor-

tality rate than white infants of mothers within the same education and age category.

Infants of white adolescent mothers are almost four times as likely to die in the first year of life as infants of a best white standard population (Figure 4). The risk increases to fivefold for infants of black teenage mothers. Also apparent are gaps between the rates of postneonatal mortality for the best stan-

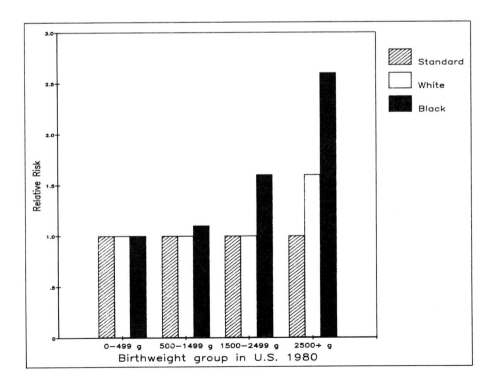

Figure 3. The relative risk of infant death by race and birth weight, United States, 1980. Comparison of BWSMR in standard populations with BWSMR in aggregated data.

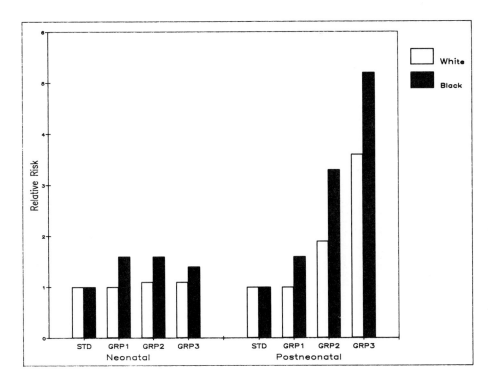

Figure 4. The relative risk of neonatal and postneonatal death for normal-birth-weight infants by sociodemographic status and race, United States, 1980. Neonatal period: birth–27 days; postneonatal period: 28 days–1 year of age. The standard (STD) is white group 1 infants. See Figure 2 for definitions of each group (GRP).

dard population and for black and white infants born to nonadolescent women who have 12 or fewer years of education: the black infants of normal birth weight born to less educated women are three times as likely to die within a month after birth, and the white infants are twice as likely to die in that time as the infants of a best standard population. The variation in mortality among groups is largely the result of different rates of infection, injury, and SIDS. This would strongly suggest that access to care and the existence of a social support system may be critical issues influencing postneonatal mortality.

Infants in all six sociodemographic groups could experience even greater reductions in mortality if preventable causes of death were eliminated from the standard population of infants born to white group I women (Figure 5). Deaths due to obstetrical trauma, hypoxia, infection, and injuries were eliminated from group I infants and the resulting rate used as the standard to demonstrate the potential reduction that could take place in all groups. Using this standard, all white infants could experience almost a threefold reduction in neonatal mortality. Postneonatal reductions in white infants would vary by sociodemographic group: white group I could experience a twofold reduction, while infants born to adolescent mothers could experience a sixfold reduction.

Blacks would experience even greater reductions. As seen in white infants, the nearly fourfold reductions would be the same across all sociodemo-graphic groups. However, the reductions in black postneonatal mortality would be greater than those for whites for all sociodemographic groups: black group I infants could experience a threefold reduction, while the reduction in infants born to adolescent mothers could be almost ninefold.

INFANT MORBIDITY

The Problem

Infant morbidity has decreased significantly in the United States since 1900. The introduction of antibiotics and the widespread use of vaccines against childhood diseases have reduced not only the mortality associated with infectious disease but also the morbidity. Today, most long-term morbidity originating in infancy involves congenital anomalies and developmental disabilities.

One fourth of congenital anomalies are known to be caused by genetic factors and one tenth by environmental factors; the causes of the remaining two thirds are unknown.[9] The reported incidence of congenital anomalies varies widely because of differences in definitions, methods of detection, demographics of the populations observed, and length of observation. According to one five-year survey, the incidence of severe congenital anomalies in the United States was 4 percent, and the incidence of total congenital anomalies (severe plus moderate) was 15 percent. Anomalies detected between birth and 5 years of age increased almost

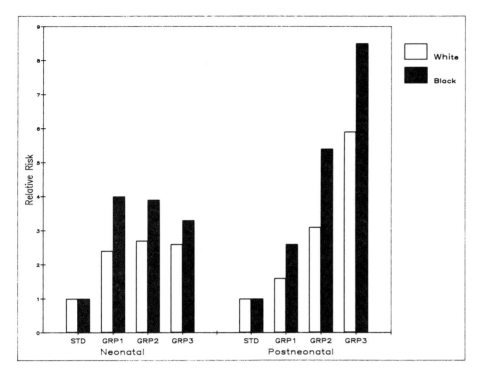

Figure 5. The relative risk of neonatal and postneonatal death for normal-birth-weight infants, by sociodemographic status and race, United States, 1980. Neonatal period: birth–27 days; postneonatal period: 28 days–1 year of age. The standard (STD) is group 1 infants with preventable causes of death excluded. See Figure 2 for definitions of each group (GRP).

fivefold. For children 5 years of age, the incidence of severe anomalies was 4.2 percent in whites and 3.9 percent in blacks.[10]

Down's syndrome occurs once in every 1,000 live births and accounts for 15–30 percent of severe mental retardation in children under 10 years of age.[9] The average survival of persons who have Down's syndrome is estimated to be 30 years[11]; thus, the 3,600 children born with Down's syndrome in 1980 will ultimately experience more than 100,000 years of disability.

Spina bifida is one of the most common serious congenital anomalies. Neurosurgical repair is necessary at birth, and despite the best treatment, affected individuals usually have loss of bowel and bladder function and leg weakness requiring braces or a wheelchair. Although the incidence of spina bifida has been declining in recent decades, improved medical and surgical care has increased survival so that the total number of persons with the disease has dramatically increased. We estimate that 4,000 infants were born with spina bifida in 1960 and 2,000, or only half as many, in 1980. In contrast, there were about 20,000 persons with spina bifida living in 1960 and 80,000 in 1980—a fourfold increase.

Most developmental disabilities, such as mental retardation, cerebral palsy, and other intractable physical and neurological impairments that require special long-term medical and educational services, originate during the prenatal or perinatal period. A small but predictable portion of mental retardation,

cerebral palsy, blindness, and deafness occurs in individuals as a complication of very low birth weight.

We estimate that 900,000 Americans now have developmental disabilities necessitating special medical or educational services and that on the average a person who has such a disability survives at least 35 years. We estimate that 15,000 newborns join this group each year.

The Cost

The costs of morbidity associated with low birth weight are less well defined than those of mortality. Low and very low birth weight are in themselves important causes of morbidity, and in the short term they account not only for longer hospital stays at birth, but also for increased frequency of hospitalization and physician visits throughout infancy.

Throughout life, the average annual medical care costs for VLBW and LBW infants are higher than the costs for normal-birth-weight babies.[12]

Of morbidities that originate in infancy, the most costly are those that necessitate long-term care: mental retardation, cerebral palsy, and congenital anomalies. An estimated $6.5–$9 billion is spent annually on the care and treatment of mentally retarded people. The annual cost for a person with a significant developmental disability ranges from $2,300 for home care to $16,300 for institutionalization.[13]

Medical care for congenital anomalies is among

the most expensive of all diseases. The National Center for Health Statistics estimated that $1.4 billion was spent for the care of congenital anomalies in 1980, 0.14 percent of all personal health care expenditures.[14] Zook and colleagues[15,16] reported that the majority of patients with congenital anomalies required repeated hospitalization, and because of this, they represented a major component of "high-cost users" of medical care—with 15 percent of patients consuming as many resources as all other patients combined.

Lifetime care for a child with spina bifida, including medical, institutional, foster care, and social, psychological, and educational services, can cost $170,000–$300,000 contrasted with $72,000 of comparable expenses for a normal child (J Lipscomb, I Kolimaga, PW Spenduto, et al., unpublished observations, 1982).

High-Risk Groups

It is difficult to define the gap between what is and what could be for morbidities originating in infancy. The problem is that far fewer data are available about morbidity than about mortality; the mortality data are also easier to quantify. Because the rate of congenital anomalies does not vary greatly between white and black infants, we believe that the gap between the mortality seen in infants born to teenage, black, or poor women and the mortality in infants born to other, less disadvantaged mothers predicts a similar gap in rates of morbidity. The gap is probably due to an excess of infection, injury, and cerebral palsy among the disadvantaged infants.

The causes of many developmental disabilities remain unknown. Although we know too little to prevent long-term morbidity, we can affect the rate of disabilities when they arise from known causes. Effective diagnostic or preventive technologies exist for certain metabolic defects (screening of newborns for phenylketonuria [PKU] and hypothyroidism), for Tay-Sachs disease (identification of carriers), for congenital rubella syndrome (immunization of mothers), for Rh disease (administration of Rh immunoglobulin), and for Down's syndrome and spina bifida (use of prenatal diagnosis).

Because many of the conditions for which there are preventive interventions (congenital rubella, PKU) are now rare in this country, we have focused on conditions that are more common but that can be prevented or detected by using current technology. These are Down's syndrome, spina bifida, and mental retardation/cerebral palsy associated with VLBW in infants.

INTERVENTIONS

Unintended Pregnancy

Education and access to appropriate health care are the two interventions that show the greatest promise for reducing the number of unintended pregnancies. To be effective, education must begin early and must stress the importance of reproductive concerns in a person's social and vocational plans. Schools, the media, and other institutions with adolescent constituencies can play vital roles in demonstrating to teenagers that their reproductive futures are in their own hands.

General information concerning the safety and efficacy of various birth control measures should be readily available to sexually active persons and those considering becoming sexually active. Such information should point out the risk of pregnancy associated with unprotected intercourse. More importantly, it should be pointed out that the health risks associated with each contraceptive method, though an important concern, are less than the risks of pregnancy.

Although we have no data on the intendedness of the pregnancy from the man's perspective, male participation in reproductive health programs is being increasingly emphasized. The fathers of children born to teenage mothers are being encouraged to become more aware of family planning practices so as to prevent future unintended pregnancies.

We can reduce the excessive number of unintended pregnancies by using known interventions. The effective contraceptive methods (pill, IUD, foam, and condom) have a combined failure rate of 6.8 per 100 women. In 1980, if all sexually active couples had routinely used one of these methods, the number of unintended pregnancies would have decreased from more than 2.4 million (JG Dryfoos, Z Stein, unpublished observations, 1976) to less than 900,000. With an expected abortion rate for contraceptive failure estimated at 62 percent, there would have been almost 1 million fewer abortions (533,000 instead of 1.5 million).

The same intervention would prevent 340,000 unintended live births. We conservatively estimate that because of the higher-risk status of this group, 5,000 infant deaths could be prevented, reducing the infant mortality rate by more than 10 percent.

In summary, more than 65 percent of all unintended pregnancies might be avoided if couples effectively controlled fertility. This could result in more than a 75 percent reduction in the total number of unintended births, including more than 100,000 unwanted births that could be prevented by increased access to sterilization. Overall, such a change would result in an increase of almost 20 percent in the proportion of wanted infants born each year. Listed below are strategies for effective methods of family planning.

Develop cooperative, broad-based educational efforts. Professional associations could disseminate to physicians and other health-care givers appropriate information on the relative risks of unintended pregnancy and effective contraception.

The mass media could make family planning information readily available. Local television broadcasting companies could receive tax incentives for developing programming in cooperation with the community's family life program and for reducing advertising that has sexual overtones. The media could give a more balanced view of the consequences of the liberated lifestyle portrayed so enticingly in many advertisements by giving more time and space to responsible pregnancy prevention.

State health departments could identify and define specific pregnancy-related programs in the state and make information about the magnitude of unintended and teenage pregnancy available to educators throughout the states.

Early work experiences that enable teenagers to feel that they play an important role in society can build self-esteem and encourage more mature decision making. State education departments should consider developing programs to increase self-responsibility and self-esteem among teenagers and to foster the peer and cross-generational communication skills that encourage mature life planning. Students would not be required to participate in these classes, and parents who elected to teach their children at home would be supplied with educational materials. But all students would be required to demonstrate their mastery of family life information by passing an examination before entering the seventh grade. School programs could be linked to accessible family planning programs, such as contraceptive services in health department clinics and at schools where the rate of unintended pregnancy is high.

Young people can be encouraged to plan their reproductive "careers" just as they plan their educational and vocational careers. Such plans include delaying the onset of sexual activity, making appropriate use of effective contraception, timing childbearing (including the interval between intended births), and timing the cessation of childbearing. School programs need to address not only the physiology of reproduction but also the individual's responsibility to himself or herself and the development of interpersonal relationships with parents and peers. Federally or locally sponsored job programs might be made available to family life pro-

gram participants who are 10–18 years of age.

Provide widely and readily available reproductive health services for women and men of all ages and from all segments of society. For some people, obtaining family planning services is difficult. The most common barriers are cost, inconvenience, and fear of the loss of privacy. All men and women need access to affordable family planning, including voluntary sterilization. Family planning services should be available in convenient locations and at hours that accommodate the schedules of teenagers, working women, and women who stay home with their small children. The confidentiality of treatment must be emphasized in all materials advertising the services of family planning clinics. States could provide funds for comprehensive health and social services for parents under 18 years of age in communities that have submitted acceptable plans for such programs.

Information on nonprescription methods of birth control, such as condoms, spermicidal foams, suppositories, and sponges, should be presented to everyone attending family planning clinics. This information could also reach the general public by television and radio advertisements and public service announcements, freely accessible printed information in pharmacies, libraries, physicians' and clinic offices, and toll-free telephone hotline services. For teenagers in particular, these educational resources can be linked under present law to easily accessible and confidential contraceptive services. Pharmacies should display nonprescription contraceptives in such a way that embarrassment about requesting them will not be a barrier to their use.

Publicly funded sterilization services could be made available to all women through fees set on a sliding scale, with women below the poverty level receiving these services free.

Develop improved methods to reduce the number of unintended pregnancies. Research on safe, inexpensive, effective, and easy-to-use methods of contraception for women and men will help develop more appropriate family planning services and education programs. Areas of research interest include (1) the development of better knowledge of the motivation and behavior conducive to appropriate family planning practices, and (2) the continued support of implementing and evaluating surveys that measure the planning of pregnancies and the incidence of unintended pregnancy.

Infant Mortality

Interventions that could reduce infant mortality are available but not universally used. We divide our recommendations into three categories: (1) interventions to reduce the number of LBW infants, (2) interventions to reduce the neonatal mortality rate, and (3) interventions to reduce the postneonatal mortality rate.

Reducing the LBWR. Interventions to reduce the excessive number of LBW infants are associated with the reduction of four risk factors: early and closely spaced childbearing, smoking throughout pregnancy, late or no prenatal care, and poor maternal nutrition.[17,18]

The maximum reduction of low birth weight could be brought about by a concerted program to persuade pregnant women to stop smoking, to seek and have available quality prenatal care beginning in the first trimester, and to practice good nutrition. We could thereby reduce the annual number of LBW infants by as much as 51,000, which could result in 4,200 (10 percent) fewer infant deaths if current mortality rates remained the same. An additional reduction of 7,400 cases of low birth weight (which would amount to 600 deaths) could be effected if the number of women below age 20 who become pregnant could be reduced 50 percent. This reduction could be most appropriately achieved by family planning services that enable women to delay the onset of childbearing and to optimally space the children they do have.

Experience suggests that the LBWR for groups II and III may be reduced 50 percent by decreasing the pregnancy rate in high-risk age groups and by encouraging all pregnant women to stop smoking, obtain prenatal care early in pregnancy, and practice good nutrition. Known interventions will affect primarily the infants who weigh 2,000–2,499 g at birth. At present, we do not know how to increase the birth weight of 80 percent of the LBW infants born each year; in short, we are now able to reduce this social problem by only 20 percent.

Interventions to detect and treat women who are in labor, or who may be at increased risk of going into labor, with a preterm fetus are being evaluated and show preliminary indications of success. However, because the efficacy of these interventions has not yet been proved, we did not use them in our estimates.

Reducing the neonatal mortality rate. We know that good intrapartum (during and just after delivery) care of mothers and early neonatal care of infants can reduce infant mortality, regardless of birth weight.[19-23] High-risk mothers, especially those with preterm fetuses, can be referred to regional centers that would provide them with quality perinatal care, including consultative and laboratory services, during the prenatal period and with specialized primary care during the intrapartum period. Such centers can also provide professional education and training programs that would improve delivery services both for normal-weight and for LBW infants. Specially trained professionals would be able to identify high-risk mothers for transfer and recognize, stabilize, and recommend transfer of sick newborns, including VLBW infants who require intensive care.

If the birth-weight- and race-specific neonatal mortality rates for all infants weighing more than 2,500 g at birth were the same as for the best standard group, the number of infants who die each year would drop by more than 4,200 (10 percent). The key to improving the neonatal mortality rate is to provide equal access to quality care for infants in all sociodemographic groups in our society.

Reducing the postneonatal mortality rate. Health professionals know as much about preventing postneonatal death as about preventing death in newborns, but their skills do not always reach the people who could benefit the most from their care. We believe that the mortality rate in the postneonatal period could be lowered if all mothers had equal access to pediatric care and possessed more parenting skills. Such changes would have the greatest impact on postneonatal infection and injury, but the burden of postneonatal illness associated with congenital anomalies and SIDS might also diminish.

If all infants had the parental care and access to health care that the infants of white educationally advantaged mothers now receive, we estimate that 7,700 fewer postneonatal deaths would occur annually. That decrease represents 60 percent of all postneonatal mortality and 20 percent of all infant mortality. Virtually all that improvement would be in older infants who had weighed 2,500 g or more at birth. In other words, the gap suggests what many have said intuitively or on the basis of individual clinical experience: good child rearing and good pediatric care are critically important even for infants who are robust at birth. Although such a reduction might be within our reach, its achievement would depend on the reduction of SIDS, which—like LBW in the neonatal period—is the chief health care problem of the postneonatal period.

Thus experience suggests that implementing the following strategies could substantially lower the overall infant mortality rate.

Reduce the low-birth-weight rate to 5 percent by the year 2000. Provide prenatal evaluation and counseling for all pregnant women during the first trimester of pregnancy. Such improved services would include (1) prenatal care followed by access to other services, as deemed appropriate for the level of risk; (2) removal of fiscal, categorical, and administrative barriers to such prenatal evaluations; and (3) counseling that includes information on the risks of smoking, of consuming alcohol and other drugs, and of exposure to environmental hazards.

Reduce the neonatal mortality of normal-birth-weight infants by 60 percent (to 0.7 per 1,000) by the year 2000. Remove barriers to quality intrapartum care, making certain that the care provided is consistent with the risk status of the mother and fetus. Efforts need to be directed particularly at those groups at greatest risk: teenage mothers, the socioeconomically disadvantaged, and black mothers regardless of age or status.

The education of professionals needs improvement in identifying, resuscitating, and stabilizing the sick neonate at delivery prior to obtaining the specialized care needed.

Reduce the postneonatal mortality rate of normal-birth-weight infants by 60 percent (to 1 per 1,000) by the year 2000. Remove barriers to preventive and curative services in the first year of life. Such barriers include race, age, residential status, and ability to pay for services.

Federal, state, and local programs should be extended to provide outpatient services to areas that now lack adequate resources.

Programs should be developed to improve parenting skills, particularly of teenage mothers, and include instruction in normal child development, injury prevention, and recognition of acute illness.

Implementation of these strategies requires support from leaders—governmental and nongovernmental—at community, state, and national levels. Such support might include:

1. Endorsing the standards for prenatal and infant care, including psychosocial support and family planning services, proposed by the Select Panel for the Promotion of Child Health.

2. Financing primary, secondary, and tertiary levels of hospital care for indigent citizens through local, state, and federal mechanisms. Regionalization is the most cost-effective way of providing highly specialized services, such as maternal, fetal, and neonatal intensive care.

3. Expanding funding mechanisms for prenatal care, delivery, and ongoing child health services for uninsured people. Expanded public programs should allow coverage of low-income, two-parent families and should cover a woman's first pregnancy regardless of income. Private insurers should provide adequate pregnancy-related and infant care benefits.

4. Providing adequate support for maternal and child surveillance activities and genetic services, including ongoing collection, tabulation, analysis, and timely dissemination of data to increase our ability to identify high-risk populations, plan interventions to reduce mortality, and evaluate intervention strategies.

Infant Morbidity

Fetuses affected by Down's syndrome can be identified by tests of amniotic fluid in the midtrimester of pregnancy. Women more than 34 years of age or who have previously had a child with Down's syndrome are at high risk for carrying an affected fetus. At present, medical practice is to inform such women of the availability of prenatal diagnosis. After prenatal diagnosis, prospective parents have the choice of planning for optimal care after birth or terminating the pregnancy.

Surveys (Centers for Disease Control, unpublished observations from surveillance of genetic services, 1980) show that 60 percent of women who are informed of prenatal diagnosis and have easy access to it elect to use it. Of those women who use prenatal diagnosis and are found to have a severely affected fetus, 95 percent elect to have an abortion. If 60 percent of all high-risk women were to use prenatal diagnosis and if pregnancy were terminated to the same extent as is now the case, 50 cases of Down's syndrome per year among blacks and 200 cases among whites would not occur. The result would be a 7 percent decrease in the incidence of Down's syndrome. Considering that the average survival of a person with Down's syndrome is 30 years, the 250 excess cases we see each year represent 7,500 years of disability.

Fetuses affected by spina bifida can also be diagnosed by tests of amniotic fluid in the midtrimester. Women who have had a child with spina bifida (or anencephaly) are at high risk for having another affected fetus. A new maternal, serum screening test can identify women in the general population who are also at high risk for carrying an affected fetus. If the serum test is positive, amniotic fluid diagnostic tests are then offered. The serum screening test (alpha-fetoprotein) has been widely available in the United States only since January 1984. We estimate that each year 660 children with spina bifida, representing 16,500 years of disability, would not be born if screening were widely available.

We further estimate that if the three main risk factors during pregnancy—smoking, lack of prenatal care, and poor prenatal nutrition—were eliminated, we would prevent 120 to 230 cases of developmental disability each year as a result of having prevented low-birth-weight babies. This would be the equivalent of eliminating 4,000–7,500 years of disability. Because we have no way of ensuring that high-risk women would stop smoking, enter prenatal care early, and obtain adequate nutrition, only one half to one third of the theoretically achievable is actually achievable.

Further limiting the ability to intervene is the recent implementation of the Diagnosis Related Group (DRG) System for hospital reimbursement, which may limit economically disadvantaged persons' access to corrective surgery for congenital anomalies. Similarly, if access to perinatal care is limited in any way, we will see an increase in infant mortality.

We recommend the following measures to limit and reduce infant morbidity:

Develop a public policy to ensure, for all citizens, the complete and unencumbered access to preventive services that will maintain the substantial reductions in morbidity already brought about by such programs as immunization and neonatal screening. We should ensure access to preventive services, particularly neonatal screening for metabolic diseases and immunizations.

SUMMARY

Each year in the United States, the following excess infant mortality and morbidity occur:

1. 7,500 deaths in infants 28 days–1 year of age (postneonatal period)
2. 4,000 deaths in infants less than 28 days of age (neonatal period)
3. 50,000 low-birth-weight infants and 4,000 infant deaths associated with low birth weight
4. 2.2 million unintended pregnancies

This excessive mortality and morbidity represent a gap between what is and what could be regarding our reproductive health. Although the gap exists at all levels of society, it is most pronounced for teenagers, blacks, the poor, and the educationally disadvantaged.

More than half of the 6 million pregnancies in the United States each year are unintended. But the risk of unintended pregnancy is not uniformly distributed. The rate of unintended pregnancy is 2.5 times as high for black women as for white women; twice as high for poor women as for those with higher incomes; and twice as high for teenagers as for older women.

Moreover, women giving birth because of an unintended pregnancy have characteristics similar to women at increased risk of experiencing an infant death. Hence, reducing unintended pregnancy among these women may also lower infant mortality. Four in 10 women become pregnant as teenagers. Early teenage childbearing usually ends schooling—often leaving young women unemployable and dependent on public welfare and public sources of medical care.

The gap in infant mortality is caused primarily by

an excess of low-birth-weight infants and an excess of postneonatal deaths among normal-birth-weight infants. White adult women with 13 or more years of education—our "best standard population"—experience the lowest infant mortality because they have low rates of low birth weight and postneonatal mortality among normal-birth-weight babies. Compared with babies of this best standard population, infants of teenage mothers are 6 to 8 times as likely to die in the postneonatal period, and infants of other white and all black mothers are 1.3 and 4 times, more likely to be of low birth weight, respectively.

Normal-birth-weight babies of mothers in the best standard population are also at less risk of dying in the neonatal period than are other infants of like weight. For example, normal-birth-weight infants of other white and all black mothers are 2.5 and 4 times more likely to die, respectively, in the first four weeks of life.

It is possible to eliminate the excessive mortality and morbidity enumerated above by the year 2000. This would mean reductions of 60 percent in postneonatal deaths, 15 percent in neonatal deaths, 20 percent in the number of infants born with low birth weight, and 65 percent in unintended pregnancy. These reductions could be achieved if interventions now available were universally used, especially within the identifiable high-risk subpopulations.

Available strategies include (1) educating potential parents on the responsibilities and risks of human reproduction, (2) making reproductive health services equally available to all men and women needing them, (3) encouraging women to lengthen the time between pregnancies, (4) ensuring that women start prenatal care in the first trimester of pregnancy, (5) improving maternal nutrition, (6) encouraging women to reduce smoking and alcohol consumption during pregnancy, (7) providing improved medical care during childbirth, (8) providing specialized neonatal care for infants who need it, (9) helping high-risk and teenage mothers improve their parenting skills, and (10) increasing access to pediatric care throughout the first year of life.

Interventions may vary from region to region, depending on the specific problem encountered. An epidemiologic assessment should be undertaken to define the health problems, describe the existing services, and provide the framework for the direction of resources. For example, providers addressing a gap in postneonatal mortality may implement (1) improved access to care for sick infants, (2) a follow-up program to support families of infants at high risk of postneonatal diseases, (3) injury control programs, and (4) public education programs to improve parenting skills.

Interventions that reduce mortality are expected to lower infant morbidity as well. Actions for reducing the burden of illness associated with congenital anomalies and developmental disabilities include (1) maintaining regional access to specialized perinatal care and corrective surgery, (2) providing pregnant women access to prenatal diagnosis for Down's syndrome and spina bifida, (3) continuing newborn screening for PKU and hypothyroidism, and (4) continuing research into the etiology of congenital anomalies and developmental disabilities and improved methods for habilitating affected infants.

Steering Committee: James Alley, M.D., M.P.H., Director, Division of Public Health, Georgia Department of Human Resources; Alfred W. Brann, Jr., M.D., Chairperson, Principal Investigator, WHO Collaborating Center in Perinatal Care and Health Service Research in Maternal and Child Health (MCH), Director, Division of Newborn Medicine, Emory University School of Medicine; Luella M. Klein, M.D., Department of Gynecology and Obstetrics, Emory University School of Medicine; and Godfrey P. Oakley, Jr., M.D., Director, Division of Birth Defects and Developmental Disabilities, Center for Environmental Health, Centers for Disease Control.

Invited Consultants: Frederick O. Bonkovsky, Ph.D., Professor of Christian Ethics, Columbia Theological Seminary, Atlanta; Ezra C. Davidson, Jr., M.D., Chairman, Department of Obstetrics and Gynecology, King/Drew Medical Center, Los Angeles; Stanley N. Graven, M.D., Department of Child Health, University of Missouri, Columbia; Nora K. Piore, Senior Program Consultant, Commonwealth Fund, New York City; Julius B. Richmond, M.D., Director, Division of Health Policy, Research, and Education, Harvard University, Boston; Jeannie R. Rosoff, President, The Alan Guttmacher Institute, New York City; and Zena A. Stein, M.A., M.B., B.C.H., Director of Epidemiology of Brain Disorders, New York State Psychiatric Institute, New York City.

Reviewers: Russell E. Alexander, M.D.; Willard Cates, M.D., M.P.H.; J. David Erickson, D.D.S., Ph.D.; Malcolm G. Freeman, M.D.; Carol Hogue, Ph.D.; Carol A. Holtzman, R.N.: Donald R. Hopkins, M.D.; James Marks, M.D., M.P.H.; Phil Nieburg, M.D., M.P.H.; Roger W. Rochat, M.D., M.P.H.; and Alison Spitz, M.P.H.

Special thanks: typing: Barbara Ervin, Ellen King, Faye McGraw; data processing: W. Scott Barton, Dwan G. Hightower, Louis Jacob, David Karan; and literature searches: Kathryn S. Deck.

REFERENCES

1. Advanced report of final mortality statistics, 1980. Hyattsville, Maryland: National Center for Health Statistics. Monthly Vital Statistics Report 1983;32(suppl):1–39.

2. Ory HW, Forrest VD. Making choices, evaluating the health risks and benefits of birth control methods. New York: Alan Guttmacher Institute, 1983.

3. Projections of the population of the United States: 1975–2000. Washington, D.C.: US Government Printing Office, 1975. (Current population report; series P-2S; no. 601).

4. Moore KA, Burt MR. Private crisis, public cost, policy perspectives on teenage childbearing. Washington, D.C.: Urban Institute Press, 1982.

5. Teenage pregnancy: the problem that hasn't gone away. New York: Alan Guttmacher Institute, 1981.

6. Lee K, Paneth N, et al. Neonatal mortality: an analysis of the recent improvements in the United States. Am J Public Health 1980;70:15–21.

7. Budetti P, Barrand N, McManus P, et al. Cost effectiveness analysis of medical technology. Background paper no. 2: Case studies of medical technologies. Case study no. 10: The cost and effectiveness of neonatal intensive care. Washington, D.C.: Congress of the US Office of Technology Assessment, 1980:19.

8. Phibbs CS, Williams R, Phibbs RH. Newborn risk factors and costs of neonatal intensive care. Pediatrics 1981;68:313–21.

9. Healthy people: the Surgeon General's report on health promotion and disease prevention. Washington, D.C.: US Government Printing Office, 1979; DHEW publication no. (PHS)79-55071.

10. Myrianthopoulos N, Chung C. Congenital malformations in singletons: epidemiologic survey. Birth Defects 1975;11(10):1–22.

11. Jones B. Years of life lost through Down's syndrome. Genetics 1979;16:379–83.

12. Boyle MH, Torrance GW, Sinclair JC, et al. Economic evaluation of neonatal intensive care of very low birthweight infants. N Engl J Med 1983;308:1331–2.

13. Conley R. The economics of mental retardation. Baltimore: Johns Hopkins University Press, 1973:311.

14. Hodgson A, Kopstein N. Personal health care expenditures according to the condition, sex and age: United States, 1980. Hyattsville, Maryland: National Center for Health Statistics, 1983.

15. Zook CJ, Moore FD. High-cost users of medical care. N Engl J Med 1980;302:996–1002.

16. Zook CJ, Savickis SF, Moore FD. Repeated hospitalization for the same disease: A multiplier of national health costs. Milbank Mem Fund Q 1980;58:454–71.

17. Reed DM, Stanley FJ. The epidemiology of prematurity. Baltimore: Urban and Schwartzenbert, 1977.

18. Gortmaker SL. The effects of prenatal care upon the health of newborns. Am J Public Health 1973;69:653.

19. Goldenberg R, Hale C, Houde J, et al. Neonatal deaths in Alabama, 1970–1980: an analysis of birth weight and race-specific neonatal mortality rates. Am J Obstet Gynecol 1983;147:687–93.

20. Guyer B, Wallach LA, Rosen SL. Birthweight-standardized neonatal mortality rate and the prevention of low birthweight: how does Massachusetts compare with Sweden? N Engl J Med 1982;306:1230–3.

21. Williams R. Measuring the effectiveness of perinatal medical care. Med Care 1979;17:95.

22. Williams RL, Chen P. Identifying the sources of the recent decline in perinatal mortality rates in California. N Engl J Med 1982;306:207.

23. David RJ, Siegel E. Decline in neonatal mortality, 1968 to 1977: better babies or better care? Pediatrics 1983;71:531–40.

Unintentional Injuries

Gordon S. Smith, M.B., Ch.B., M.P.H., and Henry Falk, M.D.

Throughout the world, including in developing countries, injuries are now the leading cause of death during half the human life span.[1,2] In the United States, injuries are the leading cause of death from the first year of life to age 44. In 1980 more than 68 million Americans were injured severely enough to require medical attention or have their daily activities restricted.[3] Disability and disfigurement are common results. Injuries are a primary cause of medical costs, losses to the economy, and human suffering. A single source of injury, the motor vehicle, cost society more than $18 billion (excluding property costs) in 1975, an amount equal to approximately 1 percent of the gross national product.[4,5]

We have the knowledge and the technology to prevent many injuries and to reduce the severity and impact of most of them. Single regulations may save thousands of lives annually, just as the 55-mph speed limit is estimated to prevent 5,000 deaths every year.[6] Each year that the available but unused standards for crashworthy automobiles are delayed, at least 9,000 lives are estimated to be lost.[6] This paper summarizes our knowledge of the main causes of unintentional injuries and identifies the gap between what is already known about controlling them and what is now being implemented.

DEFINITION OF UNINTENTIONAL INJURIES

Of all fatal injuries in the United States in 1980, 32 percent were classified as intentional (suicide and homicide) and 2 percent of unknown intent (predominantly poisoning, drowning, and injuries from firearms). The remaining 66 percent of all injury deaths were classified as unintentional according to

From the Divisions of Injury Epidemiology and Control and Environmental Hazards and Health Effects, Center for Environmental Health, Centers for Disease Control, Public Health Service, Atlanta, Georgia. Dr. Smith is now at the Department of Health Policy and Management, Johns Hopkins University School of Hygiene and Public Health, Baltimore, Maryland.

Address reprint requests to Dr. Smith, Department of Health Policy and Management, Johns Hopkins University School of Hygiene and Public Health, 615 North Wolfe Street, Rm. 4028, Baltimore, MD 21205.

the International Classification of Diseases Supplemental Classification System—External Cause (ICD-E codes). These codes classify injuries on the basis of apparent intent.

There are severe limitations to this system, especially because in many cases intent is unknown and the death is misclassified as accidental, or the information about intent is omitted from the medical record for legal, insurance, or emotional reasons. For many alcohol-related deaths, intent is difficult to determine. Who can know the mind of a drunken teenager who drives a car into a tree at 60 mph? Because our goal is to prevent such deaths, intent may not matter; a safe car design that includes air bags and automatic seat belts could prevent many such deaths, regardless of intent.

Many other injuries can also be prevented without concern for intent. For the purposes of this paper, however, only unintentional or accidental injuries as defined by the ICD-E codes will be discussed. Suicide, homicide, and other violence-related injuries are discussed in another paper. Complications of medical and surgical care and adverse reactions to drugs, although included in the total number of injuries to maintain compatibility with other published data and the ICD grouping (E800–E999), will not be discussed. A second classification system, the nature of injury codes, classifies the kind of injury or body part injured. Because these codes contain little data on cause of injury, they will not be discussed.

In determining which causes of injuries to select as high-priority problems, we encountered several difficulties, especially the fact that many of the leading causes of morbidity are not the leading causes of mortality. In a recent study comparing injury-related death with the ten leading causes of injury-related emergency room admissions, only three causes of injury—motor vehicle crashes, falls, and assaults—appeared in both groups, and only the first two of these are predominantly unintentional.[7] Cutting and piercing injuries were the second leading cause of emergency room admissions, but in 1980 they accounted for less than 0.1 percent of all injury deaths. Other injuries such as drownings have an extremely high case to fatality ratio, yet they cause little morbidity. Some types of injuries, though less common, occur in younger age groups and account for significant premature mortality (years of life lost before age 65). Other injuries, such as back injuries, are a prominent cause of outpatient morbidity and lost work days; however, relatively few of them require hospitalization, and they cause little mortality. Another difficulty is that the data on morbidity are incomplete. For example, no reliable data are available on the causes of hospitalization for injuries in this country. Because of these difficulties, we denoted as high priority every unintentional injury that causes more than 1 percent of all unintentional injury deaths in the United States.

Unless otherwise stated, the data used in the analysis for this study came from the public use data tapes from the National Center for Health Statistics (NCHS), including both mortality and hospital discharge data, and from unpublished data provided by the NCHS. All data refer to 1980, the base year for this study. The data on available interventions and their effectiveness were obtained by medical literature searches and by consultation with leading injury experts in the United States.

IMPACT ON SOCIETY

While injuries are only the fourth leading cause of death (following heart disease, cancer, and stroke), they are the leading cause of premature mortality (years of life lost before age 65) aside from infant mortality. Figure 1 shows years of life lost for the eight leading causes of death.

In 1980 unintentional injuries accounted for 105,718 deaths, 2,769,084 potential years of life lost and an estimated 48,804,537 visits to emergency rooms (see Table 1 and Figures 2 and 3 for the breakdown by cause). The National Center for Health Statistics reported that in 1980 a total of 72,715,000 injuries occurred, regardless of intent. (NCHS defines injury as that which "results in at least 1 full day of restricted activity or [requires] medical attention.") Of these, 4,392,000 were injuries sustained in motor vehicle crashes.[3] A total of 3.6 million Americans were hospitalized for injuries in 1980 requiring 27.7 million days of hospitalization. A more detailed breakdown of hospitalization by cause is not available because of poor E-coding of hospital discharge data.

Acute conditions resulting from injuries were responsible for nearly 103 million days lost from work and 480.7 million days lost from major activity (school, work, or usual daily activities). When the time lost because of long-term disability is included, the total number of days lost from major activity was 778.9 million for all injuries and nearly 145.5 million days for motor vehicle crashes alone.[3]

The financial costs of injuries, while difficult to calculate exactly, burden society and individuals alike. Cost estimates were made by extrapolating data from Hartunian's study of motor vehicle injuries and National Safety Council data.[8,9] The direct estimated costs of hospitalization, physician visits, and other professional costs, pharmaceutical costs, and expenses of home and institutional care totaled more than $19.5 billion in 1980. Indirect costs (lost wages) are estimated to add nearly $26 billion, bringing the estimated total cost of injuries to society in 1980 to almost $45.5 billion.

RISK FACTORS

In an analysis of the causes of injuries the prime consideration is the interaction of host (the person

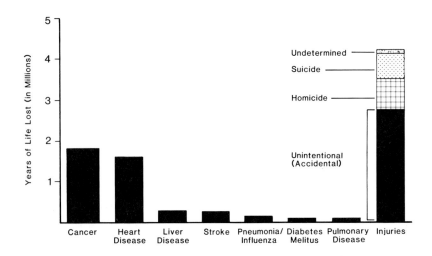

Figure 1. Potential years of life lost before age 65 from the eight leading causes of death, United States, 1980.

Table 1. Mortality and emergency room visits for unintentional injuries, United States, 1980

Specific injuries (E-codes)	Mortality[a]		Emergency room visits[b]	
	No. of deaths	Rate per 100,000 population	No. of injuries	Rate per 100,000 population
Motor vehicles (E810–25)	53,172	23.47	6,077,244	2,280
Falls (E880–8)	13,294	5.87	12,767,544	4,790
Drownings (E830,832,910)	7,257	3.20	NA	NA
Fire and flames (E890–9,924)	6,016	2.66	1,199,456	450
Poisonings (E850–69)	4,331	1.91	506,437	190
Suffocation (E911–3)	4,121	1.82	NA	NA
Natural environment (E900–9)	3,194	1.41	213,237	80
Firearms (E922)	1,955	0.86	NA	NA
Air transportation (E840–5)	1,494	0.66	NA	NA
Machinery (E919)	1,471	0.65	NA	NA
Electric current (E925)	1,095	0.48	NA	NA
Struck by falling object (E916)	1,037	0.46	NA	NA
Other	7,281	3.22	NA	NA
Total	105,718	46.67	48,804,537	18,310

[a] Data from Public Use Data Tapes—Mortality.[172]
[b] Data for emergency room rates are based on published age-specific rates from Barancik et al.[7] extrapolated to the 1980 U.S. population. Because data are not available for all categories, the number of injuries does not add up to the total shown.

injured), agent (various forms of energy—mechanical, thermal, chemical, and electrical), and environment, including the socioeconomic environment (e.g., road design or the availability and marketing of alcohol).[5] How these factors affect the human body is determined by the type of energy involved, its distribution in time and space, and the capacity of the human body to withstand the energy. For example, when energy is transferred over a small area (e.g., when the forehead strikes the rearview mirror in a crash), considerably more injury results than when the energy is spread over a larger area (e.g., when an air bag is used). Although the cause of injuries is primarily the interaction of agent, host, and environment, certain factors put people at increased risk.

Age. Injury rates vary dramatically with age, reflecting differences in activities, behavior, and injury thresholds. Mortality rates for all unintentional injuries combined are highest in the elderly: 98 per 100,000 for those over 65 and 269 per 100,000 for those over 85, compared with an overall rate of 47 per 100,000. Falls are the leading cause of both morbidity and mortality in this age group. The incidence of other nonfatal injuries also increases dramatically in the elderly.

The lowest mortality from injuries is among people 5–16 years of age. In children under 5, falls are the leading cause of nonfatal injuries, but the largest number of fatalities in this group results from motor vehicles (pedestrians and occupants), drownings, and fires (8.0, 5.0, and 5.5 deaths per 100,000, respectively).

In the 15- to 24-year-old age group, half of all deaths result from unintentional injuries. This group has especially high mortality rates from crashes, firearms, and drownings. For persons up to age 45, motor vehicles are the single largest cause of death.

Sex. Males have about 2.5 times the fatality rate

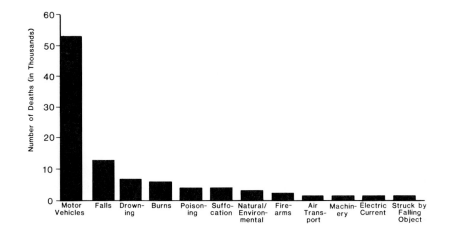

Figure 2. Number of deaths from unintentional injuries by cause, United States, 1980.

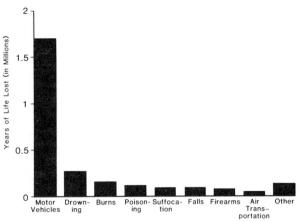

Figure 3. Potential years of life lost before age 65 from unintentional injuries by cause of death, United States, 1980.

for unintentional injuries as females. The male–female ratio of injury mortality rates varies dramatically, depending on age and the specific cause of injury, and injuries in males tend to be more severe than in females.

Alcohol. Alcohol is a major risk factor for all injuries, especially the more severe and fatal injuries. The severity of injury increases with the amount of alcohol consumed, as demonstrated with motor vehicle crashes. Approximately 10 percent of drivers in crashes that result in substantial property damage are considered impaired by alcohol, defined as blood alcohol concentration (BAC) greater than 0.05 percent; 25 percent of drivers injured in serious crashes are considered legally intoxicated, defined as BAC greater than 0.1 percent; and approximately 50 percent of all fatally injured drivers are intoxicated.[10,11] A recent study in Fulton County, Georgia, suggested that if BACs were tested on all drivers involved in fatal crashes, alcohol would be involved in considerably more cases than has been documented.[12] However, BACs were not available on all surviving drivers in this study. Among fatally injured pedestrians, one study found 39 percent to be intoxicated.[11]

Even moderate amounts of alcohol (BAC less than 0.05 percent, about one to two drinks) can impair judgment markedly,[13] but only teenagers and the elderly are at greatly increased risk of crash involvement after consuming moderate amounts of alcohol.[14,15] For adults 25–59 years of age, the majority of alcohol-related injuries do not occur among social drinkers but among persons whose BACs are 0.15 percent or higher; they represent the problem drinkers and alcoholics.[10,16–18]

The data on alcohol and nonvehicular injuries are less complete. According to one study in New York

State, 29 percent of unintentional, nonvehicular fatalities were intoxicated.[19] An emergency room breathalyzer detected alcohol in 22 percent of patients injured at home, 16 percent of those injured on the job, and 30 percent of those injured on the road.[20] In a study of occupational fatalities in Maryland, 11 percent had BACs of more than 0.08 percent at the time of death.[21] One third of the persons over 14 years of age who drowned in Maryland were found to have high BACs (greater than 0.15 percent), and 44 percent were impaired by alcohol (BACs of more than 0.05 percent).[22] Of all adults who died in house fires in Baltimore, 39 percent had elevated BACs; 50 percent of adults in cigarette-related fires had comparably elevated BACs.[23]

Although nonalcoholic drugs have not yet been shown to be a major risk factor for injury, many commonly used drugs such as barbiturates and tranquilizers increase the effect of alcohol when combined with it and have been shown to affect performance in experimental situations.[24–26] However, their exact contribution to injury causation is still to be determined.[26]

Residence, race, and socioeconomic status. Although residence, race, and socioeconomic status influence the incidence of many injuries, it is difficult to separate the effect of each factor because they are so interrelated, and published rates are not age adjusted. Native Americans have the highest death rates from unintentional injuries; they also tend to live in rural areas and to be poor. Fatal injury rates are highest in rural areas, a statistic that remains even when adjustment is made for per capita income in the area of residence. The physical environment—poor roads and emergency services and the prevalence of farm machinery and firearms—contributes to the high fatality rates in rural areas.[1] Not all people are at equal risk of being injured; house fires, because of substandard housing, are more common among the poor; private aircraft crashes produce injuries in a higher socioeconomic group. Mortality rates also vary considerably from state to state, from a low of 33 per 100,000 in New York and Hawaii to a high of 97 per 100,000 in Alaska.[1]

Occupation. Work-related injuries do not pose equal risks to all workers. Workers in mining and quarrying industries have an annual rate of 55 traumatic injury deaths per 100,000 workers; those in trade industries have a rate of only five deaths per 100,000 workers.[27] The rates for agricultural and construction workers are also high at 52 and 40 deaths per 100,000 workers, respectively. Death rates for specific occupations exhibit even higher variability, even though smaller populations are usually involved. An estimated 188–283 deaths per 100,000 workers were reported for full-time workers on active oil rigs in 1978.[28] Fire fighters have mortality rates of 75 deaths per 100,000 annually.[29]

SELECTION OF INTERVENTIONS

To determine the most effective interventions for unintentional injuries, we must consider four elements: (1) human factors, (2) active versus passive interventions, (3) analysis of the cause of injuries, and (4) the relative importance of interventions.

Human factors. Human behavior is an important cause of injuries, but attempts at changing behavior as a way of controlling injuries have met with limited success.[5,30–36] For example, in one community an intensive campaign was waged on television to increase seat belt usage, but there was no difference in usage between those who saw the messages and those who did not.[37] Programs aimed at one-time nonbehavioral changes, such as the installation of electrical outlet covers[38] and smoke detectors[39] have been somewhat more successful.

Despite the difficulties documenting successful behavioral interventions for injuries, human behaviors can change dramatically (e.g., smoking and diet) and result in substantial and measurable improvement in health outcomes (e.g., cardiovascular mortality). In addition, modifications of environments require behavioral actions by policy makers and policy implementors. More research is needed to determine the most successful means to improve the safety behavior of individuals.

Active versus passive interventions. The only effective interventions are those that accomplish what they were designed to do and are used correctly.[40] In advocating active protection (i.e., requiring the individual's active participation and cooperation), we must consider the extent to which the strategy will be used or misused. Because of the gap between design and use, interventions that have proved most effective in controlling injuries are passive: that is, they work automatically and do not call for people's repetitive, active participation.[41,42] Seat belts, for example, are an effective means of protection in frontal crashes, rollovers, and side crashes, but only about 13 percent of all drivers in the United States use them.[31] Air bags, on the other hand, protect occupants only in frontal crashes, but they function automatically and thus would protect all occupants, including those in the high-risk groups, who are less likely to use seat belts. The combined effect of seat belts and air bags is even greater, and thus seat belt use laws and other efforts to increase seat belt use will further increase the effectiveness of air bags.

Analysis of the causes of injuries. The framework developed by Haddon[43–45] is useful in analyzing the causes of injuries so that interventions can be developed. Interventions can be aimed at (1) preventing the occurrence of injury-producing events (pre-event phase), (2) reducing the extent of injury (event phase), and (3) reducing the consequences of injury (postevent phase). At each phase there are three factors that can be modified in relation to each phase: (1) human, (2) vehicles and equipment, and (3) environment. See Figure 4 for examples of possible interventions and the points at which they could act.

Phases	Factors		
	Human	Vehicles and Equipment	Environment
Pre-event	Educate public in the use of seat belts and child restraints	Safe brakes and tires	Improved road design; restrict alcohol advertising and availability at gas stations
Event	Prevention of osteoporosis to decrease likelihood of fracture	Air bags and a crashworthy vehicle design	Breakaway utility poles and crash barriers
Postevent	Treatment of hemophilia and other conditions that result in impaired healing	Safe design of fuel tank to prevent rupture and fire	Adequate emergency medical care and rehabilitation

Figure 4. Examples of injury interventions applied to the Haddon injury matrix.

Relative importance of interventions. Injury control strategies were selected after an extensive literature review and consultation with injury control experts. They were determined not necessarily by the relative importance of causative factors, but rather by the effectiveness of interventions. It has proved difficult to change some factors (a voluntary change of alcohol consumption habits is a prime example). Some interventions were selected because, although they do not have a great impact on overall mortality, they are extremely simple, safe, and effective. A good example is childproof containers for all household poisons and drugs.

GENERAL INTERVENTIONS

Corporate Action and Regulation

Traditionally, manufacturers have not focused primarily on prevention of injury that may result from their products. The Consumer Product Safety Commission estimated that more than 9 million people required emergency room treatment in 1977 for injuries received from consumer products (excluding motor vehicles, farm machinery, cigarettes, alcohol, and some other products).[5] Only a few safety standards have been self-imposed by industry. For example, hot water heater manufacturers have failed to reduce the maximum temperature setting of their product in order to prevent most tap water burns.[46]

Automotive safety standards have also suffered from the failure of industry to vigorously develop and use self-imposed standards. For example, even though the technology for air bags has been available for almost 15 years, they have been available only in luxury and selected other automobiles. (They are an option in a number of 1987 model cars.) Federal safety standards had to be imposed for brakes, restraints, door locks, fuel systems, and other features, despite the fact that these technologies were developed by the industry. These standards are credited with having saved approximately 9,000 lives annually in the mid-1970s.[47,48]

Other regulatory efforts of the federal government have not been successful, for example, regulation of the fire hazard posed by cigarettes.[49] In theory, such regulatory efforts could also be undertaken by states. Thus Maryland sought unsuccessfully to regulate the fire accelerants added to tobacco to reduce the fire hazard of cigarettes.[50] This relatively simple piece of legislation, applied nationally, could potentially save more than 2,300 lives and prevent 5,000 serious burns annually. Another failure of the legislative process to control injuries is illustrated by the widespread repeal of motorcycle helmet laws, which has resulted in approximately 1,400 additional deaths annually, 80 percent of which occur among people 15–34 years of age.[1,51]

One of the chief reasons industry has given for not implementing many safety devices is the added cost; another is that consumers should be given the freedom to buy less expensive products without safety features. However, an estimated 75–80 percent of the persons injured by motor vehicles were not the original owners or had not chosen the vehicle they were in.[52] This has important implications from a public policy standpoint. It invalidates the argument that people should be free to buy the lowest-cost product and to decide whether safety features are worth the extra cost. Their decisions affect the safety of others and as such become a public concern.

Litigation

Litigation, or the fear of it, has the potential for becoming a powerful means of affecting change. Some states have strict product liability laws that make manufacturers who do not use state-of-the-art safety designs liable for any harm that would have been prevented by such designs.[6] In several lawsuits the courts have rendered verdicts against automobile manufacturers because of a lack of safety features.[53,54] Suits against bar owners have prompted interest in and cooperation with server intervention programs, and a suit against Remington Arms Company for injuries received as a result of design faults was settled for $6.8 million.[53] Some industries have been slow to act, in spite of litigation. The Hankscraft hot water vaporizer caused severe burns, and despite several lawsuits the company did not change its design until the insurance carrier canceled their liability coverage.[53]

Clearly, there is a need to sell the idea of safety considerations to manufacturers and to devise ways of encouraging them to consider the injury-causing potential of manufactured products. One possible method of encouragement would be tax advantages for implementing new safety design changes in certain products. Such tax advantages have been effective in stimulating the solar energy industry.

Workplace Standards

The Occupational Safety and Health Act of 1970 reflected the culmination of efforts to centralize and codify design standards in the workplace. Occupational Safety and Health Administration (OSHA) regulations dictate design parameters, rules for selecting tools and equipment for safe operation, and procedures for frequent inspection and monitoring. OSHA inspections and enforcement of regulations resulted in a decrease in injuries in the year following inspection in one industry.[55] Training workers to behave safely can compensate, to a limited extent, for deficiencies in workplace design[56] but usually only for a limited time after completion of training.

Occupational safety has traditionally been governed by legislated economic and legal sanctions. In 1982 job injuries and deaths cost the nation an estimated $31.4 billion; wage losses and medical expenses alone were an estimated $5.2 billion and $3.6 billion, respectively. Thus, it is understandable that emphasis is being placed on the economic incentives in injury control. Some economists[57] have recommended injury tax laws to maximize the efficiency of such financial controls.

Medical Treatment

It is generally believed that decreasing the time from injury to emergency treatment and providing definitive care for severely injured persons decreases the risk of death.[58] Trunkey[59] described three time peaks for deaths from trauma: (1) immediate death occurs within 1 hour (accounting for more than half of all trauma deaths) and is caused by masive, generally irreversible trauma; (2) early death occurs 1–3 hours posttrauma and is largely caused by internal or other bleeding; and (3) late death occurs days or weeks after the trauma, primarily from infection or multiple organ failure. Early deaths constitute approximately 30 percent of all trauma deaths, and almost all are considered preventable through available medical procedures. Prevention of early deaths was the rationale for forming the Mobile Army Surgical Hospital (MASH) units in Korea and for developing modern emergency medical systems and major trauma units. Although it appears logical that early treatment of injuries, especially hemorrhage, should reduce the number of early deaths, considerable controversy still surrounds the effectiveness of these systems and their components.[60] A recent study of head trauma by Kraus et al.[58] found no obvious correlation between fatality rate or outcome and speed or means of transport to a hospital. Detailed evaluation of the most efficient and cost-effective methods for providing emergency care is needed.

INTERVENTION PROGRAMS

On the whole, control measures are different for each cause of injury. These measures will be dis-cussed for each of the 12 leading causes of mortality outlined in Table 1. However, in planning the implementation of specific interventions, we can consider four main intervention strategies. These four intervention strategies propose a practical way of implementing all the currently known interventions: (1) a motor vehicle safety program directed specifically at motor vehicle injuries but including many principles that apply to other transportation, such as light aircraft; (2) a home injuries control program directed at the home and the immediate environment; (3) an occupational injuries control program; and (4) an alcohol control program made up of specific countermeasures designed to reduce consumption and to separate alcohol from injury-producing situations.

Alcohol

Alcohol sales and consumption appear to be elastic: when prices increase to a certain point, consumption decreases correspondingly,[61] although the magnitude of change has not been determined.[62,63] Because alcohol taxes are not indexed to inflation, the real price of alcohol in the United States has declined almost 50 percent since 1967.[61] There is some evidence that teenagers are most sensitive to price[64]; thus price increases would have the greatest effect on this high-risk group. Researchers have suggested that the decrease in injuries and fatalities during economic recessions is caused by decreased alcohol consumption,[65] though this is uncertain. In Britain, Canada, and elsewhere, it has been shown that increasing the cost of alcohol directly reduces the occurrence of cirrhosis of the liver.[66] It is reasonable to assume from these studies that the effect of the cost of alcohol on reduced consumption may also result in fewer injuries, particularly those resulting from motor vehicle crashes.

Greater availability of alcohol may lead to increased consumption and increased injuries. Beer is marketed intensively on college campuses. According to one report, two thirds of all advertising in college newspapers ($10 million annually) is for alcoholic beverages.[67] The alcohol industry has also succeeded in decreasing the barriers to the purchase of alcohol. For example, in many states beer can now be purchased in convenience stores, fast food outlets, and gas stations, clearly linking alcohol use and the automobile and encouraging increased consumption by drivers. Wine sales in grocery stores have resulted in an increase in total wine sales, according to one report.[68]

A promising new approach to controlling drinking and driving is server intervention.[69] Several states now have laws that hold bar and restaurant owners liable for damages resulting from serving alcohol to a person who later has a crash while intoxicated. One large restaurant chain has several hundred lawsuits pending related to injuries caused by alcohol served on its premises. These suits have prompted action within the industry to control alcohol consumption in bars and restaurants.[70] Some bars are providing free transportation to patrons who would otherwise drive home intoxicated.

Effective interventions could target a specific high-risk group. One example is the current federal initiative to raise the age at which alcohol may be purchased to 21. Persons under 21 years of age are at higher risk for motor vehicle injuries. Raising the minimum purchasing age to 21 has been shown to decrease fatal nighttime crashes involving drivers under 21 by approximately 28 percent.[71] If all states raised the legal drinking age to 21, approximately 730 fatalities from nighttime crashes could be prevented annually.

Another high-risk group that should be targeted by interventions are problem drinkers. According to one study, an estimated 9 percent of all those in the drinking-age population consume 68 percent of all alcohol sold.[72] Most people who are injured after alcohol consumption are not simply social drinkers; they can be diagnosed as problem drinkers. They are often already known to community service agencies because of previous alcohol-related problems.[17,18] Identifying these people and directing alcohol treatment programs at them are likely to be more successful than directing programs at the general public. Even a small success rate for such programs would reduce injuries considerably; however, successful methods to identify and treat such people need to be developed.

Strict enforcement of safe drinking laws, including stiff penalties for violation, to prevent driving while legally intoxicated has been widely advocated. Among drivers convicted of alcohol-related traffic offenses, those whose licenses have been suspended or revoked have had fewer crashes than those who were remanded to rehabilitation programs.[73] The long-term effectiveness of drunk driving legislation needs to be examined, because although injury rates have dropped during initial enforcement, the rates have rebounded in all places evaluated. This rebound phenomenon probably occurs once people realize that the risk of being caught is small.[74]

There appears to be a general change in societal attitudes toward alcohol use. Groups such as MADD (Mothers Against Drunk Driving) and SADD (Students Against Drunk Driving) are part of a larger trend to modify the social and economic environment in which alcohol is used and to reduce its potential for becoming involved in the injury-producing event.

Motor Vehicles

Seat belts. The combined use of lap and shoulder belts reduces the likelihood of death or serious injury for all occupants by approximately 50 percent.[75] In Australia, decreases of 21–25 percent in occupant deaths were reported after seat belt use was required by law.[5,31] However, only approximately 13 percent of U.S. motor vehicle occupants now use seat belts, and the percentage is even smaller among high-risk groups. The automatic seat belt, such as that in the Volkswagen Rabbit, has been shown to be more effective overall—even though its theoretical effectiveness is approximately 5 percent less than regular three-point belts—because usage rates are 50 percent higher than for VW Rabbits with manual belts. Among those cars with automatic seat belts installed, the medical insurance claims are 14% lower than for comparable cars without automatic seat belts.[76]

Air bags. The potential effectiveness of air bags is estimated to be similar to the effectiveness of seat belts in frontal crashes and could reduce highway fatalities by approxiamtely 30 percent and serious injuries by approximately 35 percent.[75] However, they provide only minimal protection in side collisions, rollovers, and ejections. While their theoretical effectiveness is less than that of seat belts, the installation of air bags in all cars would have a far greater net impact on reducing death and injuries on the highways, because they would automatically protect everyone, even high-risk persons who are less likely to wear belts and to comply with seat belt laws. The combination of air bags and seat belts will increase protection in all motor vehicle crashes by approximately 5 percent over lap–shoulder belts alone and by about 20 percent over air bags alone.

Child restraints. Children are especially high-risk occupants in vehicles because they have traditionally been less restrained than adults. In one study only 7 percent wore seat belts or rode in infant or child restraints in areas that did not have compulsory child restraint laws. Even when the driver was belted, only 25 percent of children were restrained.[77] The effectiveness of child restraints may be similar to that of seat belts, although some estimates claim superior effectiveness—up to a 90 percent reduction in fatalities.[78] Child restraint laws have been enacted in almost every state, although enforcement is a problem. Restraint use in Tennessee was 8 percent before the law was enacted in 1979, rising to 16 percent 4 months after the law was passed and to 29 percent 3 years later.[79] Interestingly, child restraint usage in Massachusetts increased from 18 percent to 26 percent over the same period without a state child restraint law.[80] Despite what appear to be only modest increases in use rate, the law in Tennessee has been shown to reduce injuries to children in automobiles significantly.[81] Child restraint laws, like seat belt laws, are no substitute for safe vehicle design, which should include automatic restraints and other modifications to protect occupants in a crash.

Motorcycles. Motorcyclists are at high risk for serious and fatal injuries. The law requiring motorcyclists to have headlights on at all times is an attempt to increase their visibility, which appears to reduce the risk of being involved in a daytime crash by approximately 50 percent, although estimates vary considerably.[82-84] Legislation and enforcement are easy and practical means of ensuring that interventions such as this are used. However, the single most important legislative step backward in injury control occurred during the years 1976–1979, when many states repealed the laws requiring motorcyclists to wear helmets. The mortality rate among motorcyclists who do not wear helmets is almost double that of motorcyclists who do wear helmets.[51] In the states that repealed such laws, motorcycle fatalities increased 39 percent as helmet use dropped from 100 percent to 50 percent. According to the National Highway Traffic Safety Administration, the number of motorcyclists killed in 1980 was 4,960.[85] If all helmet laws were reinstated, it might be possible to reduce the mortality rate from 7.8 to 5.6 per 10,000, or approximately 30 percent. In other words, reinstatement could prevent 1,399 deaths annually; 80 percent of that number would be persons 15–34 years of age.

Bicycles. It is estimated that five of every six bicycle fatalities are caused by head and neck injuries; few of these victims have other life-threatening injuries.[86] Assuming that helmets could reduce the deaths that result from head and neck injuries by 50 percent, 402 deaths could be prevented. In 1980, 964 bicyclists were killed.[85] Extending the helmet laws to include both motorcyclists and bicyclists (few bicyclists wear helmets) could have prevented approximately 1,800 deaths in 1980, assuming 100 percent compliance with the law.

Vehicle design. Better-designed features that increase the driver's vision and improve the ability to drive safely are available. One example is the single center-mounted rear brake light at eye level, a new standard that has been shown to decrease rear-end collisions by more than 50 percent.[87,88] The design has only recently been implemented by federal regulation. A similar study has shown that modifying cars so that front and rear lights are automatically on during the day reduces the likelihood of being involved in a collision by 22 percent.[89]

The design of a motor vehicle can greatly influence its capacity to protect occupants during crashes. For example, redesigning fuel tanks so that they do not leak following a crash has greatly reduced the number of postcrash fires.[6] Numerous other design changes can vastly improve the safety of a vehicle. The Research Safety Vehicle, developed through available technology, has proved to be effective and reliable and can be produced at competitive prices. It has been estimated that 18,000 lives could be saved annually if all cars were built to the safety standards for that vehicle.[5,90]

Small cars offer less protection in both single-vehicle and multiple-vehicle crashes. This lessened protection is largely the result of the decreased auto body length, which in turn decreases the absorption of energy in an impact. Other design features of small cars, such as a decreased ability to prevent passenger ejections, also contribute to their danger. Data from Maryland show that the percentage of drivers of subcompact cars who sustained serious and fatal injuries in crashes was almost double that of drivers of full-sized cars who sustained such injuries.[91] Although simply advocating larger cars may appear an intervention, effective occupant restraint and improved car design are more logical and effective. The Research Safety Vehicle is a small car, yet its design features render it safe.

After the 55-mph speed limit law was enacted, the death rate decreased from 4.2 per 100 million miles traveled in 1973 to 3.5 per 100 million miles traveled in 1974 and subsequent years. Approximately half the reduction of 10,000 deaths annually has been attributed to the reduced speed limit.[92] If all vehicles were built so that their maximum speed could not exceed the vehicle's ability to protect occupants from fatal injury in a frontal crash, many highway deaths could be prevented.[6]

Age. It is estimated that raising the minimum driving age from 16 to 17 could reduce fatal crashes for 16-year-old drivers by 65–85 percent.[93] Assuming that the rate at which 16-year-old drivers are involved in fatal crashes in Connecticut is similar to that for the nation (26 per 100,000 population), a 75 percent decrease in fatalities would mean the prevention of approximately 815 deaths per year nationwide.

Twelve states currently have curfew laws that

prohibit 16-year-olds from driving late at night and early in the morning (usually midnight to 5 A.M.). According to a study of four of the states, crashes involving 16-year-olds were reduced by 25 percent, 40 percent, 62 percent, and 69 percent.[94] Assuming an average of an approximately 50 percent reduction in crashes nationwide, such a program would save approximately 544 lives annually.

Elderly drivers are the most likely to be involved in crashes at intersections, suggesting a loss in their ability to perceive, gauge the speed of, and respond to oncoming traffic.[1,95] Compulsory physical examinations for the elderly have been proposed by some in an effort to prohibit driving by those who are impaired. However, such screening examinations have not received broad endorsement, and there is little evidence that the elderly or those who are physically impaired cause a substantial number of serious crashes.[18]

Pedestrians. Pedestrian deaths represent the second largest category of motor vehicle deaths (8,290 in 1980). Almost half of all fatally injured adult pedestrians had BACs greater than 0.1 percent.[96] The most serious injuries result from being thrown onto the hood, windshield, or top of the car. Many fatalities can be prevented by design changes in the hood and other structures of the car.[97,98] Lowering bumper heights to less than 21 inches could significantly reduce the severity of injuries to adults (e.g., hip fractures could be reduced by 50 percent).[99]

Better separation of pedestrians from vehicles— by physical barriers and elevated walkways or underpasses, for example—will reduce the injury rate to pedestrians, although the impact of such measures is difficult to estimate. As the speed of a vehicle increases, so does the ratio of deaths to injuries (e.g., the ratio increases 10-fold in areas that have 55-mph speed limits in comparison with areas that have 30-mph speed limits), and the likelihood of being struck is greater in higher speed zones.[1] The strict enforcement of speed limits in high-risk areas and more traffic lights, stop signs, and pedestrian over- or underpasses are likely to reduce the injuries to pedestrians greatly.

Road design. Mortality rates per vehicle mile traveled on interstate highways are one third the rates on other roads, primarily because of improved road design, which eliminates intersections and better separates the lanes of oncoming traffic.[9] Highway design often determines whether a crash will result in injury or death. That 16,000 motor vehicle occupants are killed in single-vehicle crashes every year attests to the importance of designing roadsides so that straying cars can be brought to a

stop without causing deaths or severe injuries. Placing roadside structures at a safe distance from traffic lanes or using only structures that decrease crash forces, such as breakaway light poles and barrels filled with energy-absorbing materials, have been shown to greatly reduce injuries in a crash.[100] Fatalities can also be reduced by redesigning a relatively small number of easily identifiable hazardous corners, downgrades, bridge abutments, and utility poles.[6,101] Vehicle rollovers, which occur in about 46 percent of single-vehicle crashes, happen most often on horizontal left-hand curvatures greater than 6 degrees.[102] On the basis of this finding, reflector markers were placed on the centerlines of all these high-risk curves in Georgia, producing a 20 percent reduction in nighttime crashes compared with daytime crashes at these curves.[103]

In 1980, 2,197 fatalities occurred at intersections controlled by traffic lights. Simply increasing the duration of the yellow phase of traffic signals could greatly reduce intersection conflicts, probably as much as 50 percent.[104,105] Assuming that fatal crashes would be proportionately reduced, approximately 1,000 lives could be saved annually by the universal adoption of a longer yellow signal.

Designing roads so that emergency vehicles can easily reach crash sites could greatly increase the speed with which victims receive medical treatment. Fatality rates in rural areas are more than twice those in urban areas.[1] Although much of this difference reflects different crash patterns, some of the difference reflects the delay in appropriate medical care for the victims.

Reduced travel. Reducing the number of miles traveled by private automobile considerably reduces the risk of injury, as injury rates vary greatly according to type of transportation. The death rate for vehicle occupants per 100 million miles traveled is 21 for motorcycles, 14 for general aviation, 13 for automobiles, 0.15 for buses, and 0.07 for passenger trains. The safest form of travel is a scheduled commercial airplane—0.04 deaths per 100 million miles traveled.[1]

Falls

The elderly have the highest fatality rates from falls, primarily as a result of complications after the fall. The largest single cause of hospitalizations and injury-related deaths in this category is hip fracture. Although modern treatment for hip fracture has reduced the time of hospitalization, functional impairment, and fatalities,[106] preventive measures can further reduce complications and perhaps even reduce the rate of fractures. For example, impaired vision and disturbances of gait and balance are responsible for many falls by the elderly; correcting these problems should reduce the risk.

Osteoporosis in postmenopausal women greatly increases the risk of fracture and complications. Current research suggests that fluoride, calcium, or estrogen therapy may strengthen bones and decrease osteoporosis,[107,108] although concern has been expressed about the side effects of estrogen therapy. Exercise has also been suggested as a means of increasing muscle tone and confidence; it may also help prevent osteoporosis.[18]

It has been estimated that two of every three falls among the elderly involve some environmental cause, such as an unsafe staircase, faulty steps, or inadequate lighting.[109] Proper illumination, handrails, childproof barriers and walkways, and nonskid surfaces on stairs and bathtubs would provide a safer environment for everyone, including the elderly.[110]

Falls from hospital beds are common. In one hospital it was estimated that during an average stay of 20 days, 1 patient in 40 fell out of bed.[111] One author suggested that certain types of rails on hospital beds actually increased the number of falls by creating a hazard over which people had to climb.[112] Placing beds closer to the floor could minimize injuries caused by falls from beds, especially for the elderly.

Sharp edges and corners are a common cause of injury during a fall. According to one study of childhood falls, furniture caused half the injuries, and coffee tables were responsible for 85 out of 193 injuries.[113] Designing houses and furniture with consideration for their potential for injury could substantially reduce the number of injuries.

Hard surfaces such as concrete playground surfaces and wood floors increase the likelihood of injuries. Providing sand playground surfaces and padded floors in homes, hospitals, and nursing homes would reduce the number and extent of injuries. (New York State stipulates that the floors of boxing arenas be padded to protect boxers; no such regulation exists for nursing home floors.)

In many instances an older person who has fallen is unable to get up off the floor. One study showed a significant increase in fatalities and complications in persons who were rescued more than 1 hour after the injury had occurred.[114] Providing alarms at floor level or devices that could be worn on the body could reduce this risk.

Falls from heights cause many deaths and severe injuries. A program in New York City called Children Can't Fly has been actively supported by the legislature and directly aided by the city, which has provided window bars in high-rise buildings. Deaths resulting from young children's falls from windows decreased from 57 in 1973 to 37 in 1975[115] and to 4 in 1980.[116] However, according to a recent article in the *New York Times*,[117] 25 children died in 1983 as a result of falling from windows, suggesting that the effect of the program has worn off. The history of this program indicates that direct passive interventions in which the environment is modified could reduce deaths up to 90 percent but that efforts must be maintained if the effect is to continue.

The wearing of helmets by horseback riders and the use of safety nets or harnesses in certain settings are interventions that will reduce or abolish many serious injuries. Protective clothing, such as the leather jackets worn by motorcyclists, can reduce the impact of a fall.

Drownings

Most drowning victims are young people; the rates are especially high for children 1–2 years of age and for males 17–20 years of age.[1] The principal sites are natural bodies of water (oceans, lakes, rivers), swimming pools, and bathtubs.[118]

Much effort has been focused on providing swimming instruction for children, including infants. Although this strategy seems reasonable, it has not been demonstrated to decrease the number of drownings, and some concern has been expressed that swimming instruction may give a young child a false sense of security in a hazardous situation.[6] The occurrence of water intoxication as a result of teaching infants to swim is also a concern.[119]

It was estimated that almost 20 percent of drownings in one study[22] could have been prevented by modifying the physical environment. These modifications include the placement of physical barriers along riverbanks, bridges, wharves, swimming pools, and roads bordering ditches and waterways. Posting signs about depth, undertow, or slippery banks at natural bodies of water may also be effective.

Approximately 250 children 1–4 years of age drown in swimming pools every year in the United States.[118] We recommend the development of standards to govern safe swimming pool design. Licenses could be a prerequisite for private and public pool construction, and pool owners should be required to install certain safety features, including adequate fences with self-latching gates and accessible rescue and resuscitation equipment. According to an evaluation of fencing around swimming pools in Australia, the drowning rate for children in Canberra, where fences are required, was one ninth the rate for children in Brisbane, where fences are not required.[120] Slip-resistant surfaces around swimming pools and bathtubs and adequate lighting around and under pools have also been suggested.[22]

Restricting the sale of alcoholic beverages in boating, pool, and beach areas and imposing penalties on drunken boat drivers would potentially reduce drownings in adults and teenagers. Of water fatalities in persons over 15 years of age, 44 percent had BACs greater than 0.05 percent, and 33 percent had very high levels—more than 0.15 percent.[22]

Building and modifying boats so that they are stable, have adequate lighting, and contain appropriate safety devices such as flotation equipment could significantly reduce boat-related drownings.[22] The federal flotation and other safety standards established in 1972 are apparently responsible for the drop in fatalities associated with motorboats—from 19.2 per 100,000 boats in 1970 to 7.9 per 100,000 in 1982.[121] The use of lifelines for workers near the water would also reduce fatalities.

Increasing the public's knowledge of cardiopulmonary resuscitation techniques is likely to greatly affect survival because drowning victims could be resuscitated immediately by a friend, family member, or passerby in the near vicinity.

Fire and Flames

Most intervention efforts to prevent burns have consisted of educational safety programs centered on safe storage and handling of flammable materials and matches, installation of smoke detectors and fire extinguishers, and the use of tight-fitting clothing. One-time actions, such as installation of smoke detectors,[39] and specifically targeted programs[122,123] may be effective, but general efforts produce little benefit.[124]

According to a recent study, smoke detectors reduced the potential for death in 86 percent of fires and the potential for severe injuries in 88 percent.[125] Their effectiveness was increased if sprinkler systems were also used. Installing automatic sprinkler systems in all new and existing houses could dramatically reduce the spreading of a fire. Because this would involve considerable expense, priority should be given to high-risk buildings, such as old wooden apartment houses. However, the use of new sprinkler pipe materials such as plastics can considerably reduce the cost.

Building codes produce specific benefits: fire doors and fire walls to prevent the spread of fire, clearly marked exists and fire extinguishers in public buildings, and sprinkler systems.[126] Many old apartment buildings have only one means of egress. According to a study in Baltimore, two thirds of those who died in house fires had tried to escape.[92] Modern houses are considerably less flammable than most older houses because of the flame-retardant materials used in construction and the improved standards for heating and electrical systems. Enforcement of building codes in existing buildings, especially in high-risk areas, could dramatically reduce deaths and severe injuries.

Cigarettes are estimated to cause about half of all deaths from house fires,[23] or approximately 2,300 deaths annually. Most cigarettes made in this country contain additives both in the paper and in the tobacco that cause the cigarette to burn for as long as 28 minutes, even if left unattended.[59] Without the additives a cigarette will self-extinguish in less than 4 minutes—less than the time in which most furniture, upholstery, and mattresses will ignite. More than 19 existing patents would increase the self-extinguishing capabilities of a burning cigarette still further.[127] If even a 50 percent reduction in cigarette-related fires could be achieved by a single law requiring safety standards for cigarettes, an estimated 1,000 lives would be saved annually.

Matches that burn at a lower temperature and self-extinguish when dropped have been developed. This feature, combined with a feature that makes them more difficult for children to light, could prevent some of the fires caused by matches.

Ignited clothing, formerly a common cause of burns in children and the elderly, now accounts for only 5 percent of all burn deaths, three fourths of which are persons over age 65 (311 deaths in 1980). Fabrics today are less flammable, and flammability standards for children's sleepwear have been developed. These two improvements have resulted in a drop from an average of 12 admissions annually for sleepwear-related burns in one pediatric burn unit to 3 admissions in 1975 and only 1 in 1976.[128] The original efforts to extend flammability standards to all clothing for high-risk groups were hampered because one commonly used retardant was found to be carcinogenic. Current efforts are directed at encouraging the elderly to wear tight-fitting clothing, since they are now the group at highest risk. The use of flame-retardant material for drapes and wall coverings could also reduce the incidence of house fires.

Burns from hot water taps are estimated to cause 1.9 hospitalizations per 100,000 population, with an average hospitalization time of 16.7 days.[44] Of these injured persons, 50 percent are children under the age of 5, and 27 percent are persons over 60 years of age. Reducing water heater temperatures to below 130°F (preferably 120°F) could virtually eliminate burns from hot water taps, 95 percent of which occur in the home.[92] Voluntary adjustments by hot water heater manufacturers or regulations mandating that water heaters be preset to 120°–130°F, rather than the common setting of 150°F, would result in decreased morbidity.[129] At 160°F full-thickness burns occur after a 1-second exposure, whereas a 30-second exposure is necessary to cause the same burn at 130°F and a considerably longer exposure time at 120°F.[130] Assuming a 90 percent reduction in scald burns from tap water if temperature settings in all water heaters were lowered, we estimate that 16–46 lives a year would be saved, and hospitalizations would be reduced from more than 61,000 to approximately 57,000 annually.

A common cause of scalds in children could be prevented by modifications in coffee filters, as demonstrated by the Burn Institute of Copenhagen.[131] Guards on heating stoves, childproof switches on cooking stoves, and wide-bottomed pots that are less likely to tip over are other safeguards.

State regulations governing the use of fireworks dramatically affect fireworks injuries. In Washington State the injury rate from fireworks doubled within a year after the laws were relaxed.[132]

Public knowledge about the immediate treatment of burns, that is, using cold water to reduce the depth of the burn, would considerably reduce the morbidity from burns and might also have some effect on mortality.

Modern treatment in specialized burn centers can greatly improve the survival rate of the seriously injured and decrease the length of hospitalization.[133,134]

Poisoning

Chemicals known to be hazardous should be analyzed to determine whether their potential for harm outweighs their benefits and whether safer substitutes can be used. For example, replacing barbiturates with less toxic hypnotics such as the benzodiazepams resulted in an almost threefold decrease in barbiturate fatalities between 1970 and 1980.[135]

Reducing the contents of packages containing toxic substances (for example, limiting the number of baby aspirin tablets in a bottle to less than the fatal dosage) is also an effective intervention. Restricting antidepressant prescriptions to nonlethal quantities could significantly reduce the ever-increasing number of deaths from antidepressant overdose. Single-dose packaging of potentially lethal drugs is another possible intervention.

Small subtherapeutic doses of an emetic might be added to drugs to prevent poisoning. The emetic would be harmless when the tablets were taken in normal doses but would cause vomiting if excessive quantities of the drug were ingested.[6] Unfortunately, the potential hazards to overdose patients may limit this approach.

Poisoning deaths in children under the age of 5 have declined dramatically since 1960, largely because of changes in formulation and packaging of poisonous agents.[1,136] From 1973, when the Poison Prevention Packaging Act became law, to 1976, there was a 50 percent decrease in drug poisonings of children under the age of 5. This was a substantially greater decrease than that in poisonings by other substances, most of which were not required to be packaged in childproof containers. Packaging dangerous household products in unit doses is an intervention that could further reduce the poisoning of small children: the container, once it had been opened and the contents had been used, would be thrown away.

Between 1947 and 1980, unintentional deaths from domestic gas leaks decreased 96 percent, and poisonings from gas declined a total of 72 percent.[1] The decrease was primarily because of changing from coal gas, which is higher in carbon monoxide, to natural gas. Similar changes occurred in Britain, where suicides from gas poisoning dropped correspondingly, without any increase in suicides by other means.[137,138]

Improved design of motor vehicle bodies and exhaust systems to prevent holes that allow fumes to leak into the car would greatly reduce the number of deaths caused by carbon monoxide poisoning.[139] Some cars have been designed so that, when the engine is running, a slight flow of air through the inside prevents the buildup of exhaust gases.[1] Automatic warning devices that detect abnormal carbon monoxide levels and are linked to a fail-safe device that turns off the engine would prevent most carbon monoxide deaths. Finally, regular safety inspections to check the integrity of the vehicle body and the exhaust system could also reduce the incidence of carbon monoxide poisoning.

Poison control centers all over the country have greatly improved the treatment of victims and provide valuable advice on the toxicity of compounds. Although their impact has not been precisely evaluated, the centers have no doubt contributed to the steady decline in poisoning deaths during the last 20 years.[1]

Suffocation

Fatal choking in children typically involves round objects. The foods most commonly reported in choking incidents are pieces of hot dog, candies, nuts, and grapes[140,141]; round or pliable objects, such as undersized infant pacifiers, small balls, and uninflated or underinflated balloons, are the most commonly reported nonfood items. Parents should be advised of the potential of common foods and objects to cause choking, and they should be taught the Heimlich maneuver.[142] Labeling of the foods that are hazardous for young children, such as the labeling used by Giant Foods, would reinforce parental awareness.[141]

The small parts standards of the Consumer Product Safety Commission (CPSC) preclude the manufacture of products for children under 3 if parts of the broken object could obstruct the airway (i.e., are less than 33 mm in diameter). Balloons, which cause 14 percent of children's deaths from choking on small objects, are excluded from this standard. However, including a 33 mm ring inside the balloon could prevent most of these deaths.

According to one study,[141] 64 percent of all choking in children was caused by vomitus or regurgitated food. This may mask the true underlying cause of death and often reflects other medical conditions.

The term *cafe coronary* describes sudden deaths that occur in adults when food, most often large pieces of meat, lodges in the airway. These deaths often occur in restaurants, where alcohol use and a reluctance to remove unchewable food from the mouth probably play a role.[1] Other contributing factors are drug intoxication, inadequate dentition, and, in the elderly, debilitation.[143] Early recognition and simple first aid by the public can greatly increase survival from such incidents, reducing the number of deaths by perhaps 25 percent for all ages.

Mechanical suffocation and strangulation deaths occur primarily in children. Suffocation is caused by plastic bags and sheeting, plastic sides of playpens and cribs, entrapment in refrigerators and other appliances, and burial under falling earth and other materials.[144] Strangulation is caused by hanging from pacifier cords, clothing, and high chair straps; wedging the head between crib slats or between the mattress and bed frame; and from catching the head in electrically operated car windows. Deaths from suffocation in refrigerators decreased more than 80 percent for units sold in the period 1978–1981 compared with the years 1966–1968. This decline was the result of redesigning refrigerator interiors so that children can escape if trapped inside.[144] Similar reductions might also occur as a result of other design changes, such as designing plastic garment bags with holes, spacing crib slats so they could not cause strangulation, and erecting barriers around sites of potential cave-ins. CPSC now has regulations concerning crib design, but because cribs are typically used for such a long time, it may take some years for the safety regulation to become fully effective.

Natural Environment

In 1980, environmental factors as a cause of death included excessive cold (707 deaths), excessive heat (1,700 deaths), exposure and neglect (415 deaths), reactions to venomous plants and animals (47 deaths), other animal-inflicted injuries (107 deaths), lightning (94 deaths), and cataclysm (tornado, flood, earthquake, etc.; 118 deaths). Although not large, the numbers are subject to wide annual variation and to excessive publicity in comparison with publicity about the number of deaths from other injuries. The 3,194 deaths from natural and environmental factors in 1980 compared with a 12-year average (1968–1980) of 1,270 deaths annually. The high number was a consequence of the "great heat wave" of 1980, which resulted in 1,700 deaths from heatstroke—up from an annual average of approximately 200.[145] Natural and environmental agents are largely unpredictable and difficult to prevent; however, much can be done to minimize the injuries that result.

Modern Doppler radar makes it possible to warn people about approaching tornadoes and hurricanes.[146] Despite the better warnings, tornadoes in the South cause more deaths than in the North, apparently because people do not trust organized warning systems and do not take evasive action.[147] Adequate warnings of flash floods can reduce deaths by 60 percent; monitoring dams regularly during heavy rains is another important source of warnings.[148]

According to studies of tornadoes,[149] the rate of serious injury or death for people in apartment buildings was 1.3 per 1,000 occupants; the rate for people in single-family homes was 3.2 per 1,000; and the rate for people who attempted to flee the storm in cars was 23.2 per 1,000. The highest risk was among residents of mobile homes, whose rate of serious injury or death was 85.1 per 1,000 occupants. Seeking shelter in large, solid buildings thus considerably reduces the risk of injury in tornadoes.

Earthquake prediction is still an evolving science, but with early warning it may be possible to reduce injuries by mass evacuation or by injecting fluids into the ground to build up stress so that the quakes are minor instead of major destructive ones.[150,151] In China, early prediction and relocation of people away from dangerous structures before the earthquakes of 1975 and 1976 are credited with having saved many lives.[152] Volcanic eruptions can now also be predicted with some reliability.[153] In most ski resorts, avalanche control is widely practiced.[154]

According to studies of the 1976 Guatemala earthquake,[155] all deaths and serious injuries occurred in adobe houses, even though 15 percent of the homes in the area were of the traditional wood-and-cornhusk construction. Strengthening existing buildings and enacting stringent building codes for new buildings in high-risk areas, such as California, would significantly reduce injuries from earthquakes. Unfortunately, the costs of these changes often limit their use, especially in less affluent areas where the risks of injury are higher.[18]

Hypothermia primarily occurs in winter and is more common in elderly and debilitated individuals, who often have a decreased perception of cold.[156] Little is known about strategies for preventing hypothermia. Many city governments have tried to reduce the incidence of hypothermia by helping low-income persons pay their winter heating costs. The number of deaths from myocardial infarction increases following major blizzards[157]; however, no specific risk factors have been identified on which to base any preventive recommendations.[158]

In a study of the 1980 heat wave,[145] it was found that people who had 24-hour air conditioning suffered 98 percent fewer heatstrokes than neighbors who had no air conditioning. Spending even part of the day in an air-conditioned building reduced the risk of heatstroke by one fourth; electric fans, however, did not significantly reduce the risk. Persons at high risk, such as the elderly and infirm, should be taken to air-conditioned heat wave shelters for part of the day.

Little is known about the prevention of lightning-related deaths, 28 percent of which occur in open fields, 14 percent under trees, 5 percent in or near water, 4 percent on golf courses, 3 percent at telephones, and 43 percent in unknown locations.[159]

Considerable attention has been directed at planning and managing emergency and rehabilitative efforts to reduce the impact of natural disasters.[160] Recent efforts have also been directed at reducing the psychological and physical problems that follow natural disasters and the problems of relocation.[161]

Firearms

Firearms are second only to motor vehicles as a cause of injury death in the United States. In 1980 almost 34,000 deaths from firearms occurred, of which unintentional ("accidental") deaths represent only 7 percent.

About one half of the 1,955 unintentional firearm deaths in the United States occur in the home,[92] and approximately one in five households has a handgun.[162] Our recommendations for legislation and control are directed primarily at handguns, not all guns. Handguns account for only 20 percent of the firearms in use today, but they are involved in the majority of both criminal and unintentional firearm injuries.[163] An increasing number of local communities are proposing handgun control laws. However, the problem has lain in documenting how well local handgun laws work. Some states, such as New York, have strict laws on ownership but cannot prohibit the importation of handguns from other states.

Possible options for preventing unintentional gun injuries are (1) reducing the availability of guns, especially easily concealed handguns, through federal gun control laws; (2) locking up guns and keeping them out of the reach of children; (3) fostering the use of single-shot guns, which must be reloaded between firings, to reduce the likelihood of accidental firings; (4) requiring hunters to wear bulletproof vests and helmets; (5) minimizing the possibility of inadvertent discharge by better gun design (thus making it more difficult for a child to fire a gun); and (6) using less harmful ammunition in handguns.[1]

Air Transportation

Of any mode of transport, scheduled plane service has the lowest fatality rate per 100 million person miles traveled, a reflection of the success of stringent safety standards and regulations. The high fatality rate in light airplane crashes, however, has received little attention. Of all light aircraft, 60 percent can be expected to crash during the typical 20-year life expectancy for these planes.[164] Adverse weather conditions obviously contribute, though their exact role has not been determined. Postcrash fires, which cause considerable morbidity and mortality, could be prevented by designing more crash-worthy fuel systems, using cabin furnishings that do not ignite easily and will not emit toxic fumes on burning, and devising an improved means of escape from damaged aircraft.[164,165] It is estimated that if planes were designed on the same crash principles as those developed for the automobile, 75 percent of airplane crash fatalities could be prevented (RG Snyder, personal communication, 1984).

Machinery

Of the 1,471 machinery-related deaths in 1980, the vast majority were clearly occupational in origin. Experience, training, and supervision are considered fundamental factors in most occupational safety and accident prevention programs.[166] However, safety training appears to have had only limited effectiveness, and specific factors associated with machine operations in industry seem to be more important. Ergonomic design features of both machines and tasks interact with human behavioral factors, often encouraging risk-taking behavior. For example, wage incentives such as those found in piece rate operations increase injury risks: in order to work faster, the machine operator sometimes deactivates a safety device that normally prevents exposure of the worker's hands to hazardous parts of the machine.

Built-in safety devices will continue to influence the risk of machine injury dramatically. Guards that permit machine operation but do not allow workers to put their hands into hazardous areas are now commonplace. The National Institute for Occupational Safety and Health is conducting research on presence-sensing guard systems that deactivate machinery when hands are placed near hazardous zones.[167] Robotics promises to dramatically reduce workers' exposure to certain machines that have been reponsible for a large number of amputations, lacerations, and fractures.

Many physical features of the work site, as well as elements of the job itself, determine the level of risk. Features such as lighting, climate, and noise indirectly contribute to some injuries. Noise, for example, may mask warning sounds from machines and increase the risk of injury.

Critical to the prevention of one class of job fatalities are the workplace layout and the work practices associated with "lockout/tagout."[168] Fatal injuries occur regularly when an employee begins maintenance or clean-up work on a piece of equipment and a second employee inadvertently starts up the machine. Lockout/tagout procedures are one way of controlling such incidents, but worksite layout may also be altered so that nothing blocks the operator's view of the hazardous part of the machine.

Lack of roll-over protective structures is responsible for approximately 50 percent of the deaths on tractors.[169] Other workplace vehicles that need such safety features include self-powered industrial trucks and construction equipment.

Many large companies have excellent first aid and medical treatment facilities, and medical personnel are available. In these plants, injuries can be treated immediately, but medical treatment services are notably absent from many smaller plants.

Electric Current

Of the 1,095 deaths from electrocution in 1980, about one third occurred in the home.[1] An esti-
mated 600 work-related electrocutions occur each year to workers in agriculture, construction, transportation, and public utilities.[26,170] Contact with high-energy power lines appears to be the leading cause. Prevention includes burying transmission lines, using shorter lengths of irrigation pipes in agriculture, insulating equipment that is likely to come in contact with live wires, and installing ground fault interrupters.[1] Devices exist that can detect electrical fields and either warn equipment operators or immobilize the equipment (e.g., crane booms) so that workers cannot contact live wires.

Being Struck by a Falling Object

Little information is available about the specific cause of these injuries. Fatalities caused on the job by falling objects occur primarily in the timber and logging industries when woodsmen are struck by falling trees and limbs.[171] Logging hazards are doubly threatening because of the remoteness of the typical logging work site and lack of ready access to emergency medical services. Education, enforcement of safety rules, an alertness are the keys to avoiding these injuries. Protective equipment, including adequate head protection, is probably of limited benefit in logging injuries but offers significant protection from most falling objects.

SUMMARY

Injuries make a substantial impact on the duration and quality of our lives. To many people, injuries are considered the result of accidents. The definition of *accident* implies inevitability or carelessness, raising the concept of blame or fault. However, injuries are not simply the outcome of accidents; rather, they are often highly predictable events. We already know much about the causes of injuries and risk factors—such as characteristics of time, place, and person—and numerous effective preventive measures exist. We have identified four mixed-intervention strategies that, based on our estimates, could prevent more than half of all injury-related deaths (Figure 5). They include the following.

1. *Motor vehicle safety program.* We estimate that a broad-based mixed strategy could reduce motor vehicle fatalities, injuries, and costs by as much as 75 percent. This program would include installation of air bags, enactment and enforcement of seat belt and child restraint laws, control of vehicle speed, improved road design, and the maximum use of available technology to design a safe, crashworthy vehicle.

2. *Home injury program.* Approximately 23,000 deaths from unintentional injuries occur in the

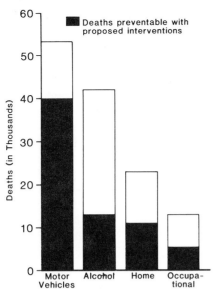

Figure 5. Total number of deaths from unintentional injuries and deaths preventable by proposed interventions.

home annually[9]: 6,700 from fatal falls, 4,400 from burns and fires, 3,100 from poisonings, 2,400 from suffocation, 1,100 from unintentional firearms injuries, 900 from drownings (largely children under 5 years of age), and 4,400 from other causes. It was estimated that a targeted intervention program directed at these and other home injuries could reduce all home-based injuries by approximately 50 percent.

3. *Occupational injury control program.* Of the estimated 13,000 occupational injury deaths that occur annually, one third are caused by motor vehicle crashes, 75 percent of which we estimate to be preventable. The remaining two thirds of the fatalities are from falls, industrial equipment, being struck by falling objects, electrocutions, and firearms. Using what little data are available, we estimate that 25 percent of the other occupational injury deaths (i.e., the two thirds not related to motor vehicles) could be prevented. This percentage might be increased significantly if basic prevention principles are applied to the occupational setting and further injury control research is done. For all causes combined, we estimate that about 40 percent of the deaths and serious injuries from occupational injuries could be prevented, resulting in about 5,200 fewer deaths annually.

4. *Alcohol intervention program.* If a broad-based societal approach to alcohol usage were initiated, a reduction of about 25 percent in all fatal and serious injuries could probably be achieved. Other injury control measures such as seat belts and air bags would also reduce alcohol-related injuries. A program specifically targeted at problem drinkers must

be an essential component of any effort to control alcohol use. Any program that reduces unintentional alcohol-related injuries will also greatly reduce the incidence of alcohol-related diseases.

We believe that the gap between what is and what could be is larger for unintentional injuries than for any single disease. Unfortunately, many of the interventions proposed are likely to encounter considerable political barriers from special interest groups. And yet, if we are to increase life expectancy and "close the gap" in the United States, the most effective means, using the technology we have, is through intensive injury control programs such as those we propose. Implementing these measures will demand the concerted efforts of local, state, and federal governments, corporations, health care systems, private organizations, and perhaps most of all, individuals.

Pat Coleman, Ph.D., Division of Safety Research, National Institute for Occupational Safety and Health, Morgantown, West Virginia, assisted with the occupational injuries section. Lawrence Budnick, M.D., and Edwin Kilbourne, M.D., both with the Special Studies Branch, Chronic Diseases Division, Center for Environmental Health, Centers for Disease Control, assisted with the sections on drowning and environmentally related injuries, respectively.

REFERENCES

1. Baker SP, O'Neill B, Karpf RS. The injury fact book. Lexington, Massachusetts: Lexington Books, 1984.

2. Wintemute GJ. The size of the problem. In: Wintemute GJ, Baker SP, Baker D, et al., eds. Principles for injury prevention. New York: World Health Organization, 1985:217–40.

3. Current estimates from the National Interview Survey: United States, 1980. Hyattsville, Maryland: National Center for Health Statistics, 1981; DHHS publication no. (PHS)82-1567. (Vital and health statistics; Series 10; no. 139).

4. Faigin BM. 1975 societal costs of motor vehicle accidents. Washington, D.C.: Department of Transportation, report no. DOT-HS 802 119, 1976.

5. Haddon W Jr, Baker SP. Injury control. In: Clark D, MacMahon B, eds. Preventive and community medicine. 3rd ed. Boston: Little, Brown, 1981:109–60.

6. Robertson LS. Injuries: causes, control strategies, and public policy. Lexington, Massachusetts: Lexington Books, 1983.

7. Barancik JI, Chatterjee, Greene YC, et al. Northeastern Ohio trauma study. I. Magnitude of the problem. Am J Public Health 1983;73:746–51.

8. Hartunian NS, Smart CN, Thompson MS. The incidence and economic cost of cancer, motor vehicle injuries, coronary, heart disease, and stroke: a comparative analysis. Am J Public Health 1980;70:1249–60.

9. Accident facts. Chicago: National Safety Council, 1981.

10. Jones RK, Joscelyn KB. Alcohol and highway safety 1978: a review of the state of knowledge. Washington,

D.C.: Department of Transportation, report no. DOT HS-803 764, 1978.

11. Fell JC. Alcohol involvement in traffic accidents: recent estimates from the national center for statistics and analysis. Washington, D.C.: Department of Transportation, report no. DOT HS-806 269, 1982.

12. Berkelman RL, Herndon JL, Callaway JL, et al. Fatal injuries and alcohol. Am J Prev Med 1985;1:21–8.

13. Cohen J, Dearnaley EJ, Hansel CEM. The risk taken in driving vehicles under the influence of alcohol. Br Med J 1958;1:1438–42.

14. Hyman MM. Accidental vulnerability and blood alcohol concentrations of drivers by demographic characteristics. Q J Stud Alcohol 1968;29(4):34–57.

15. Zylman R. Age is more important than alcohol in the collision—involvement of young and old drivers. J Traffic Safety Educ 1972;20(1);7–8,34.

16. Baker SP, Spitz WU. Age effects and autopsy evidence in disease in fatally injured drivers. JAMA 1970;214:1079–88.

17. Waller JA. Identification of problem drinking among drunken drivers. JAMA 1967;200:114–20.

18. Waller JA. Injury control: a guide to the causes and prevention of trauma. Lexington, Massachusetts: Lexington Books, 1985.

19. Alcohol and violent death—Erie County, New York, 1973–1983. Morbid Mortal Weekly Rep 1984;33:226–7.

20. Wechsler H, Kasey EH, Thum D, et al. Alcohol level and home accidents. Public Health Rep 1969;84:1043–53.

21. Baker SP, Samkoff JS, Fisher RS, et al. Fatal occupational injuries. JAMA 1982;248:692–7.

22. Dietz PE, Baker SP. Drowning—epidemiology and prevention. Am J Public Health 1974;64:303–12.

23. Mierley MC, Baker SP. Fatal house fires in an urban population. JAMA 1983;249:1466–8.

24. Joscelyn KB, Maickel RP. Report on an international symposium on drugs and driving. Springfield, Virginia: National Technical Information Service, report no. DOT HS-4-00994-75-1, 1975.

25. Moskowitz H. Introduction to special issue on drugs and driving. Accident Anal Prev 1976;8:1.

26. Moskowitz H. Introduction to special issue on drugs and driving. Accident Anal Prev 1986;17:281–2.

27. Leading work-related diseases and injuries—United States. Morbid Mortal Weekly Rep 1984;33:213–5.

28. Occupational mortality in the oil industry—Louisiana. Morbid Mortal Weekly Rep 1980;29:230–1.

29. 1980 annual death and injury survey. Washington, D.C.: International Association of Fire Fighters, 1980.

30. Robertson LS, Zador PL. Driver education and fatal crash involvement of teenaged drivers. Am J Public Health 1978;68:959–65.

31. Robertson LS. Estimates of motor vehicle seat belt effectiveness and use: implications for crash protection. Am J Public Health 1976;66:859–64.

32. Robertson LS, Haddon W Jr. The buzzer-light reminder system and safety belt use. Am J Public Health 1974;64:814–5.

33. Robertson LS. Crash involvement of teenage drivers when driver education is eliminated from high school. Am J Public Health 1980;70:599–603.

34. Robertson LS. Insurance incentives and seat belt use. Am J Public Health 1984;74:1157–8.

35. Reisinger KS, Williams AF. Evaluation of program designed to increase the protection of infants in cars. Pediatrics 1978;62:280–7.

36. Reisinger KS, Williams AF, Wells JK. Effect of pediatricians' counseling on infant restraint use. Pediatrics 1981;67:201–6.

37. Robertson LS, Kelley AB, O'Neill B, et al. A controlled study of the effect of television messages on safety belt use. Am J Public Health 1974;64:1071–80.

38. Derschewitz RA, Williamson JW. Prevention of childhood household injuries: a controlled clinical trial. Am J Public Health 1977;67:1148–53.

39. Miller RE, Reisinger KS, Blatter MM, et al. Pediatric counseling and subsequent use of smoke detectors. Am J Public Health 1982;72:392–3.

40. Robertson LS. Present status of knowledge in childhood injury prevention. In: Bergman AB, ed. Preventing childhood injuries: report of the twelfth Ross roundtable on critical approaches to common pediatric problems. Columbus, Ohio: Ross Laboratories, 1982:1–13.

41. Haddon W Jr, Goddard JL. An analysis of highway safety strategies. In: Passenger car design and highway safety. New York: Association for the Aid of Crippled Children and Consumers Union of the US, 1961.

42. Robertson LS. Behavioral research and strategies in public health: a demur. Soc Sci Med 1975;9:165.

43. Haddon W Jr. Options for prevention of motor vehicle injury. Isr J Med Sci 1980;16:45–65.

44. Haddon W Jr. Advances in the epidemiology of injuries as a basis for public policy. Am J Public Health 1980;95:411–21.

45. Haddon W Jr. A logical framework for categorizing highway safety phenomena and activity. J Trauma 1982;12:193–207.

46. Baptiste MS, Feck G. Preventing tap water burns. Am J Public Health 1980;70:727–9.

47. Robertson LS. Automobile safety regulations and death reductions in the United States. Am J Public Health 1981;71:818–22.

48. Effectiveness, benefits, and costs of federal safety standards for protection of passenger car occupants. Washington, D.C.: Department of Transportation, 1976.

49. McGuire A. Cigarettes and fire death. NY State J Med 1983;83:1296–7.

50. Teret SP, DeFrancesco S. The Cigarette Safety Bill: a case study in injury control advocacy. J Public Health Policy 1983;4:440–6.

51. Watson GS, Zador PL, Wilks A. The repeal of helmet use laws and increased motorcyclist mortality in the USA: 1975–1978. Am J Public Health 1980;70:579–85.

52. Baker SP. Who bought the cars in which people are injured? an exploratory study. Am J Public Health 1979;69:76–8.

53. Teret SP. Injury control and product liability. J Public Health Policy 1981;2:49–57.

54. Insurance Institute for Highway Safety. Woman sues automaker for failure to install air bags. Status Rep 1984;19(11):5.

55. Robertson LS, Keeve JP. Worker injuries: the effects of workers compensation and OSHA inspectors. J Health Polit Policy Law 1983;8:581–97.

56. Margolis B, Kroes W. The human side of accident prevention. Springfield, Illinois: Charles C Thomas, 1975.

57. Smith RS. The feasibility of an injury tax approach to safety. Law Contemp Prob 1974;38:730–44.

58. Kraus JF, Black MA, Hessol P, et al. The incidence of acute brain injury and serious impairment in a defined population. Am J Epidemiol 1984;119:186–201.

59. Trunkey DD. Trauma. Sci Am 1983;249(2):28–36.

60. Smith JP, Bodai BI. The urban paramedic's scope of practice. JAMA 1985;235:544–8; and responding letters in JAMA 1986;225:609–12.

61. Mosher JF, Beauchamp DE. Justifying alcohol taxes to public officials. J Public Health Policy 1983;4:422–39.

62. Alcohol and health: fourth special report to the US Congress. Rockville, Maryland: US Dept of Health and Human Services, National Institute on Alcohol Abuse and Alcoholism, 1981.

63. Miller PE, Nirenbert TD, McClure G. Prevention of alcohol abuse. In: Tabakoff B, Sutken PB, Randall CL, eds. Medical and social aspects of alcohol abuse. New York: Plenum, 1983.

64. Warner KE. Smoking and health implications of a change in the federal cigarette excise tax. JAMA 1986;255:1028–32.

65. O'Neill B. Recent trends in motor vehicle crash deaths. Presented at the meeting of the American Association for Automotive Medicine, San Antonio, Texas, 1983.

66. Cook P. The effect of liquor taxes on drinking, cirrhosis, and auto accidents. In: Moore MH, Gersteion DR, eds. Alcohol and public policy: beyond the shadow of prohibition. Washington, D.C.: National Academy Press, 1981.

67. Council on Alcohol Policy. Q Newsletter 1984;3:1–7.

68. Holder HD, Blose JO. Reduction of community alcohol problems: a community solution. Presented at the 111th annual meeting of the American Public Health Association, Dallas, Texas 1983.

69. Mosher JF: Server intervention: a new approach for preventing drinking and driving. Accident Anal Prev 1983;15:483–97.

70. Mosher JF: Server intervention: present status and future prospects. Presented at the Research Workshop on Alcohol and the Drinking Driver, National Institute of Alcoholism and Addiction and the meeting of the National Highway Traffic Safety Administration, Bethesda, Maryland, 1984.

71. Williams AF, Zador PL, Harris SS, et al. The effects of raising the legal minimum drinking age on fatal crash involvement. J Leg Stud 1983;12:169–79.

72. Hammond R. Moderate alcohol use threat to liquor industry. Alcoholism: the national magazine 1983 Jan–Feb:63.

73. Ross HL. Deterring the drinking driver: legal policy and social control. Lexington, Massachusetts: Lexington Books, 1982.

74. Ross LR. The Scandinavian myth: the effectiveness of drinking-and-driving legislation in Sweden and Norway. J Leg Stud 1975;4:285–310.

75. Report of NHTSA Task Force to Analyze the Effectiveness of Various Restraint Systems. Washington, D.C.: Department of Transportation, 1984.

76. Losses, personal injury protection coverages: injury claim frequencies for Volkswagen Rabbits with automatic and manual seat belts, 1981 and 1982 models. Washington, D.C.: Highway Loss Data Institute Insurance, report no. HLDIA-21, 1984.

77. Williams AF. Observed child restraint use in automobiles. Am J Dis Child 1976;130:1311–7.

78. American Academy of Pediatrics, Committee on Accident and Poison Prevention: Automatic passenger protection systems. J Pediatr 1984;74:146–7.

79. Williams AF, Wells JK. The Tennessee child restraint law in its third year. Am J Public Health 1981;71:163–5.

80. Williams AF, Wells JK: Evaluation of the Rhode Island child restraint law. Am J Public Health 1981;71: 742–3.

81. Decker MD, Dewey MJ, Hutcheson RH Jr, et al. The use and efficacy of child restraint devices. JAMA 1984;252:2571–5.

82. Hurt HH, Ouellet JV, Thom DR. Motorcycle accident cause factors and identification of counter measures, vol. 1. Springfield, Virginia: National Technical Information Service, report no. DOT HS-805-862, 1981.

83. Muller A. An evaluation of the effectiveness of motorcycle headlight use laws. Am J Public Health 1982;72:1136–41.

84. Zador P. How effective are daytime motorcycle headlight use laws? Am J Public Health 1983;73:808.

85. Fatal accident reporting system, 1980. Washington, D.C.: Department of Transportation, report no. DOT HS-805-953, 1981.

86. Fife D, Davis J, Tate L, et al. Fatal injuries to bicyclists: the experience of Dade County, Florida. J Trauma 1983;23:745–55.

87. Malone TB, Kirkpatrick M, Kohl JS, et al. Field test evaluation of rear lighting systems. Springfield, Virginia: National Technical Information Service, 1978.

88. Rausch A, Wong J, Kirkpatrick M. A field test of two single center, high mounted break light systems. Accident Anal Prev 1982;14:287–91.

89. Stein H. Fleet experience with daytime running lights in the United States—preliminary results. Washington, D.C.: Insurance Institute for Highway Safety, 1984:26.

90. DiNapoli N. Research safety vehicle phase LI: comprehensive technical results, vol. II. Springfield, Virginia: National Technical Information Service, 1977.

91. Insurance Institute for Highway Safety. A special issue: small car deaths, injuries worst; models vary greatly. Status Rep 1982;17(20):1–11.

92. Baker SP, Dietz PE. Injury prevention. In: Healthy People: The Surgeon General's Report on Health Promotion and Disease Prevention: Background Papers. Washington, D.C.: US Government Printing Office, 1979: DHEW publication no. (PHS)79-55071A.

93. Williams AF, Karpf RS, Zador PL. Variations in minimum licensing age and fatal motor vehicle crashes. Am J Public Health 1983;73:1401–3.

94. Preusser DF, Williams AF, Zador PL, et al. The effect of curfew laws on motor vehicle crashes. Law Policy 1983;6:115–28.

95. Williams AF, Karpf RS. Teenage drivers and fatal crash responsibility. Law Policy 1984;6:101–13.

96. Baker SP, Robertson LS, O'Neill B. Fatal pedestrian collisions. Am J Public Health 1974;64:319–25.

97. Ashton SJ. Vehicle design and pedestrian injuries. In: Chapman AJ, Wade FM, Foot HC, eds. Pedestrian accidents. New York: Wiley, 1982.

98. Ashton SJ, Pedder JB, Mackay GM. Pedestrian leg injuries, the bumper and other front structures. Presented at the third International Conference on Impact Trauma of the International Research Committee on the Biokinetics of Impacts, Berlin, 1977.

99. Weiss EB Jr, Pritz HB, Hassler CR. Experimental automobile–pedestrian injuries. J Trauma 1977;17:823–8.

100. Kelley AB, Hebert R. Boobytrap! 16 mm teaching film. New York: Harvest A-V Inc., 1972.

101. Wright PH, Robertson LS. Priorities for roadside hazard modification. Washington, D.C.: Insurance Institute for Highway Safety, 1976.

102. Wright PH, Zador P. A study of fatal overturning crashes in Georgia. Transport Res Rec 1981;819:8–17.

103. Zador PL, Wright PH, Karpf RS. Effect of pavement markers on nighttime crashes in Georgia. Transport Res Rec (in press).

104. Stimpson WA, Zador PL, Tarnoff PJ. The influence of the time duration of yellow traffic signals on driver response. Inst Transp Eng J 1980 Nov:22–9.

105. Zador P, Stein H, Shapiro S, Tarnoff P. The effect of signal timing on traffic flow and crashes at signalized intersections, Res Rec 1985.

106. Waller JA. Falls among the elderly—human and environmental factors. Accident Anal Prev 1978;10:21–33.

107. Riggs BL, Hodson SF, Hoffman DL, et al. Treatment of primary osteoporosis with fluoride and calcium. JAMA 1980;243:446–9.

108. Weiss NS, Ure CL, Ballard JH, et al. Decreased risk of fractures of the hip and lower forearm with post menopausal use of estrogen. N Engl J Med 1980;303;1195–8.

109. The epidemiology of accident traumas and resulting disabilities. Report on a World Health Organization Symposium. Euro Reports and Studies 57, 1982.

110. Haddon W Jr. Energy damage and the ten countermeasure strategies. J Trauma 1973;12:321.

111. Grubel F. Falls: a principal patient incident. Hosp Manage 1959;88:37–8,137.

112. Rubenstein HS, Miller FH, Postel S, et al. Standards of medical care based on consensus rather than evidence: the case for routine bedrail use for the elderly. Law Med Health Care 1983 Dec:271–6.

113. Hongladarom GC. Analysis of the causes and prevention of injuries attributed to falls. Olympia, Washington: Department of Social and Health Services, 1977.

114. Wild D, Nayak US, Isaacs B. How dangerous are falls in old people at home? Br Med J [Clin Res] 1981;282:266–8.

115. Speigel CN, Lindaman FC. Children can't fly: a program to prevent childhood morbidity and mortality from window falls. Am J Public Health 1977;67:1143–7.

116. Bergner L. Environmental factors in injury control: preventing falls from heights. In: Bergman AB, ed. Preventing childhood injuries. Report of the Twelfth Ross Roundtable on Critical Approaches to Common Pediatric Problems. Columbus, Ohio: Ross Laboratories, 1982;57–60.

117. Safety in summer: window guards. NY Times 1984 July 14:48.

118. Metropolitan Life Insurance Company. Accidental drowning by cause and site. Stat Bull 1977;58(June):9–11.

119. Kropp RM, Schwartz JF. Water intoxication from swimming. J Pediatr 1982;101:947–8.

120. Pearn J, Nixon J. Prevention of childhood drowning accidents. Med J Aust 1977;1:616–8.

121. US Coast Guard. Boating Statistics 1982. Washington, D.C.: Department of Transportation, report no. COMDTINST M16754.1D, 1982.

122. Berger LR. Childhood injuries: recognition and prevention. Curr Probl Pediatr 1981;12:1–59.

123. Garner LM, Lowe DM, Jones SB. A community action approach for prevention of burn injuries: Missouri Division of Health. Washington, D.C.: US Government Printing Office; DHEW publication no. (HSM)72-10008, 1972.

124. McLoughlin E, Vince CJ, Lee AM, et al. Project burn prevention: outcome and implications. Am J Public Health 1982;72:241–7.

125. US Fire Administration. An evaluation of residential smoke detector performance under actual field conditions: final report. Emmitsburg, Maryland: Federal Emergency Management Agency, 1980.

126. Clarke FB, Birky MM. Fire safety in dwellings and public buildings. Bull NY Acad Med 1981;57:1047–60.

127. McLoughlin E. The Cigarette Safety Act. J Public Health Pol 1982;3:226–8.

128. McLoughlin E, Clarke M, Stahl K, et al. One pediatric burn unit's experience with sleepwear-related injuries. Pediatrics 1977;60:405–9.

129. Wilson RP Jr, Lee WD, Ashley LE. The feasibility of lowering water heater temperature as a means of re-

ducing scald hazards. Cambridge, Massachusetts: Arthur D. Little, 1977.

130. Mortiz AR, Henriques CF Jr. Studies in thermal injury. II. The relative importance of causation of cutaneous burns. Am J Pathol 1947;23:695–720.

131. Sørensen B. Prevention of burns and scalds in a developed country. J Trauma 1976;16:249–56.

132. Harris JR, Kobayashi JM, Frost F. Injuries from fireworks. JAMA 1983;249:2460.

133. Feller I, Tholen D, Cornell RG. Improvement in burn care, 1965 to 1979. JAMA 1980;244:2074–8.

134. Demling RH. Burns (medical progress). N Engl J Med 1985;313:1389–98.

135. Oliver RG, Hetzel BS. Rise and fall of suicide rates in Australia: relation to sedative availability. Med J Aust 1972;2:919–23.

136. Walton WW. An evaluation of the Poison Prevention Packaging Act. Pediatrics 1982;69:363–70.

137. Alphey RS, Leach SJ. Accidental death in the home. R Soc Health J 1974;94:97–102.

138. Hassall C, Trethowan WH. Suicide in Birmingham. Br Med J 1972;1:717–8.

139. Baker SP, Fisher RS, Masemore WC, et al. Fetal unintentional carbon monoxide poisoning in motor vehicles. Am J Public Health 1972;62:1463–7.

140. Baker SP, Fisher RS. Childhood asphyxiation by choking or suffocation. JAMA 1980;244:1343–6.

141. Harris CS, Baker SP, Smith GA, et al. Childhood asphyxiation by food: a national analysis and overview. JAMA 1984;251:2231–5.

142. Koop CE. The Heimlich maneuver. Public Health Rep 1985;100:557.

143. Mittleman RE, Wetli CV. The fatal cafe coronary: foreign body obstruction. JAMA 1982;247:1285–8.

144. Kraus JF. Effectiveness of measures to prevent unintentional deaths of infants and children from suffocation and strangulation. Public Health Rep 1985;100:231–40.

145. Kilbourne EM, Choi K, Jones TS, Thacker SB. Risk factors for heat stroke: a case control study. JAMA 1982;247:3332–6.

146. Kerr RA. Doppler radar: new look into violent weather. Science 1978;202:1172–4.

147. Sims JH, Bauman DD. The tornado threat: coping styles of the North and South. Science 1972;176:1386–92.

148. French J, Ing R, Von Allmen S, et al. Mortality from flash floods: a review of National Weather Service reports, 1969–81. Public Health Rep 1983;98:584–8.

149. Glass RI, Craven DJ, Bregman DJ, et al. Injuries from the Wichita Falls tornado: implications for prevention. Science 1980;207:734–8.

150. Harlow DH, White RA, Cifuentes JL. Quiet zone within a seismic gap near western Nicaragua: possible location of a future large earthquake. Science 1981;213:648–51.

151. Raleigh CB, Healy JH, Bredehaeft JD. An experiment in earthquake control at Rangely, Colorado. Science 1976;191:1230–7.

152. Shapley D. Chinese earthquakes: the Maoist approach to seismology. Science 1976;193:656–7.

153. Kerr RA. Mount St. Helens: an unpredictable foe. Science 1980;208:1446–8.

154. Hartline BK. Snow physics and avalanche protection. Science 1979;203:346–8.

155. Glass RI, Urrutia JJ, Sibony S, et al. Earthquake injuries related to housing in a Guatemalan village. Science 1977;197:638–43.

156. Milner JE. Hypothermia [Editorial]. Ann Intern Med 1978;89:565–7.

157. Glass RI, Zack MM. Increase in deaths from ischaemic heart disease after blizzards. Lancet 1979;1:485–7.

158. Glass RI, Weisenthal AM, Zack MM, et al. Risk factors for myocardial infarction associated with the Chicago snowstorm of Jan 13–15, 1979. JAMA 1981;245:164–5.

159. Vigansky HN. General summary of lightning. Storm Data 1982;24(12):40–6.

160. Emergency health management after national disasters. Washington, D.C.: Pan American Health Organization, scientific publication no. 407, 1981.

161. Longue JN, Hansen H, Struening E. Some indications of the long-term health effects of a natural disaster. Public Health Rep 1981;96:67–79.

162. Alviana JD, Drake WR. Handgun control: issues and alternatives. Presented at the 43rd annual meeting of the United States Conference of Mayors, Washington, D.C., 1975.

163. Crime in the United States, 1979: FBI Uniform Crime Reports. Washington, D.C.: Department of Justice, 1979.

164. Snyder RG. Survival in airplane crashes. University of Michigan Transportation Research Institute Res Rev 1983;13:1–11.

165. Snyder RG. Comparison of automobile and airplane crashes: implications for preventing injuries. In: Proceedings of the American Medical Association Conference on Prevention of Disabling Injuries. Chicago: American Medical Association, 1983.

166. Accident prevention for industrial operations. Chicago: National Safety Council, 1982.

167. Barash M, Etherton J. Experimental self-tripping systems for semi-automated metal stamping: design safety, reliability, and quality. In Proceedings of the Sixth International System Safety Conference, Houston, Texas, 1983.

168. Pettit T, Concha S, Linn H. Application and use of interlock safety devices. Hazard Prev 1983 Nov–Dec:4–9.

169. Simpson S. Farm machinery injuries. J Trauma 1984;24:150–2.

170. Occupational injuries and illnesses in the United States by industry, 1981. Washington, D.C.: Department of Labor, 1981.

171. Frazier T, Coleman P. Job injuries among loggers. Washington, D.C.: US Government Printing Office; DHHS publication no. 83-104, 1983.

172. Public use data tapes—mortality. Hyattsville, Maryland: National Center for Health Statistics, 1980.

Violence: Homicide, Assault, and Suicide

Mark L. Rosenberg, M.D., Richard J. Gelles, Ph.D.,
Paul C. Holinger, M.D., M.P.H., Margaret A. Zahn, Ph.D.,
Evan Stark, Ph.D., Judith M. Conn, M.S.,
Nancy N. Fajman, M.M.Sc., and Trudy A. Karlson, Ph.D.

Violence poses a new challenge for public health in the United States. Defined here as the use of force with the intent to harm oneself or another, violence is not a medical or public health problem in the traditional sense, nor is it a problem that can be prevented or treated by medical means alone. It is, however, an appropriate and important focus for public health, in concert with allied disciplines such as sociology, criminology, economics, law, public policy, psychiatry, anthropology, and education. Modern-day public health is not powerless against violence, and, in fact, plays a key role in the coalition of contributing disciplines. Knowledge from all relevant fields can be applied to new programs in police departments, welfare and child protective services, shelters for battered women, rape crisis centers, health care facilities, and the courts.

This study focuses on homicide, assault, and suicide. Better data are available for fatal outcomes than for nonfatal injuries; nevertheless, this study also examines aggravated assault and the abuse of women and children, because the health and social costs of these forms of violence are so high. The costs of all three forms of violence are measured in terms not only of morbidity and mortality but also of the impact they can have on the quality of life and the drain on health care resources.

Because the lives lost to violence are so often those of young people, homicide and suicide rank fourth and fifth, respectively, among all health problems for years of potential life lost. The abuse of women may be the most frequent cause of physical injury for which women seek medical attention —more common than automobile injuries, rape, and mugging combined. In 1980 alone, suicide, homicide, and aggravated assault taken together accounted for more than 50,000 deaths, 1.3 million years of potential life lost, 1.8 million hospital days, and $754 million in health care costs.

DEFINITIONS

Homicide, criminal or noncriminal. The latter category includes justifiable or excusable homicides (such as those committed in self-defense or in the line of duty by a police officer) and negligent homicides.

Domestic violence, assault or homicide. Injuries inflicted on one member of a family by another family member. Since the Uniform Crime Reports data do not indicate whether the victim and perpetrator lived together—a common criterion for definitions of "domestic" violence—we use the surrogate term "family" violence to denote acts in which the victim and perpetrator are blood relatives, married, or ex-husband/ex-wife.

Friends' and acquaintances' homicides. A known, nonfamilial relationship between victim and offender. The category "friend" includes persons who are acquainted (including boyfriend/girlfriend), work together, or are known to each other.

Stranger homicides. Murders in which the victim and killer are known not to have had a prior relationship.

Aggravated assaults. These are defined by the Federal Bureau of Investigation as one of the following: (1) an attack with a weapon, regardless of whether injury resulted; (2) an attack without a

From the Division of Injury Epidemiology and Control, Center for Environmental Health and Injury Control, Centers for Disease Control, Atlanta (Rosenberg and Conn), the Department of Community Medicine, Emory University School of Medicine, Atlanta, (Fajman), the Faculty of Arts and Sciences, University of Rhode Island, Kingston (Gelles), the Department of Psychiatry, Michael Reese Hospital, Rush–Presbyterian–St. Luke Medical Center, Chicago (Holinger), the Department of Sociology, Temple University, Philadelphia (Zahn), the Department of Public Administration, Rutgers University, Newark, New Jersey (Stark), and the Center for Health Systems Research and Analysis, University of Wisconsin, Madison (Karlson).

Address reprint requests to Dr. Rosenberg, Division of Injury Epidemiology and Control, CEHIC, Koger F-36, CDC, 1600 Clifton Road, Atlanta, GA 30333.

weapon, resulting either in serious injury (e.g., broken bones, loss of teeth, loss of consciousness) or in undetermined injury necessitating two or more days of hospitalizations; or (3) an attempted assault with a weapon.

Suicide attempts. Nonfatal outcomes of intentional self-destructive acts.

Suicides. Fatalities resulting from intentional self-destructive acts.

DATA SOURCES

The true incidence of violence is difficult to determine. Morbidity, particularly that related to domestic violence, often goes unreported. Suicides and suicide attempts are underreported, either deliberately (to "spare" the family or to avoid losing life insurance benefits) or unintentionally. Lack of uniformity in data collection results in underestimated homicides.

The following sources supplied the majority of our data. Each source is briefly described, and its limitations are noted.

Federal Bureau of Investigation Uniform Crime Reports (UCR) (1980). Over 15,000 city, county, and state law enforcement agencies report the number of "actual offenses known" to the FBI–UCR program for (1) the crimes of murder and nonnegligent manslaughter, rape, robbery, aggravated assault, burglary, larceny–theft, motor vehicle theft, and arson; and (2) the noncriminal acts of justifiable homicide and negligent manslaughter.

Data are forwarded to the FBI one month after the reported occurrence. For all reported homicides, information is included on the age, race, and sex of the victim, the relationship of the offender to the victim, and other information on the victim and offender in the Supplementary Homicide Report (SHR). For cases that are "unsolved" at that one-month mark, the relationship between perpetrator and victim is listed as unknown. Although this relationship may subsequently be clarified, the initial report ("relationship unknown") stands and is counted in the final statistics for the year. Each year, data are incomplete for approximately 5–10 percent of the total murder and nonnegligent manslaughter cases because (1) SHRs are not submitted by the reporting agency or (2) the agency did not submit reports to the UCR program for all or part of the year. In the second instance, the UCR program estimates the number of cases based on data from the months for which reports were actually received or based on the crime rate for all agencies with the same jurisdiction size. For the present study, infor-

mation on the age, race, sex, and relationship of the offender and victim was obtained from the SHR for murder and nonnegligent manslaughter and justifiable homicide.

No federal laws require reporting to the FBI–UCR program, but 39 states have their own mandatory state reporting requirements.

National Crime Survey (NCS) (1980). Survey estimates of aggravated assaults are obtained from a stratified, multistage cluster sample of approximately 62,000 households. All persons 12 years of age or over within each selected household are eligible to be interviewed. The incidence of victimization—along with information on medical treatment, property loss, characteristics of the victim, relationship of the victim to the offender, whether the police were notified, and other pertinent details of each event—is obtained from each respondent.

Any estimate of the amount of crime that is based upon either the UCR or the NCS (victimization surveys) will undercount the amount of actual crime. This is partially because neither source can include "hidden" crimes. The UCR cannot include crimes unless they come to the attention of the police, and one recent study based on hospital emergency room records showed that four times as many aggravated assaults were reported to the hospital than were reported to the police;[1] the NCS cannot include information about incidents unless a victim is both willing and able to report. An additional source of undercounting results from the crime hierarchy that these systems use (rape, robbery, aggravated assault, burglary, larceny, and motor vehicle theft). Thus, a person who was robbed and assaulted would be classified only as a robbery victim, and the robber/assaulter's arrest would be classified solely as a robbery arrest in the UCR.

National Study of the Incidence and Severity of Child Abuse (1979–1980). National estimates were made from a stratified random sample of 26 counties clustered within the ten states of Arizona, California, Georgia, Illinois, Kansas, Missouri, New Hampshire, New York, Ohio, and South Carolina. The cases of child abuse and neglect for this study were all confirmed child abuse and child neglect cases received by (1) the County Child Protective Services agency between May 1, 1979, and April 30, 1980, excluding reports immediately referred to other agencies; (2) other agencies that may have statutory authority for investigating or treating situations involving child abuse or neglect (e.g., county sheriff's department, juvenile court, county public health department); and (3) institutions and agencies whose staff may encounter abused or neglected children (e.g., public schools, short-stay general hospitals). Information on age, severity of injury, type of abuse or neglect, and annual family income was obtained for each confirmed case in the study.

National Center for Health Statistics (NCHS) Mortality Data Tape (1980). NCHS compiles information from death certificates, which probably underestimates the true number of suicides by at least 25–40 percent. All deaths for which the cause was determined to be a self-inflicted injury (ICD-9 codes E950–E959) were used in this report to estimate the number of suicides that occurred in 1980.

Suicide attempts. There are no adequate data on the national incidence or characteristics of suicide attempts. We estimated the number and characteristics of suicide attempters from a variety of relatively small studies reported in the medical literature.

HOMICIDES AND AGGRAVATED ASSAULTS

Impact on Health

Mortality. Homicide is not distributed evenly throughout the population. It takes its greatest toll among minorities, males, and the young. In 1980 approximately 78 percent of homicide victims were male, and nearly 59 percent were males between the ages of 15 and 34, even though that age group constitutes only 35 percent of the population. Blacks and other racial minorities, who make up only 17 percent of the total population, were the victims of approximately 46 percent of homicides. Among children, those under 3 and over 14 years of age are most vulnerable to murder; again, black and other nonwhite males are at greatest risk.

Geographically, the highest homicide rates occur in a band of southern states stretching from California to North and South Carolina. Homicide rates are generally higher in urban than in rural areas, and the rates for young black males are highest in large cities in the north central part of the nation.[2]

In 1980 homicides in the United States accounted for at least 23,970 deaths and more than 690,000 potential years of life lost before age 65. The toll may be greater because some homicides are misclassified as accidents or listed as "cause of death unknown." In potential years of life lost, homicide ranked fourth among all causes of death. Homicide was 11th on the list of causes of death for all races; for black and other nonwhites 15–34 years of age, it was the leading cause of death.

Males are 3.5 times more likely to be murdered than females and are at higher risk in each category of victim–offender relationship. Black and other nonwhite males have higher death rates than do white males. The rates of death for nonwhite males ranged from a high of 17.7 per 100,000 for murder by a friend or acquaintance to a low of 2.7 per 100,000 for justifiable homicide—a category in which blacks and other nonwhite males constitute 53.7% of all victims. Black and other nonwhite women consistently have higher homicide rates than white women, and they are more likely to be killed by a family member or friend than are white males.

Of all murders in the United States in 1980 for which the FBI had adequate information, 32.9 percent were of friends and acquaintances; 15.8 percent were within families; and 12.8 percent were of strangers. In the remaining 34.4 percent, the relationship between victim and offender was unknown.[3]

The overall death rate for homicides was 10.6 per 100,000 in 1980. In cases in which the relationship between offender and victim was known, murder by a friend or acquaintance accounted for the greatest number of homicide deaths (7,504), a rate of 3.3 per 100,000. Murder by a family member accounted for 3,607 deaths in 1980 (1.6 per 100,000), and murder by a stranger resulted in 2,911 deaths (1.3 per 100,000). Of all 1980 homicides, approximately 45 percent were committed by persons known to the victim; nearly one third of those homicides were committed by family members. Justifiable homicide by police offenders and citizens resulted in 926 deaths in 1980, a rate of 0.4 per 100,000.

Most family homicides involve spouses, occur in the home, and occur after a series of assaultive incidents.[4,5] Analysis of FBI data[6] indicates that approximately 55 percent of family homicide victims are white and 43.7 percent are black. The median age is 33 for victims and 32 for offenders. The weapon used to kill is a handgun in 40 percent of the cases, followed by other guns (24 percent), knives (17 percent), and other means (18 percent).

Murders of persons less than 18 years old by a family member or other person accounted for 93,000 years of potential life lost in 1980. Family members committed 501 child homicides during that year. For child homicides, black and other nonwhite male children were at highest risk: 6.8 per 100,000, or 467, deaths in 1980, followed by black and other nonwhite females (3.3 per 100,000) and white males (2.3 per 100,000).

When homicide risk is plotted against age for these children, the result is a U-shaped curve on which children under 3 and over 14 years of age are at greatest risk and children 6–11 years of age at lowest risk. In 1980 children under 2 years of age accounted for 24 percent of all child homicide deaths. The 419 homicide deaths in that age group yielded a rate of 4.2 per 100,000, but some cases may have gone unreported.

In cases where the victim is an acquaintance of the offender, the typical victim is younger and more likely to be male and black than in cases where offender and victim are family members. In 1978, 53.3 percent of the victims of acquaintance homicides were black, and 45.2 percent were white. Offenders, whose median age is 23, are usually younger than their victims. Handguns were the weapon of choice in 48.6 percent of all cases; knives were used in 19.6 percent. Acquaintance homicides are most likely to occur on the street. A higher percentage occurs in bars than is true for other types of killings.[6]

Most victims and offenders of stranger homicides are men, and the median age of victims (31 years) is greater than that of offenders (25 years). Most such killings involve firearms—53 percent handguns, 13.9 percent another type of gun. Overall, 43.2 percent of stranger homicides are associated with another crime, often robbery (32 percent). In urban areas, 57 percent of these killings are associated with another crime, with robbery again being the most common.[6]

In many murders the relationship between perpetrator and victim is unknown. The data suggest, however, that many homicides classified as unknown are really murders of strangers, because murders that occur between intimates are usually solved and appropriately classified.

Morbidity. Aggravated assaults, or "incomplete homicides," can be used to measure morbidity associated with homicide. For Americans over the age of 12, 1.6 million incidents of aggravated assault occurred in 1980, a rate of 892 per 100,000.[3] Males were 2.7 times more likely to be victims than females, with men 20–24 years of age being at greatest risk (3,115.5 per 100,000). At least 355,500 victims were hospitalized, and hospital costs (for those who survived assaults plus those who eventually died as a result of aggravated assault) totaled approximately $606 million. The cost of physician visits raised that cost to $638 million. No data are available for the costs of emergency room treatment, pharmaceuticals, extended care after initial hospitalization, or the treatment of offenders who were injured in aggravated assaults.

Aggravated assaults accounted for more than 8 million days lost from activities such as paid work, school, or child rearing; at least 4,718,200 of those were paid workdays. Because a large percentage of victims are women who are economically dependent on their husbands, it is likely that a great deal more time was lost from major nonpaying activity such as child care and housekeeping. No data are available on time lost by children from school or preschool because of domestic violence, child abuse, and neglect.

The geographic distribution of domestic violence shows the highest reported rates in the West and Midwest. Reported rates are lower in rural areas and higher in cities.

Assault results in a wide range of possible disabilities. In the absence of detailed data, we assumed that 70 percent are psychological; sensory and musculoskeletal disabilities (each 15 percent) account for the balance.[1] The average cost of losing one's vision or of the incapacitating fear that prevents one from returning home after a life-threatening attack there is incalculable.

Projections based on the NCS indicate that in 1980 there were approximately 192,000 assaults or attempted assaults by family members, a rate of 99.4 per 100,000 U.S. population (not the population within those families). Other estimates of the number of women beaten each year range from 1.8 million[7] to 3–4 million.[8] Assaults within families represent at least 21,000 hospitalizations, 99,800 hospital days, 28,700 emergency room visits, and 39,900 physician visits. Total health care costs incurred for domestic assaults have been estimated to be at least $44,400,000.

Assaults within families accounted for at least 175,500 days lost from paid work in 1980. Of all the emergency room visits made by women seeking treatment for injury, 19 percent involved battering. Battered women use medical and psychiatric services many times more frequently than other women, sometimes in lieu of other refuge. Visits motivated by battering may be even more common at such nontrauma sites as the maternity clinic or ambulatory care service.[8]

Quality of Life. Interpersonal violence may result in only a minor physical injury but have a devastating impact upon the victim's life in terms of fear, anxiety, and subsequent restrictions in activities and movements. Victims may become quite isolated, and the changes they make in their job, home, or pattern of activities may markedly constrict their freedom and lower the quality of their lives. The changes remind them of the new fears that have become part of their lives. Homicide can have a crippling effect on surviving family members that affects several generations.

Research indicates that children who are victims

of violence suffer delays in physical, social, and emotional development. Many children who witness violence suffer from posttraumatic stress disorders, conditions frequently made worse when they must participate as official witnesses in court.[9]

Battered women are at greatly elevated risk of alcoholism, drug abuse, attempted suicide, abusing their children or having them abused, rape, and mental health problems, including severe depression and even psychosis.[8,10]

Family violence is one of the four most common reasons cited for divorce, and although divorce may solve the immediate problem, it may also result in increased economic deprivation for women and children.

The threat of violent attack may be as damaging as the attack itself. Battered spouses and children may focus all their energies on reducing the chance that a partner or parent will explode in violent rage, and it is impossible to calculate the potential achievements and creativity lost in such situations.

The Possible Causes

In general, researchers view aggravated assault and homicide as outcomes of similar types of behavior and see homicide as an infrequent climax to aggravated assault, or a "completed" aggravated assault. It is generally presumed that strategies that would reduce aggravated assault would reduce homicides as well.

Research and thinking about the causes of aggravated assault and homicide fall into three broad categories: biological, psychological, and sociological.

Biological traits (male sex and young age) or conditions (temporal lobe epilepsy and major affective disorders, for example) can be important risk factors for homicide victimization or perpetration.[11] However, it is difficult to separate the biological and cultural components of those risk factors.

Psychological hypotheses about violence emerge mainly from studies of learning theory and developmental theory. Learning theory suggests that violence is learned from role models and reinforced by rewards and punishments provided by others.[12,13]

The sociological literature yields three main theories about the causes of violence. According to cultural theory, certain subgroups have higher rates of homicide because they accept violence as a cultural norm. Structural theory holds that homicide rates are largely influenced by large social forces—lack of opportunity, racism, and poverty—rather than by individual cognition. Interaction theory focuses on a series of events between perpetrator and victim and on how those interactions escalate into a homicide. Arguments that threaten sexual identity or

self-esteem, for example, may lead to murder.

Associated Factors

Certain factors are empirically associated with the occurrence of homicide and assault. These factors vary for different victim–offender relationships (Tables 1–4).

Poverty is associated with the murder of friends and acquaintances, children and spouses, and with the robbery-associated murder of strangers.[14–16] It is more strongly associated with murders of family members and friends than of acquaintances.[17] The ideology of male dominance is associated with killings of strangers, friends and acquaintances, and spouses.[15,16,18] Racism and racial discrimination are associated with killings of strangers and friends or acquaintances.[6,14,15,19–21] Increased population density is associated with robbery-motivated homicide.[17,21,22]

Alcohol and drug consumption are associated with all types of homicide except child murder.[5,19,23,24] Alcohol is also frequently linked with episodes of family violence, but there is no proof that alcohol consumption causes family violence or homicides. Many violent men abuse women whether or not they have consumed alcohol; in some cases, alcohol may be an excuse for behavior that has already been decided upon.[5]

Finally, the most likely victims of wife and child abuse are pregnant women and unwanted children.[25,26] While most research shows that battered women have the same average number of children as nonbattered women, battered women are pregnant more often and abort more frequently.[8] In addition, parents' unrealistic expectations about children contribute to the use of inappropriate and abusive disciplinary techniques.[27,28]

The interaction of four factors may precipitate homicide or nonfatal violence among family members. The first is the cultural belief that it is appropriate or morally correct to strike children or women either to achieve some goal ("instrumental violence") or to express one's feelings ("expressive violence").

The second factor is structural stress, which results when an adult family member has appropriate goals but lacks the psychological, economic, and social resources to attain those goals.

A third factor is social isolation, although it is not clear whether the isolation is a "cause" or a consequence of battering. Families may be cut off from resources of help for coping with structural stress and from people who might be able to calm a potentially violent situation.[29]

The fourth factor is the availability of protective

Table 1. Factors that may predispose a person to kill a friend or acquaintance, and proposed prevention strategies

Structural	Cultural	Interactionist	Biological
Factors			
Poverty/unemployment[14–17]	Male belief in physical prowess, search for thrills and action[15,16]	Drug and alcohol consumption[5,19,23,24]	Male sex[15,19]
Ideology that masculinity means a dominant male social role[15,20,42,65]	Underdeveloped verbal skills[15]	Weapons possession[66–68]	Youth (20–29 years of age)[67,69,70]
Racial segregation and discrimination[14–16,19,42,65]	Belief that one should not intervene in another's fights[19]		
	Televised violence and media support[14]		
	Encouragement of fighting by bystanders[19]		
Prevention strategies			
Eliminate poverty and unemployment	Reduce media violence	Reduce alcohol and drug consumption	
Change conceptions of masculinity	Increase community and witness intolerance of violence	Reduce firearm injuries	
Reduce racial segregation and discrimination		Teach conflict resolution skills for young males	

Adapted from Rosenberg ML, Stark E, Zahn MA.[78]

Table 2. Factors that may predispose a person to kill or abuse a child, and proposed prevention strategies

Structural	Cultural	Interactionist	Biological	Psychosocial
Factors				
Poverty and/or unemployment	Belief in violence and/or physical punishment as socializing agent[71,72]	Lack of adequate support facilities	Young parental age	Parents abused as children
Too many and/or unplanned-for children	Belief that parents have ultimate right to do what they want with child		Physical or mental disabilities of child	Parents had violent role model
Lack of education about child rearing	Parents' unrealistic expectations of children (especially children with mental or physical disabilities)			
Parental dominance ideology (see Cultural)				
Prolonged marital stress				
Social isolation of nuclear family				
Prevention strategies				
Eliminate poverty from families	Establish alternate ways to socialize child	Establish community/ neighborhood intervention centers and hot lines	Prevent/treat childhood disabilities	Treat identified abused children
Reduce isolation of nuclear family	Provide high-quality child care facilities to reduce parental stress			
Educate about planned parenthood and child rearing	Aid handicapped children			
	Change parental expectations of children			

Adapted from Rosenberg ML, Stark E, Zahn MA.[78]

Table 3. Factors that may predispose a person to kill his/her spouse, and proposed prevention strategies

Structural	Cultural	Interactionist
Factors		
Poverty[14–17]	Male belief in physical prowess, toughness, that he is "head of house" and has control over females[15,16]	Alcohol and drug consumption[5,19,23,24]
Male dominance over females[15,19,20,42]		Weapons possession[66–68]
Isolation of nuclear family[5]	"Hands-off" view of domestic disputes by criminal justice system[72,73]	Male use of force to compensate for verbal disadvantage[15]
	Televised violence and other media supports[74]	No safe place for women to go
Prevention strategies		
Eliminate poverty for men and women	Increase verbal ability and means of problem solving	Reduce alcohol and drug consumption
Eliminate sexual inequality (especially in child rearing and employment) and notions that masculinity requires dominance	Initiate criminal justice and social service interventions	Reduce firearm injuries
	Reduce media violence	Teach how to "fight fair" and resolve conflicts nonviolently
Reduce isolation of nuclear family		Teach how to walk away from a potentially violent situation

Adapted from Rosenberg ML, Stark E, Zahn MA.[78]

services to victims of domestic violence. Service institutions may be unresponsive or may actively promote the feeling that the victims of violence have somehow provoked or deserved this response.

When all four factors are present, the rewards of being violent may outnumber the costs.[29] The reward for domestic violence is power: controlling other family members, punishing them, and getting one's own way. Moreover, the permissive posture of the criminal justice system toward domestic violence means that violent family members will experience few costs such as arrest or removal from the home.

SUICIDE

Impact on Health

Mortality. In 1980 there were 26,689 suicides in the United States, a rate of 11.9 per 100,000, corresponding to 619,532.5 years of potential life lost before age 65. Suicide ranks fifth on the list of causes of premature years of life lost. The rate of suicide is greatest among the young—the rate has tripled among people 15–24 years of age since the mid-1950s—and among the old.[30] It is the third leading cause of death for persons 15–34 years of age.

In 1980 half of all suicides occurred among persons 15–39 years of age.[31] This marked shift downward in the age of persons committing suicide represents a fundamental change in the nature of suicide in this country. Most of our notions about persons at highest risk for suicide, their reasons for committing it, and how to prevent them from doing it were based on suicide as primarily a problem of older persons. These notions now must be thoroughly reassessed. The groups now at greatest risk for suicide are young white men 20–24 years of age and men over the age of 65. Among persons 20–24 years of age, the ratio of men to women who commit suicide is greater than four to one.

Cohort studies suggest that the baby-boom generation has higher rates of suicide and depression and is therefore a high-risk group. We do not know whether those proportionally higher rates will persist or whether this generation's suicide rates will level off and then decrease.[32,33] It is also possible that these high rates reflect an independent trend toward higher rates among young people rather than a cohort effect. Previously attempted suicide is also a risk factor for suicide; approxi-

Table 4. Factors that may predispose a person to commit a robbery-motivated killing, and proposed prevention strategies

Structural	Cultural	Interactionist	Biological	Psychosocial
Factors				
Poverty[14–17]	Materialism	Lack of criminal justice and legal prosecution[56]	Male sex[15,19]	From disorganized home
Ideology that masculinity means a dominant male[15,20,42,65]	Male belief in thrills and action[15,75,76]	Alcohol and drug consumption[5,19,23,24]	Youth (teenagers)[66–68]	Developmental lack of empathy[13]
Racial segregation and discrimination[14–16,19,42,65]	Belief that perpetrator will not be caught or severely punished[56]	Weapons possession[66–68]		
Lack of role models for adolescents	Criminal way of life condoned, and opportunities provided to engage in it[77]			
Urban (population) density[17,22,69]	Belief that victims are not real and are to be used			
	Externalization of blame			
	Televised violence and media support for "bad guy"[74]			
Prevention strategies				
Reduce poverty	Reduce media violence	Reduce alcohol and drug consumption		
Reduce racial segregation	Increase empathy	Reduce firearm injuries		
Create integrated, meaningful role for adolescents	Increase community intolerance of robbery	Educate potential victims		
	Swift, sure criminal justice response to robbery and special handling of offenders who injure	Initiate witness cooperation and assistance programs		
		Have "defensible space construction" (i.e., light streets, construct safer places)		
		Initiate new patterns of police surveillance		

Adapted from Rosenberg ML, Stark E, Zahn MA.[78]

---

mately 1–10 percent of suicide attempters subsequently commit suicide.[34,35]

Morbidity. Although suicide attempts are frequently seen as unsuccessful suicides, there are strong indications that the two represent epidemiologically distinct phenomena. For example, the higher incidence of suicide (and its most dramatic increase) is among white males, who show a suicide rate three times that of females[31]; on the other hand, females attempt suicide up to three times more often than males.[34]

It has been estimated that suicide attempts are eight times more common than suicides.[34,35] This means that the ratio of attempts to completed suicides is about 25 to 1 for females and 3 to 1 for males. Using these figures, we estimate that approximately 210,000 attempts occur each year. Assuming that 20 percent of all suicide attempters were hospitalized and that the average length of hospitalization was six days, we estimate that these attempts account for 259,200 hospital days, 43,200 hospitalizations, 155,500 physician visits, and 631,900 days lost from work or major activity. The cost of health care for treating suicide attempts includes approximately $110.2 million in hospital costs and $6.2 million for physician visits. Lacking precise data, we estimate that 5 percent of suicide attempts (10,800 cases per year) result in a permanent disability.

Because approximately 15 percent of all people

who have a major depressive disorder commit suicide, one might argue that part of the costs of treating those disorders could be designated as costs for suicide prevention. The total costs for treating depression have been estimated at $2 billion per year, so it might be appropriate to say that 15 percent of that cost, or $300 million per year, is related to preventing suicide and treating suicide attempts (see also the paper on "depression").

Quality of Life. Suicide has a tremendous impact on the surviving family members, who must bear the guilt and social stigma of suicide by a family member. Guilt and blame may produce psychological symptoms or physical illness that impair the functioning of the family and may lead to divorce or long-standing psychological scars in parents or siblings. In addition, many families are fearful that another family member will commit suicide. This fear is well founded: members of families in which a suicide has occurred are themselves at higher risk for suicide.[36]

The quality of life for survivors is also affected economically if the suicide was by a wage earner or if survivors are unable to collect life insurance benefits.

Families of attempters, like families of suicides, have to contend with the stigma and with the fear of another—possibly successful—suicide attempt. The family may also be burdened with the cost of mental health care and possibly medical care for the attempter. Only a small percentage of people who attempt suicide incur permanent physical disabilities, such as crippling or disfigurements. Nevertheless, a scar on the wrist or the neck may evoke painful memories. A suicide attempt may also limit the person's employment opportunities for many years.

Frequent suicide attempts elevate the level of anxiety within a community. One young person's suicide may precipitate similar suicides ("cluster suicides") and attempts among friends or acquaintances. "Suicide contagion" may threaten the community, its schools, and its social services.

The Possible Causes

Biological. Of the almost 27,000 persons who commit suicide each year, an estimated 5,000–12,400 may be persons diagnosed as having affective disorders and an estimated 4,000–7,000 as schizophrenics.[37–39] Thus approximately 14,000 suicides, or 50 percent, occur among persons who have major psychiatric disorders. In addition, an estimated 7,000–13,000 suicides each year are linked to alcoholism.[38]

Psychological. Previous suicide attempts, family history of suicide or of physical or sexual abuse, and recent loss of a spouse (through divorce or death), a parent, or a job have been identified as risk factors for suicide.

Sociological. Social isolation, homelessness, unemployment, and drug and alcohol abuse all contribute to suicide.

A detailed examination of the epidemiology of suicide in the United States from 1900 to 1980 reveals that suicide rates fluctuate with war and peace, population shifts, and the state of the economy.[40] Historically, the changes in rates associated with those factors affect both sexes and all age groups and races.

Like suicides, suicide attempts may be motivated by job stress, family conflict, or the loss of a loved one. Young black women—reported in some studies to be a very high-risk population for suicide attempts—often cite family violence as a precipitating factor.[41] A history of depression, alcoholism, or battering is also associated with such attempts. Contagion from another suicide, either within the family or the community, may also be associated with suicides and suicide attempts.

INTERVENTIONS

Homicide, Assault, and Child Abuse

Despite the extensive literature on violence and homicide, few authors have concerned themselves specifically with prevention. The only national effort to develop prevention policies was the establishment of the National Commission on Violence in 1966.[13] In a recently compiled bibliography on homicide, only 17 (4 percent) of the 364 bibliographic items directly dealt with prevention,[42] and only one book dealt solely with this topic.[43] The following interventions have been identified by research as those most likely to reduce homicide, assault, and child abuse (see also Tables 1–4).

Decrease the cultural acceptance of violence. Society must assure women of equal access to jobs and financial security and provide protection. This will ensure that they seek help and eliminate one of the chief reasons many women remain in homes where they or their children are subjected to violence.

Reduce racism. In young black men a cultural acceptance of violence seems to be linked with low self-esteem and low valuation of human life, especially that of other blacks.[15,44,45]

Forbid the use of corporal punishment of children. Conduct public awareness campaigns that outline the extent, seriousness, and consequences of violence in the family and community. Violence in the home should not be considered a private family matter.

Regulate children's television programming. Without censoring programming, regulatory agencies could mandate that children's programming (especially afternoon and Saturday morning programs) be nonviolent. Noncommercial time slots for children's programs should be considered. When violence is depicted for audiences of adults as well as children, it should not be portrayed as a proper solution to human problems.

Develop strategies to reduce firearms-associated injuries. Proposals include (1) licensing provisions; (2) prohibitions against buying, selling, or possessing guns; (3) prohibitions against carrying guns (but not against owing them)[46]; (4) mandatory penalties for the use of a gun in a felony; and (5) mandatory prison sentences for carrying nonlicensed firearms. Case studies of four such approaches have suggested that such measures can reduce killings of spouses and reduce homicide among young men.[47–50]

We calculated that in 1980, if all handgun deaths had been prevented, 10,533 lives would have been saved. However, we assumed that another weapon would have been substituted in at least 20 percent of the murders of family, friends, and unknowns and in 10 percent of the murders involving strangers. Thus, approximately 8,600 lives might have been saved if handgun deaths had been prevented, a total reduction of 36 percent in homicide deaths.

Of all the strategies we considered, limiting access to firearms is likely to have the most dramatic effect on spouse, friend, and robbery-related stranger murders. It would not, however, affect the rate of child homicide to as great an extent.

Coordinate health care with social services. • Increase education in family life, family planning, and child rearing. This would appear to hold considerable promise for reducing family stress and violence.[51]

• Expand support for families through community-based services. Programs that help reduce violence include self-help groups for shelters for abused women and children, home health visitors for expectant and recent parents, and free transportation to health clinics. Tax and welfare policies that divide families should be reexamined.

• Develop education programs for conflict resolution. Schools, churches, and other community agencies could teach nonviolent conflict resolution to high-risk groups such as young black men.

• Improve the ways the health care system recognizes and manages cases of violence.[52] Problems in the system include the failure to recognize injuries caused by violence, the failure to report such injuries, the use of pejorative trems to label abused women, disincentives for health care personnel to become involved with such cases, and the failure to follow up violent assault cases.

• Educate health care providers in the recognition, diagnosis, management, and reporting of problems of violence. Education for professionals should also focus on the assessment and treatment of psychiatric trauma.

• Expand the network of trauma treatment centers so that care is available to residents of high-risk areas, to children who are victims of physical or sexual abuse, and to those who witness violence.[9]

• Strengthen programs for the detection and treatment of child abuse. Because intervention cannot take place until abused children are identified, reporting and treatment programs should be expanded through public awareness campaigns that educate people about child abuse and how to report it.

• Investigate abuse reports with a multidisciplinary team based in a local hospital, clinic, or other agency.

• Enable child welfare agencies to provide immediate shelter for children who are in danger. These facilities should be linked to medical and psychological services within the community.

• Increase funding for child protective services and decrease caseloads.

• Expand and strengthen programs and shelters for battered women. Shelters where women and their children who are victims of battering can seek refuge are considered the single most important intervention for battered women.

• Coordinate the efforts of health care facilities, social service agencies, schools, and police departments in recording, preventing, and intervening in violent incidents.

• Promote employment for high-risk adolescents.

• Reduce the consumption of alcohol and other drugs.

Alter practices of criminal justice. Police and citizen intervention teams should be trained to mediate disputes and refer troubled people to social service agencies.

Crisis intervention units run by civilians may be even more effective than units staffed by police officers. In addition to providing backup to the police when rape and assault victims or relatives of homicide victims require support, such crisis units can be called in before volatile situations turn violent.

Police should treat family assaults as criminal behavior. It is critical that police respond to domestic assaults as criminal acts, not private family matters.

Numerous factors influence what the police do, such as whether both partners are present when the police arrive, whether alcohol is involved, and how willing the victim is to sign an arrest warrant.[53,54] However, recent research indicates that when police have reason to believe an assault has been committed, arresting a violent husband reduces the chances of future wife assault.[55]

Arrest should be used as in any other assault, not as a last resort. The complainant should not be encouraged to "kiss and make up." Victims of family violence should be accorded the same representation and support as victims of stranger assault. Police should also keep thorough records of domestic violence to ensure that victims have proof of victimization should they need it for legal action.

Linkages between police and social services should be improved. Many poor people at high risk, particularly women and blacks, have no contact with anyone except police officers when they are victimized by violence. Police need to be able to make appropriate and effective referrals to health and social service agencies.

More citizen surveillance, victim assistance, and silent witness programs should be initiated. Most crimes are solved because someone witnessed the event, an informant told the police, or the victim identified the offender.[56]

Prosecutors, judges, and juries should be better educated about woman battering and child abuse. Moreover, courts and laws should treat domestic violence as criminal behavior. Reporting of wife abuse should be mandatory in every state. Courts should not hesitate to use protective orders, temporary restraining orders, and peace bonds to keep violent offenders from attacking partners or children. Such access is especially needed in rural areas.

Change environmental factors. Architectural and social planning principles can be used to create safer domestic environments. Changes might range from improving lighting in high-density neighborhoods to ensuring that all Americans have secure homes. Research could define high-risk occupations and settings and determine ways of improving safety for high-risk groups. Police officers and cab drivers, for example, are at high risk for assault and murder. Intervention might include bulletproof vests for police officers and protective barriers for cab drivers.

Suicide

Two issues influence the effectiveness of the proposed interventions that follow. First, global factors such as war, the economy, and shifts in population have a striking impact on suicide rates. Second, solid data about how various interventions might affect suicide rates are sparse.

We have concentrated on mortality in this section, although morbidity calculations have been included when appropriate. To calculate morbidity, we made the following assumptions: eight suicide attempts occur for each completed suicide; 50 percent of those who are kept from attempting suicide because of a specific intervention will attempt suicide by another means; 20 percent of the attempters are hospitalized for an average stay of six days per attempt; attempters' hospital costs average $400 per day.

Limit the availability of lethal agents. Guns were used in 57.3 percent of all suicides in 1980. Although it has not been demonstrated that limiting the use and availability of firearms can prevent suicides,[57] limiting their availability to people at high risk of suicide should be considered.

For the population at large, we estimated that 60 percent of suicides involve firearms, that 70 percent of these potential suicide victims could not or would not obtain guns if the access of the general population to firearms were effectively reduced, and that 50 percent of the potential victims unable to obtain guns would use another method. According to those calculations, firearms regulations for the general population would prevent approximately 20 percent of all suicides and save 5,370 lives a year. In terms of morbidity, we estimate that 21,600 attempts could be prevented, 25,900 hospital days prevented, and $10.4 million in hospital costs saved.

Alternatively, access to firearms might be limited only for persons with major psychiatric disorders. Our projections for members of this high-risk group are based on the following assumptions: persons with major psychiatric disorders constitute 50 percent of all suicides; 60 percent of these suicides involve firearms; 40 percent of these potential suicide victims could not or would not obtain guns if there were firearm regulations for high-risk groups; and 50 percent of the potential victims would use another method if a gun was unobtainable. Regulations applying only to persons in these high-risk groups could thus prevent approximately 4 percent of all suicides, saving approximately 1,100 lives a year. In terms of morbidity, we estimate that 4,320 attempts could be prevented, 5,180 hospital days could be avoided, and over $2 million in hospital costs could be saved.

Poisoning by a solid or liquid, usually a prescription medication, was the second most common means of suicide in 1980, accounting for 11.3 percent of all suicides. Several measures could limit the potential lethality of these drugs: First, restricting the number of tablets or capsules in each prescription might decrease suicide rates.[58,59] Second, because many potential suicide victims stockpile medications prescribed by several physicians, computer networks might be used to give pharmacists or physicians access to information about a person's recent purchases of medication from more than a single source.

To calculate the effectiveness of intervening in medication, we assumed that the amounts of medication that could be prescribed at a given time would be limited and that stockpiling could be detected and used to identify very-high-risk patients. We estimate that these combined strategies might prevent 50 percent of the suicides in which medications are used, but that 50 percent of the victims who were diverted from using drugs would find another means. Therefore, we might prevent approximately 2.8 percent of all suicides each year, saving approximately 750 lives.

Increase affective awareness. In the ordinary course of things, neither parents-to-be nor children are taught very much about the range of feelings and emotions common to human beings. Yet the inability to recognize and communicate those feelings or affects—joy, anger, disgust, fear—may play an important part in the etiology of suicide. We recommend that parent education, teacher training, and school curricula for children place greater emphasis on the recognition and expression of feelings. Developing affective awareness in children could decrease suicides by 20 percent, saving approximately 5,000 lives each year. Such education could prevent 21,600 suicide attempts and therefore avoid 25,900 hospital days and save over $10.4 million in hospital costs.

"Gatekeepers," people who are likely to have contact with persons who are suicidal, represent a diverse group; e.g., members of the clergy, primary care physicians, teachers, coaches, guidance counselors, and even hairdressers and bartenders. Members of these groups should be trained to identify and assess self-destructive behavior and to intervene when appropriate. Even psychiatrists need additional training in the recognition and treatment of persons who are suicidal. For example, despite mounting evidence that antidepressant drugs are often effective treatments for major depression, many psychiatrists continue to rely on "talking therapies" alone.[60]

To calculate the effect of this intervention, we assumed that 50 percent of all suicide victims would make their intentions clear to a gatekeeper at a time when intervention would be possible; that education would enable 50 percent of gatekeepers to intervene (and that they could not do so without education); that 15 percent of potential suicide victims would follow up on the intervention[61]; and that 75 percent of those who followed up on the intervention would be saved. We calculate that gatekeeper education would prevent approximately 2.8 percent of all suicides per year, saving about 750 lives. In terms of morbidity, this intervention could prevent 3,024 attempts, avoid 3,630 hospital days, and save almost $1.5 million in hospital costs.

Predict and respond to changes in suicide incidence. When the population of young people increases, the suicide rates among the young also increase.[32,33,62] In contrast, suicide rates for adults and older people increase when the proportion of adults and older people begins to decrease in the population.[32] Better responsiveness to such demographic changes by government, educational institutions, and private corporations could improve the timeliness and effectiveness of interventions.

Increases in suicide incidence should also be accompanied by a corresponding expansion of programs directed toward the survivors (family and friends) of people who commit suicide. A special type of intervention may be necessary for adolescents whose friend or classmate commits suicide. Schools, student bodies, and small communities may be particularly vulnerable to suicide clusters,[63] and public health and mental health workers must develop enough of an understanding of suicide "contagion" to identify and recommend appropriate responses by school and community leaders.

The impact of such an approach is difficult to assess, but we assume that an estimated 15 percent of the approximately 5,500 suicides and 7.5 percent of the attempts by persons under the age of 25 could be prevented by better application of population data, survivor programs, and school-based interventions. This could prevent 825 suicides and 8,450 attempts, avoid 10,100 hospital days, and save nearly $4.1 million in hospital costs.

Increase the services of suicide prevention centers. Suicide prevention centers attempt to respond to persons in a suicidal crisis by offering services such as 24-hour telephone hot lines, individual and group psychotherapy or referral, and counseling for survivors. According to one study, such centers consistently reduce the suicide rates of young white women by approximately 1.75 per 1,000,000.[64] If we assume that young white women have a suicide rate of 5.25 per 100,000, this would amount to a reduction of approximately 3.3 percent.

Focus on high-risk groups. Practical intervention

might include targeting high-risk individuals for prevention when they are seen at nonpsychiatric facilities. For example, intervention to assess and reduce suicide rates might be appropriate for alcoholics who come to detoxification centers, for battered women who seek obstetrical or trauma care, or for young men with aggressive behavior disorders who are arrested for the first time.

SUMMARY

Although interpersonal violence has many forms, we have, for a variety of reasons, focused on homicide, assault, and suicide. We believe that violence among members of a family or household deserves special attention. In particular, we believe that the abuse of women and children should be a focus of national attention.

Three broad problems recur throughout the literature on homicide, assault, and suicide: (1) poverty, racial discrimination, and sex discrimination; (2) cultural acceptance of violence; and (3) ready availability of lethal agents. The intervention for which we project the greatest impact is limiting the availability and use of lethal agents (firearms and medications). However, we recognize the equal importance of reducing social inequities and reeducating both the potential perpetrators and the victims.

We estimate that a total of 31,000 fatalities from homicide and suicide could be prevented every year. By enacting and enforcing firearms controls, 8,600 homicides and 5,370 suicides could be avoided. Limiting the availability of firearms could also prevent injuries from 21,600 suicide attempts.

Despite the absence of a consistent policy and analytic framework, we have tried to present a well-constructed set of interventions for each type of violence studied. We hope that this initial effort to identify appropriate interventions will be followed by further interdisciplinary efforts to determine which generic changes in current policy and practice will have the most significant effects.

Many people helped in assembling and reviewing parts or all of this paper. We wish to acknowledge their valuable contributions: Mary Pat Brygger, Director, Domestic Abuse Project, Inc., Minneapolis; E. Michael Gorman, Ph.D., M.P.H. (Medical Anthropologist), Violence Epidemiology Branch, Center for Health Promotion and Education, CDC; David Hemenway, Ph.D. (Health Economist), Dept. of Health Policy and Management, Harvard School of Public Health, Boston; Gus Kaufman, Ph.D. (Clinical Psychologist), Men Stopping Violence, Atlanta; Thomas Lalley, Assistant Chief, Center for Antisocial and Violent Behavior, National Institute of Mental Health; James A. Mercy, Ph.D. (Sociologist), Assistant Branch Chief, Violence Epidemiology Branch, Center for Health Promotion and Education, CDC; Jill D. Rosenberg, M.S.W. (Educational Consultant), Masters of Public Health Program, Department of Community Medicine, Emory School of Medicine, Atlanta; Linda E. Saltzman, Ph.D. (Criminologist), Violence Epidemiology Branch, Center for Health Promotion and Education, CDC; Jack C. Smith, M.S. (Statistician), Chief, Research Statistics Branch Division of Reproductive Health, Center for Health Promotion and Education, CDC; Dennis D. Tolsma, Director, Center for Health Promotion and Education, CDC.

The following persons helped tremendously in the preparation of this manuscript: Amelia E. Bass (Typist, Violence Epidemiology Branch), Christine S. Fralish (Technical Information Specialist, Educational Resources Branch), and Donna C. Hiett (Secretary, Violence Epidemiology Branch) of the Center for Health Promotion and Education, CDC; and Anne D. Mather (Editor), Mather Medical Editorial Services, Marietta, Georgia.

REFERENCES

1. Barancek JI, Chatterjee BF, Green YC, et al. Northeastern Ohio trauma study. I. Magnitude of the problem. Am J Public Health 1983;73:746–51.

2. Homicide surveillance, 1970–78. Atlanta, Georgia: Centers for Disease Control, 1983.

3. Crime in the United States: FBI Uniform Crime Reports. Washington, D.C.: Department of Justice, 1980.

4. Luckenbill DF. Criminal homicide as a situated transaction. Soc Prob 1977;25:176–86.

5. Gelles RJ. The violent home. Beverly Hills, California: Sage Publications, 1974.

6. Riedel M, Zahn MA. The nature and patterns of American homicide. Washington, D.C.: National Institute of Justice, 1983.

7. Straus MA, Gelles RJ, Steinmetz SK. Behind closed doors: violence in the American family. Garden City, New York: Doubleday, 1980.

8. Stark E, Flitcraft A, Zuckerman D, et al. Wife abuse in the medical setting: an introduction for health personnel. Washington, D.C.: Office of Domestic Violence, monograph no. 7, 1981.

9. Eth S, Pynoos R. Bearing witness: a model for research and intervention. Presented at the 138th annual meeting of the American Psychiatric Association, Anaheim, California, 1984.

10. Gelles RJ, Cornell CP. Intimate violence. Beverly Hills, California: Sage Publications, 1984.

11. Mednick SA, Pollock V, Volavka J, et al. Biology and violence. In: Wolfgang ME, Weiner NA, eds. Criminal violence. Beverly Hills, California: Sage Publications, 1982: 21–80.

12. Meargee EI. Psychological determinants and correlates of criminal violence. In: Wolfgang ME, Weiner NA, eds. Criminal violence. Beverly Hills, California: Sage Publications, 1982: 81–170.

13. Mulvihill DJ, Tumin MM, eds. Crimes of violence: a staff report submitted to the National Commission on the Causes and Prevention of Violence, vol. 12. Washington, D.C.: US Government Printing Office, 1969.

14. Rose HM. Lethal aspects of urban violence. Lexington, Massachusetts: Lexington Books, 1979:4–5.

15. Curtis LA. Violence, race and culture. Lexington, Massachusetts: Heath, 1975.

16. Wolfgang ME, Ferracuti F. The subculture of vio-

lence: towards an integrated theory in criminology. London: Tavistock, 1967.

17. Smith MD, Parker RN. Types of homicide and variation in regional rates. Soc Forces 1980;59:136–47.

18. Jackson T. Violence and the masculine ideal: some qualitative data. In: Steinmetz S, Strauss M, eds. Violence in the family. New York: Harper & Row, 1974.

19. Wolfgang ME. Patterns in criminal homicide. New York: Wiley, 1958.

20. Steinmetz SK, Straus MA. Violence in the family. New York: Harper & Row, 1974.

21. Cook PJ. Robbery in the United States: an analysis of recent trends and patterns. Washington, D.C.: National Institute of Justice, 1983.

22. Shichor D, Decker DL, O'Brien RM. Population density and criminal victimization: some unexpected findings in central cities. Criminology 1979;17:184–93.

23. Collins J. Drinking and crime. New York: Guilford, 1981.

24. Zahn MA, Snodgrass G. Drug use and the structure of homicide in two US cities. In: Flynn EE, Conrad JP, eds. The new and the old criminology. New York: Praeger, 1978.

25. Gelles RJ. Child abuse as psychopathology: a sociological critique and reformulation. Am J Orthopsychiatry 1973;43:611–21.

26. Gelles RJ. Power, sex, and violence: the case of marital rape. Fam Coord 1977;26:339–47.

27. Galdston R. Observations of children who have been physically abused by their parents. Am J Psychiatry 1965;122:440–3.

28. Steele B, Pollock C. A psychiatric study of parents who abuse infants and small children. In: Helfer R, Kempe C, eds. The battered child. Chicago: University of Chicago Press, 1968:103–47.

29. Gelles RJ. An exchange/social control theory. In: Finkelhor D, Gelles R, Straus M, et al., eds. The dark side of the family: current family violence research. Beverly Hills, California: Sage Publications, 1983.

30. Youth suicide surveillance. Atlanta, Georgia: Centers for Disease Control, 1985.

31. Suicide surveillance, 1970–80. Atlanta, Georgia: Centers for Disease Control, 1985.

32. Holinger PC, Offer D. Prediction of adolescent suicide: a population model. Am J Psychiatry 1982;139: 302–7.

33. Holinger PC, Offer D. Toward the prediction of violent deaths among the young. In: Sudak HS, Ford AB, Rushford NB, eds. Suicide among children and adolescents. New York: Wright, 1984.

34. Wexler L, Weissman MM, Kasl SV. Suicide attempts 1970–75: updating a United States study and comparisons with international trends. Brit J Psychiatry 1978;132: 180–5.

35. Kennedy P, Kreitman N, Ovenstone IMK. The prevalence of suicide and parasuicide ('attempted suicide') in Edinburgh. Brit J Psychiatry 1978;132:180–5.

36. Paykel E, Dienelt M. Suicide attempts following acute depression. J Nerv Ment Dis 1971;153:234–43.

37. Waltzer H. Suicide risk in young schizophrenics. Gen Hosp Psychiatry 1984;6:219–25.

38. Miles CP. Conditions predisposing to suicide: a review. J Nerv Ment Dis 1977;164:231–46.

39. Pokorny AD. Prediction of suicide in psychiatric patients. Arch Gen Psychiatry 1983;40:249–57.

40. Holinger PC. Violent deaths in the United States, 1900–1980. New York: Irvington (in press).

41. Stark E. The battering syndrome: social knowledge, social therapy, and the abuse of women [Dissertation]. Binghamton, New York: State University of New York, 1984:590.

42. Riedel M, Zahn MA. The nature and patterns of American homicide: an annotated bibliography. Washington, D.C.: National Institute of Justice, 1982.

43. Allen NH. Homicide: perspectives on prevention. New York: Human Sciences Press, 1980.

44. Poussaint AF. Black-on-black homicide: a psychological–political perspective. Victimology 1983;8:161–9.

45. Bulham HA. Franz Fanon and the psychology of oppression. New York: Plenum, 1985.

46. Moore MH. The bird in hand: feasible strategy for gun control. J Policy Anal Manage 1983;2:185–95.

47. Geisel MS, Roll R, Weltick RS Jr. The effectiveness of state and local regulation of handguns: a statistical analysis. Duke Law J 1969;647–76.

48. Pierce GL, Bowers WJ. The Bartley–Fox gun law's short term impact on crime in Boston. Ann Am Acad Pol Soc Sci 1981;455:120–37.

49. Jones ED III. The District of Columbia's firearms control regulations act of 1975: the toughest handgun control law in the United States—or is it? Ann Am Acad Pol Soc Sci 1981;455:138–49.

50. Loftin C, Hill RH. Regional subculture and homicide: An examination of the Gastil-Hacknew thesis. Am Sociol Rev 1974;39:714–24.

51. Ross CJ, Zigler E. An agenda for action. In: Gerbner G, Ross CJ, Zigler E, eds. Child abuse: an agenda for action. New York: Oxford University Press, 1980:293–304.

52. Klingbell K. Comprehensive model to detect, assess, and treat assaultive violence in hospital settings. In: Task force on black and minority health. Washington, D.C.: US Government Printing Office, 1985.

53. Berk S, Loseke D. "Handling" family violence: the situated determinants of police arrest in domestic disturbances. Law Soc Rev 1980;15:317–46.

54. Parnas R. The police response to domestic disturbance. Wisc Law Rev 1967;914–60.

55. Sherman LW, Berk RA. Deterrent effects of arrest for domestic violence. Am Sociol Rev 1984;49:261–72.

56. Greenwood PW. The violent offender in the criminal justice system. In: Wolfgang M, Weiner NA, eds. Criminal violence. Beverly Hills, California: Sage Publications, 1982:320–46.

57. Boyd JH. The increasing rate of suicide by firearms. N Engl J Med 1983;308:872–4.

58. Oliver RG, Hetzel BS. An analysis of recent trends in suicide rates in Australia. Int J Epidemiol 1973;2:91–101.

59. Goldney RD, Katsikitis M. Cohort analysis of suicide rates in Australia. Arch Gen Psychiatry 1983;40:71–4.

60. DiMasio A, Weissman MM, Prusoff BA, et al. Differential symptom reduction by drugs and psychotherapy in acute depression. Arch Gen Psychiatry 1979;36:1450.

61. Souris M, Elefteriadis C. The practitioner and suicide prevention: an inquiry. Bibl Psychiatr 1982;162:33–41.

62. Holinger PC, Offer D. The epidemiology of suicide, homicide, and accidents among adolescents: trends in self-destructiveness and the potential for prediction. In: Feldman RA, ed. Advances in adolescent mental health. Greenwich, Connecticut: JAI Press (in press).

63. Holinger PC, Offer D. Perspectives on suicide in adolescence. In: Simmons R, ed. Social and community mental health, vol. 2. Greenwich, Connecticut: JAI Press 1981:139–257.

64. Miller HC, Coombs DW, Leeper JD, et al. An analysis of the effects of suicide prevention facilities on suicide rates in the United States. Am J Public Health 1984;74:340–3.

65. Klebba AJ. Homicide trends in the United States, 1900–1974. Public Health Rep 1975;90:195–204.

66. Zimring FE. Determinants of the death rate from robbery: a Detroit time study. In: Rose HM, ed. Lethal aspects of urban violence. Lexington, Massachusetts, Lexington Books, 1979:31–50.

67. Block R. Violent crime. Lexington, Massachusetts, Lexington Books, 1977.

69. Cook PJ. The effect of gun availability on violent crime patterns: gun control. Ann Am Acad Polit Soc Sci 1981;455:49–89.

69. Cook PJ. The influence of gun availability on violent crime patterns. In: Tomy M, Morris N, eds. Crime and justice, an annual review of research, vol. 4. Chicago: University of Chicago Press, 1983.

70. Fox JA. An econometric analysis of crime data [Dissertation]. Philadelphia: University of Pennsylvania, 1976.

71. Erlanger H. The empirical status of the subculture of violence thesis. Soc Prob 1974;22:280–91.

72. Robin GD: Justifiable homicide by police officers. J Crim Law Criminol Police Sci 1970;8:48–56.

73. Lundsgaarde HP. Murder in space city. New York: Oxford University Press, 1977.

74. Cook TD, Kendzierski DA, Thomas SV. The implicit assumptions of television research: an analysis of the 1982 NIMH report on television and behavior. Public Opinion Q 1983;47:161–201.

75. Curtis LA. Criminal violence—national patterns and behavior. Lexington, Massachusetts: Lexington Books, 1974.

76. Silberman CE. Criminal violence and criminal justice. New York: Vintage, 1978.

77. Smith ME, Thompson JW. Employment, youth and violent crime. In: Feinberg KR, ed. Violent crime in America. Washington, D.C.: National Policy Exchange, 1983.

78. Rosenberg ML, Stark E, Zahn MA. Interpersonal violence: homicide and spouse abuse. In: Public health and preventive medicine. 12th ed. Norwalk, Connecticut: Appleton-Century-Crofts, 1406–9.

Commentary and Intervention Strategies

Cross-Sectional Analysis: Precursors of Premature Death in the United States

Robert W. Amler, M.D., and Donald L. Eddins

From 1900 to 1980, the average life expectancy in the U.S. increased from 47.3 to 73.7 years at birth, an increase of 26.4 years in 80 years.[1] This substantial improvement was the result primarily of achievements in infectious disease prevention and control and general improvements in public health. For example, tuberculosis, dysentery, and diphtheria—leading causes of death in 1900—are now rare and even more rarely fatal. Smallpox has been eradicated and measles nearly eliminated through immunization. In most instances, control has resulted less from breakthrough cures than from intervention against precursors of fatal disease that could be eliminated or reduced with existing technology.

The old killers are so readily prevented today that any deaths they do cause are considered unnecessary, or premature. Likewise, the leading killers of the 1980s, though not entirely preventable today, cause many deaths that can be considered premature because of known precursors that are preventable. Such precursors impose a double burden on our people and our health care system: they afflict patients and families directly, and they consume resources that otherwise could be devoted to health problems for which reliable preventive strategies are not yet known.

The purpose of the present study is to determine the leading precursors of premature death in the U.S., from illnesses of diverse etiology and to quantify their health impact.

DEFINITIONS

Access to care. The proportion of persons afflicted with a health problem who obtain specific clinical services of such quality, quantity, and frequency as to avoid or minimize adverse outcomes (i.e., complications, continued illness, and death) to the fullest extent possible, according to nationally recognized standards of care.

Burden. The combined health, economic, and social impact of a health problem or precursor.

Cascade model. The method used in this study to attribute more than one precursor to the burden of a health problem. Example: Precursor *A* accounted for 60 percent of deaths from health problem *X*, Precursor *B* accounted for 50 percent, and Precursor *C* accounted for 10 percent. This model attributed deaths from health problem *X* in the following manner:

Precursor *A:* 60 percent

Precursor *B:* 20 percent (50 percent of the remaining 40 percent)

Precursor *C:* 2 percent (10 percent of the remaining 20 percent)

Direct personal health care costs. The sum of three costs: (1) short-term inpatient hospitalization; (2) physician, dentist, and other professional care; (3) pharmaceuticals, medical appliances, and sundries.

Gap. The burden of unnecessary illness, computed as the difference between the current burden of health problems and the lesser burden that is achievable with knowledge already at hand.

Gaps in primary prevention. Missed opportunities and inadequate access to personal and community-based activities, services, utilities, and health care that operate prior to the onset of illness in a person and effectively prevent illness. This definition includes such diverse activities as disease surveillance, nutritional guidance, vector control, immunization, fluoridation, pasteurization, sanitation, health risk appraisal, prenatal care, health education, and various environmental controls.

Incidence rate (annual). The number of new cases of a health problem in a year, divided by the total population.

Overnutrition. Obesity, high serum cholesterol, or both.

Precursor. Risk factor (risk indicator), health care problem, or preventive strategy that, if reduced,

From the Centers for Disease Control, Atlanta.

Address reprint requests to Dr. Amler, Centers for Disease Control, Atlanta, GA 30333.

ameliorated, or more fully implemented, respectively, would result in a lower rate of death or illness caused by different etiologies.

Period prevalence rate. The total number of cases of a health problem in a specified period divided by the total population at the midpoint of the period.

Point prevalence rate. The total number of cases of a health problem at a specified point in time divided by the total population at the same point in time.

Screening. Tests, protocols, or procedures that are (1) intended to clearly identify persons in an apparently healthy population who are at higher than average risk for specific health problems which are more amenable to correction if detected during an early stage, and (2) effective and beneficial.

Years of potential life lost before the age of 65. Data class in use since 1982[2] that measures the impact of diseases that kill people before the customary age of retirement. It is computed as the sum of products over all age groups up to the age of 65, each product being the annual number of deaths in an age group multiplied by the average number of years remaining before the age of 65 for that age group.

METHODS

Selection of Health Problems

Our principal data sources were studies commissioned for "Closing the Gap" and reported throughout this volume that quantified the impact of major health problems in the U.S. with emphasis on precursors that might be amenable to prevention (see "Introduction and Methods"). The problems were selected in September 1983 by an expert panel, using methods previously described,[3] from conditions listed in the *International Classification of Diseases, Ninth Revision.* The panel used five selection criteria: (1) point prevalence and secular trends, (2) severity of health impact and cost, (3) sensitivity to intervention using current scientific or operational knowledge, (4) feasibility of such intervention, (5) generic applicability of such intervention to other health problems.

Altogether, 15 broad health problems were studied (Table 1).

Analyses of Data

Data were abstracted and classified according to years of potential life lost before the age of 65 and annual totals of deaths, incidence and prevalence data, days of hospitalization, and direct personal

health care costs, when available. The same data classes were used to determine the preventable burden, by each precursor, of each studied health problem. The total preventable burdens of each health problem were not compared; instead, the total "gap" in each class was computed in cross-section for each precursors.

Data classes were defined and standardized to allow comparisons between different reports, and revisions were made to minimize duplicate counts of deaths or cases. The resulting estimates were compared with other published data[4] and with additional estimates provided by the National Center for Health Statistics (NCHS).[1] All rates were age adjusted to the 1980 U.S. resident population, 227,156,000.[1] Rates estimated for years other than 1980 were projected to 1980 using short interval trends, which were assumed to be linear.

Preventable precursors identified in the studies conducted for "Closing the Gap" were ranked and cross-tabulated by the same data classes over all studied health problems. A cascade model was used to attribute morbidity and mortality to precursors that overlapped.

Rounding Protocol and Significant Digits

Estimates were reported with all digits shown precisely as they were computed, although the authors concluded from numerous manipulations that most estimates had no more than three significant digits. This protocol was established to make it easier to replicate all computations and ensure correct documentation of the cross-sectional analysis. Thus, rounding was avoided as much as possible, with full recognition of the undesirable effect, a false appearance of precision.

RESULTS

Background Summary Data

In 1980 the U.S. resident population was approximately 227,156,000.[1] There were an estimated 3,612,258 births[1] and 1,995,000 deaths.[1] Nearly 46,000 deaths were infants under 1 year of age—an infant mortality rate of 12.6 per 1,000 live births.[10] The average life expectancy at birth in 1980 was 73.7 years (females 77.5 years, males 70.0 years), a gain of 26.4 years since 1900.[1] Premature death resulted in the loss of 11,897,174 potential years of life before the age of 65. Life expectancy for persons at the age of 65 translated to an average longevity of 81.4 years (females 83.3 years, males 79.1 years), a gain of only 4.5 years since 1900.[1]

In 1980, patients received approximately

Table 1. Studied health problems and major precursors, United States, 1980

Studied health problems	Quantified precursors	Other identified precursors
Alcohol dependency and abuse	Alcohol	Gaps in screening, gaps in primary prevention
Arthritis and musculoskeletal diseases	Gaps in primary prevention	Socioeconomic level
Cancer	Tobacco, alcohol, occupation, gaps in screening, dietary fat, inadequate dietary fiber, gaps in primary prevention	Socioeconomic level
Cardiovascular diseases	Tobacco, high blood pressure, overnutrition, diabetes	Inadequate physical activity, socioeconomic level
Dental diseases	Gaps in primary prevention, tobacco, inadequate access to care	Socioeconomic level
Depression	None	Gaps in primary prevention, alcohol, inadequate access to care
Diabetes mellitus	Overnutrition, tobacco, inadequate access to care	Socioeconomic level
Digestive diseases	Alcohol, tobacco, gaps in screening, gaps in primary prevention	None
Drug dependence and abuse	None	Gaps in primary prevention, inadequate access to care, socioeconomic level
Infectious and parasitic diseases	Gaps in primary prevention, gaps in screening, inadequate access to care	Tobacco, alcohol, occupation
Respiratory diseases	Tobacco	Occupation, inadequate access to care
Unintended pregnancy and infant mortality and morbidity	Tobacco, gaps in primary prevention, inadequate access to care	Alcohol, socioeconomic level
Unintentional injury	Alcohol, injury risks exclusive of alcohol, tobacco, handguns	Socioeconomic level
Violence: homicide, domestic violence, and suicide	Alcohol, handguns, gaps in primary prevention, gaps in screening, inadequate access to care	Socioeconomic level

274,508,000 days of inpatient hospitalization in nonfederal, nonpsychiatric, short-stay hospitals, corresponding to 37.8 million patient discharges exclusive of newborn infants.[5] The total health expenditure was $249 billion,[5] of which $219.4 billion (88.1 percent) was expended for direct personal health care. This total includes hospital care ($100.3 billion); physician, dentist, and other professional care ($67.7 billion); nursing home care ($20.7 billion); drugs and drug sundries ($19.4 billion); and eyeglasses, appliances, and other ($11.0 billion).[5]

Health Problems and Precursors

The broad health problems covered by "Closing the Gap" accounted for approximately 1,883,000 deaths in 1980 (94.4 percent of the total), according to mortality data from the National Center for Health Statistics. This estimate corresponds to approximately 9,372,676 years of potential life lost before the age of 65 (78.1 percent of the total). The consultants estimated a total of 207,856,924 (75.7 percent) days of hospital care and $176.6 billion (80.7 percent) in direct personal health care costs. Major precursors associated with these health problems are summarized in Table 1.

Defining the Gap

In 1980 the adjusted number of deaths in the United States resulting from quantifiable precursors was 1,258,867, 63.1 percent of the deaths that occurred in that year (Table 2). This estimate corresponds to 8,425,932 potential years of life lost before the age of 65 (70.8 percent of the total) and 82,056,240 days of hospital care (29.9 percent of the total).

Tobacco accounted for the greatest number of deaths (338,022) in this model (Figure 1). High blood pressure (297,162) and overnutrition (289,502) were also important precursors of death. These three precursors together accounted for 73.5 percent of preventable causes of death.

The leading precursor of premature death (Figure 2) measured by potential years of life lost before age 65, was non-alcohol-related injuries (1.8 million). Alcohol and tobacco each accounted for 1.5 million, and gaps in primary prevention accounted for 1.3 million potential years of life lost before age 65. The four precursors together accounted for 75.0 percent of the total.

The leading precursor of hospitalization (measured by days of care) was non-alcohol-related injuries (25.5 million days). Overnutrition accounted for 17.1 million days, tobacco 16.1 million, and high blood pressure 9.8 million. The four precursors combined accounted for 82.4 percent of the total.

Major Precursors

Tobacco. As the leading precursor of death, tobacco was also one of the major precursors of potential years of life lost before the age of 65 and days of hospital care (Figure 3). The primary cause of death resulting from using tobacco (162,564 deaths)

was cardiovascular diseases (heart attack, stroke, and diabetes), but tobacco-related cancer deaths (124,534) were also prominent. The increased prevalence of female smoking resulted in a dramatic increase in lung cancer rates in women through 1980. It can be expected that this trend will continue in the foreseeable future and that lung cancer deaths among women will exceed breast cancer deaths by 1985. In addition, tobacco caused an estimated 42,547 deaths from lung disease, 4,200 infant deaths related to low birth weight, 2,300 deaths from fires, and 1,897 deaths from peptic ulcer disease.

Injury risks. Both alcohol-related and non-alcohol-related injuries were the leading precursor of years of life lost before the age of 65—a total of 3,252,926 years lost (38.6 percent of the preventable total, 27.3 percent of the U.S. total). Numerous precursors were identified for various non-alcohol-related injuries (see "Unintentional Injuries").

Alcohol. Alcohol was a leading precursor of premature death (Figure 4), primarily because of its role in the occurrence of fatalities, both from motor vehicles (26,589 deaths) and from numerous other types of injuries (27,094), such as falls and drownings. Noninjury deaths resulting from alcohol use included 26,048 from cirrhosis and 19,516 from cancer.

Gaps in primary prevention. This precursor accounted for 15.1 percent of premature death (Figure 5), primarily because of the large number of infant deaths (12,500) potentially preventable through improved prenatal care and reproductive health ser-

Table 2. Major precursors of premature death, United States, 1980: attributable deaths, years lost before age 65, and days of hospital care

Precursor	Deaths	Potential years lost before age 65	Days of hospital care
Tobacco	338,022	1,497,161	16,098,587
High blood pressure	297,162	340,752	9,781,647
Overnutrition	289,502	292,960	16,306,194
Alcohol			
total	99,247	1,795,458	3,348,354
(injury)	(53,683)	(1,497,206)	(2,229,824)
(other)	(45,564)	(298,252)	(1,118,530)
Injury risks (excluding alcohol)	64,169	1,755,720	25,470,176
Gaps in screening	56,592	172,793	3,647,729
Gaps in primary prevention	54,027	1,273,631	4,651,730
Inadequate access to care	21,974	324,709	2,141,569
Occupation	16,807	102,065	581,740
Handguns	13,365	350,683	28,514
Unintended pregnancy	8,000	520,000	n/a
Total preventable	1,258,867	8,425,932	82,056,240
(percentage)	(63.1)	(70.8)	(29.9)
Total all causes	1,995,000	11,897,174	274,508,000

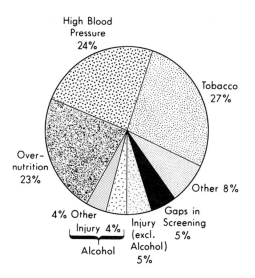

Figure 1. Premature deaths. Three precursors—tobacco, high blood pressure, and overnutrition—account for 73.5 percent of premature deaths in the U.S.

vices and the substantial numerical impact of each infant death on the measurement of years of life before age 65. Other causes of death potentially amenable to primary prevention (after excluding, by means of cascade, deaths triggered by other precursors) included infectious diseases and suicide. In addition, a substantial number of cancer deaths were potentially preventable through screening.

Unintended pregnancy. A leading precursor of premature death, unintended pregnancy accounted for an estimated 8,000 infant deaths (less than 1 percent of the preventable total), largely from infec-

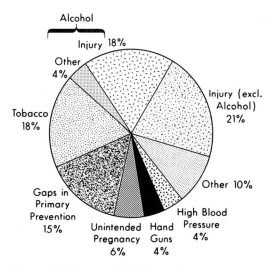

Figure 2. Years of life lost. Four precursors—injury risks, alcohol, tobacco, and gaps in primary prevention—account for 75 percent of years of potential life lost before the age of 65 in the U.S.

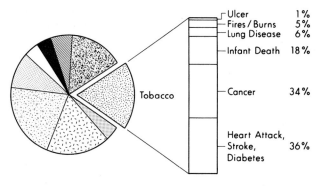

Figure 3. Years of life lost, tobacco. Years of life lost before the age of 65 were attributed to tobacco, based on age-specific mortality rates from different causes of death. Besides cardiovascular diseases and cancer, infant death and other causes were prominent.

tious etiologies. However, because of the substantial numerical impact of each infant death, this corresponded to 520,000 years of life lost before the age of 65 (6.2 percent of the preventable total).

High blood pressure. High blood pressure was a leading precursor of death, accounting for 295,162 deaths from cardiovascular diseases (Figure 1). Because of the age distribution of deaths attributed to high blood pressure, this precursor was less prominent as a cause of years of life lost before age 65, 4.0 percent of the preventable total (Figure 2).

Overnutrition. A pattern similar to that observed for high blood pressure emerged for overnutrition. It was a leading precursor of death, accounting for 289,502 deaths from cardiovascular diseases (Figure 1). Because of the age distribution of deaths attributed to overnutrition, this precursor was less prominent as a cause of years of life lost before age 65, 3.5 percent of the preventable total (Figure 2).

Other precursors. While making less overall im-

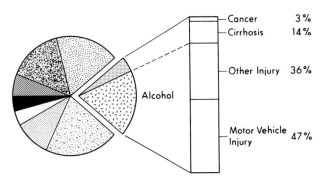

Figure 4. Years of life lost, alcohol. Years of life lost before the age of 65 were attributed to alcohol, based on age-specific mortality rates from different causes of death. Injuries, both motor vehicle and non-motor-vehicle related, were the most prominent.

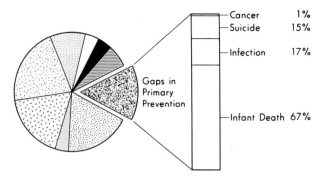

Figure 5. Years of life lost, gaps in primary prevention. Years of life lost before the age of 65 were attributed to gaps in primary prevention, based on age-specific mortality rates from different causes of death. Infant death and infection were the most prominent.

pact than those mentioned above, other precursors were nonetheless important as potential areas for effective intervention (Table 2). These included handguns, inadequate access to care, and occupational hazards.

DISCUSSION

Methodologic Issues

Four important assumptions underlie the present study and the broad spectrum of health problems it encompassed. First, most of the reports in "Closing the Gap" indicated that mortality data are more accessible than morbidity data. Mortality data are also easier to compare across different diseases. Although the emphasis on mortality certainly influenced our analyses, in most cases the same precursors seemed to be operative for morbidity. Nevertheless, the burden of some conditions—arthritis, dental diseases, and depression—manifested almost entirely as morbidity and was thus probably understated.

Second, the reports were developed by different panels of consultants working separately. For this reason, caution is required in combining results from different studies. For example, some consultants studied the total burden of a broad health problem (e.g., unintentional injuries), while others studied only selected diseases (e.g., lung cancer, breast cancer) within a broad health problem (e.g., cancer). Some consultants were able to quantify the impact of such precursors as physical inactivity and nutritional problems, while others were not. In addition, the impact of occupational and environmental hazards was not studied directly. Therefore, it did not seem appropriate to rank broad health problems by deaths or by any other data class.

In several instances consultants used different as-

sumptions, and such differences were not always obvious. Health care cost categories, in particular, were often defined differently. Therefore, the computation of direct health care costs was not completed in the present study.

A third concern was the use of different disease models by different consultants, however appropriate to their own specialty. For example, some consultants modeled a health problem only as a single underlying cause of death, some only as one of multiple causes of death, and some both ways. Probably the burden of a health problem (and the impact of its precursors) is somewhat underestimated by the first model and somewhat overestimated by the second.

The second model is attractive from two standpoints of risk computation: (1) most persons, at the time of death, have many serious health problems that likely add to the probability of death, and (2) a life can be saved in more than one way. Unfortunately, this model also brings additional uncertainties in coding for cause of death and attribution of precursors. For example, how reliably does controlling a well-documented, modifiable precursor (e.g., high blood pressure) prevent the death of a person who is diagnosed as having many serious problems, some of which are preventable by other means and some not? Moreover, if this second model is used, the computed annual number of lives potentially saved in the future can easily exceed the total annual number of deaths in the future. For this reason, most consultants to "Closing the Gap" chose the first model.

Finally, there were occasional discrepancies between the consultants' findings and previously published estimates of mortality, morbidity, and cost. Most discrepancies were easy to reconcile, but some were not, because of differences such as diagnostic criteria, population groupings, and geographic clusters. In a few such cases, these differences prompted the authors to substitute a published estimate. Nevertheless, the present study broadly assumed that "Closing the Gap" studies contained the best current estimates of burden, precursors, and prevention opportunities. Therefore, these estimates were usually preferred.

Cross-sectional Strategy

Despite the methodologic issues noted above, the fundamental strategy of the present study was to combine precursor data from health problems in different specialties in cross section. Many precursors were commonly associated with one or two health problems, but certain precursors attained greater importance because they affected many different (in some cases, nearly all) health problems. Often the seriousness of such precursors could not be fully recognized when only one health problem was considered. For example, the burden of alcohol could not be fully measured only by deaths from liver disease, by years of life lost from drunk driving, by hospitalization in detoxification units, or by the economic cost of alcoholism.

Thus, the results of the present study lack the precision that the full-digit estimates would appear to claim, and the model lacks the sophistication that ideally would account for adverse effects of interventions, incomplete population coverage, interactions between precursors, or competing causes or death. However, the findings presented here are robust and should be useful in their simplicity as a clear departure point for more advanced studies of our opportunities as a nation to close the gap.

Key Findings

Whether measured by crude deaths or by years of life lost before the age of 65, approximately two thirds of deaths in the United States are attributable to a preventable precursor and thus are potentially unnecessary, or premature (Table 2). The major precursors differ somewhat in rank between the two measures, but the similarities are more striking than the differences.

There are relatively few major precursors of premature death in the United States. In the present study, six precursors accounted for three fourths of crude deaths, three fourths of years of life lost before age 65, and three fourths of hospital days from preventable causes. The six precursors were tobacco, alcohol, injury risks, high blood pressure, overnutrition, and gaps in primary prevention. Of these six, tobacco had the greatest effect; it was a leading precursor in all three data classes.

CONCLUSIONS

The burden of premature death in the United States in the 1980s is large and, in large measure, preventable. The analyses performed for "Closing the Gap" identified a small number of precursors responsible for two thirds of all deaths occurring annually in this country; all those precursors are potentially preventable.

The public health revolution of the early twentieth century brought unprecedented benefits to the U.S. population and economy. The evidence from the present study suggests that opportunities exist to achieve additional, comparable gains at the present time.

The authors acknowledge the guidance of William H. Foege, M.D., and technical assistance from the following individuals: Michael K. Berry, M.P.H., Norman L. Collin, Nancy N. Fajman, M.P.H., Ronald E. Hewett, Thomas O'Brien, Nancy D. Pearce, James S. Marks, M.D., Craig C. White, M.D., and Ronald W. Wilson. "Closing the Gap" was supported by the Culpeper Foundation, the Henry J. Kaiser Family Foundation, and the Robert Wood Johnson Foundation.

REFERENCES

1. Health, United States, 1983. Hyattsville, Maryland: National Center for Health Statistics, 1984; DHHS publication no. (PHS) 84-1232.

2. Centers for Disease Control. Premature mortality in the United States: public health issues in the use of years of potential life lost. Morbic Mortal Weekly Rep 1986;35 (suppl):2S.

3. Foege WH, Amler RW, White CC. Closing the gap: Report of the Carter Center health policy consultation. JAMA 1985;254:1355–8.

4. Centers for Disease Control. Annual summary 1980: reported morbidity and mortality in the United States. Morbid Mortal Weekly Rep 1981;29:54.

5. Health, United States, 1982. Hyattsville, Maryland: National Center for Health Statistics, 1983; DHHS publication no. (PHS) 83–1232.

Intervention Strategies: Reports of the Working Groups

Each of the 15 chapters in *Closing the Gap* provides a close look at a specific problem that affects the nation's health. The organizers of the consultation realized that several common threads connect the different health problems, and they reasoned that recommendations for interventions could be best coordinated by looking at "generic" precursors and interventions.

Some precursors were obvious from the beginning. Tobacco use is clearly implicated in cancer, cardiovascular disease, and respiratory disorders. But what relationship does violence, for example, have with other health problems? A cross-match of all the risk factors revealed some interesting connections. The link between violence and dental disease, diabetes, and several other problems is inadequate preventive care. Ranked according to their impact on morbidity and mortality, six major precursors were identified (Table 1).

Six working groups were assembled to explore these precursors for the purpose of devising interventions. Each group was composed of representatives from the fields of health, business, insurance, education, and government. This diversity was intended to promote a crosscutting exchange of ideas and to avoid confounding, subtle professional biases. Their work identified numerous opportunities for prevention. Their suggested intervention strategies target education, the media, industry, the workplace, agriculture, the health care system, and local, state, and federal governments. Their findings imply that shared responsibility is crucial if our nation's health is to improve.

It should be noted that socioeconomic level was not addressed separately, even though it was identified as a precursor for several health problems. However, the working groups acknowledged that lack of readily available and easily accessible health care is most critical among persons of low socioeconomic status. This recognition is implicit in the discussion of gaps in preventive services, which are cited as an important precursor in 12 of the 15 health problems.

Although the working group reports are critical of many existing systems, their recommendations are positive. The ultimate message is that by selecting our goals and working cooperatively, we can ensure a healthier future for the entire nation.

TOBACCO

Chairperson: Jesse Steinfeld, M.D.
Rapporteur: Craig White, M.D.

In 1964 a group of consultants, all of whom were considered by the tobacco industry to be impartial and many of whom were heavy smokers, submitted a report to the Surgeon General indicating that cigarette smoking was a causative or associated factor in several diseases, including many cancers and cardiovascular and lung diseases. Literally hundreds of thousands of reports citing statistical, epidemiologic, and pathologic evidence have subsequently confirmed the Surgeon General's report. Cigarette smoking has emerged as the single greatest public health hazard in the United States. This is not surprising when one considers that the human body is equipped neither immunologically nor biochemically to handle the more than 6,000 chemicals in cigarette smoke—many of which are toxic.

Approximately 53 million Americans now smoke—a reduction in the overall prevalence of smoking compared with 1964. Efforts to curtail smoking over two decades have resulted in about 37 million Americans quitting. Without the antismoking programs and public education already implemented, we would now be a nation of 90 million smokers of nonfiltered, high-nicotine, high-tar cigarettes.

Nonetheless, the actual number of smokers in the United States has remained essentially the same because of the increasing total population and high smoking rates among the young. Of those still smoking, the percentage who smoke 25 or more cigarettes a day has increased markedly.

While the prevalence of cigarette consumption is declining in the developed nations, we are greatly concerned about the rapid increase in tobacco use and tobacco-associated diseases in developing countries. It is accurate to say that tobacco is one of the most significant health problems in the world today.

Address reprint requests to Daphna W. Gregg, 325 Brooks Avenue, Atlanta, GA 30307.

Table 1. Working groups on intervention strategies: selected generic precursors

Generic risk factors
   Tobacco use
   Injury risks
   Alcohol overuse
   Unintended pregnancy

Generic problems
   Gaps in prevention
   Violence, depression, and substance abuse

More than 350,000 people in the United States still die from smoking-related diseases every year. This is equivalent to four wide-body jets crashing every day with no survivors. We would not tolerate such a waste of life from airplane crashes, and yet we accept tobacco, with its monumental risks, as a pervasive element in our society.

Recent surveys reveal that although most people know tobacco is harmful, well over half do not associate smoking with heart disease. They may associate smoking with cancer, but many do not realize that the cancer it causes is largely incurable and may be deadly. Understanding of the dangers of smokeless tobacco is probably even more limited. Perhaps listing all tobacco-related deaths in a separate section in the obituary pages would help disseminate information on the health risks. In addition, we could report the use of tobacco on death certificates as we do the heavy use of alcohol.

As a nation, we should restrict the promotion of tobacco products, including smokeless tobacco, by either banning the promotion of all tobacco products or requiring the industry to conform to its own advertising standards, which prohibit ads that suggest smoking is essential to social prominence or sexual attraction or that portray smokers participating in strenuous physical activity. We must work with the media to increase coverage of smoking, tobacco, and health issues. Equal space and time should be requested to counteract the effect of advertisements.

Recently, the U.S. District Court in New Jersey gave us a powerful tool in combating tobacco use: litigation. The judge ruled that people injured by smoking tobacco and who claim the warnings on cigarette packs are not adequate are entitled to present their claims for adjudication. Although extremely controversial, this tool could be influential. If a number of lawsuits are successful, the tobacco industry may find, as the asbestos industry did, that it cannot afford to manufacture cigarettes because the cost is too high.

We believe that the sale of cigarettes should be restricted to retail outlets only; sale at all health care institutions should be prohibited. Physicians should be better trained about the hazards of tobacco and encouraged to refer patients to smoking cessation programs. We should work with insurance companies to establish and expand nonsmoker differentials on insurance policies.

We could increase the federal excise tax on cigarettes and eliminate the price support and allotment programs for tobacco. Since this would pose an economic dilemma for the small tobacco farmer, programs should be developed to encourage the transition to nontobacco crops.

Attempts to reduce the prevalence of smoking have focused almost exclusively on the individual. In an effort to consider both societal as well as individual approaches, we have grouped our recommendations for strategies to reduce smoking prevalence into four basic categories: education and information, economic incentives, restrictive policies, and system intervention. The categories themselves are not particularly important; they simply provide a general framework in which to group strategies for discussion purposes. Specific interventions and efforts appropriate to each category use existing knowledge and resources and link the efforts of health professionals, educators, legislators, and professional organizations.

Education and Information

1. Mass media efforts
   a. Increase public knowledge of the hazards of smoking and tobacco
   b. Encourage and promote smoking cessation
   c. Provide incentives for nonsmokers (especially youths) not to start
   d. Coordinate efforts among various agencies and organizations involved in antismoking activities
   e. Stimulate public participation in programs to reduce smoking
   f. Specifically target interventions on activities of high-risk groups, including minorities, pregnant women, and the poor
2. National health education efforts
   a. Promote educational activities in primary and secondary schools
   b. Promote educational activities in the community
3. Labeling: Develop an index of mutagenicity for printing on all cigarette package labels

Economic Incentives and Disincentives

1. Subsidies
   a. Eliminate the federal price support programs

for tobacco in order to discourage production and consumption

b. Provide subsidies, low-interest loans, or other incentives for farmers (small and possibly even large) to grow crops other than tobacco

2. Insurance

a. Expand discounts, rebates, and benefits on health and life insurance to nonsmokers

b. Consider reductions in home, property, and auto insurance coverage for nonsmokers

3. Federal excise tax on cigarettes

a. Continue current tax authorization and make tax reflect inflation

b. Increase tax amounts to be commensurate with the direct health care costs attributable to tobacco (approximately $1 per pack). Channel these revenues into Medicare/Medicaid to offset smokers' higher medical care expenses

Restrictive Policies on the Marketing, Promotion, and Use of Tobacco

1. Restrict marketing of tobacco products

a. Approve sale only at licensed retail outlets

b. Prohibit sale of cigarettes from vending machines (to make cigarettes less easily available to minors)

c. Prohibit sale of cigarettes in hospitals, nursing homes, other health care facilities, and pharmacies

2. Restrict promotion of tobacco products

a. Ban all advertising of tobacco products if possible (including sponsorship of sporting and cultural events, complementary cigarettes)

b. At the least, prohibit the use of advertising suggesting that cigarette smoking is essential to social prominence or social attraction, or portraying smokers participating in physical activity requiring stamina or athletic conditioning beyond normal recreation

c. If advertising is to continue, require compensatory time and space for antismoking health education messages

d. Require that advertising of tobacco products strictly comply with "truth in advertising" ethics and codes

e. Immediately require that the promotion of smokeless tobacco products conform to the standards for advertising and promotion of cigarettes

Integrate Intervention Activities into Existing Social Systems

1. Health care systems

a. Prohibit smoking in all health care institutions

b. Take responsibility for providing either direct aid for smoking cessation or appropriate referral to persons or programs offering such aid

c. In the education of health professionals, stress the health hazards of smoking and provide complete information regarding the health consequences of smoking and methods for smoking cessation

d. Stress the importance of professionals' serving as role models by refraining from using tobacco themselves

2. Workplace

a. Provide appropriate guidelines that discourage smoking in the workplace and support nonsmokers' rights

b. Make smoking cessation and education programs available to all employees

c. Provide incentives for nonsmoking in the workplace (bonuses, vacations, dinners, etc.)

d. Generate support for antismoking policies and efforts

3. Educational system

a. Prohibit tobacco use in schools

b. Stress the importance of teachers' serving as role models by refraining from using tobacco themselves

c. Make cessation aid available for faculty, staff, and students

4. Voluntary agencies

a. Coordinate a professional media campaign to discourage smoking

b. Coordinate cessation activities at appropriate sites

c. Act as a referral network for professionals and the public regarding cessation programs, and establish guidelines and standards for programs

5. Public areas: Restrict smoking in all public areas

UNINTENTIONAL INJURIES

Chairperson: Susan Baker, M.P.H.
Rapporteur: Dan Horth

Injuries impose a greater burden on modern society than any disease, but this burden is not shared equally. Rather, it rests heavily on the poor, teenagers, young children, and the elderly. Mortality from injuries is a leading cause of years of life lost prematurely. When injuries are not fatal, they can result in serious and permanent morbidity and disability.

Unlike many other major health problems, injuries can be prevented by a variety of measures already available and inexpensive in relation to their benefits. Yet, tragically, these measures are not applied.

Injuries from motor vehicles account for more deaths before age 65 than any other single cause. Measures to prevent these injuries exist but are not being applied. Safer vehicle design with automatic restraints represents the single largest opportunity to close the gap of preventable injuries and deaths. In addition, seat belt use is vitally important. Seat belt laws should be promoted in all states in a form that will not jeopardize or delay standards for passive restraints.

Because of the extremely high death and injury rates involving teenage drivers and occupants, states should develop strategies to reduce teenagers' exposure to high-risk driving situations such as night driving and alcohol-impaired driving. Such measures include increasing the driving age and restricting driving privileges to daylight hours.

Alcohol contributes to at least half of all motor vehicle-related deaths. We recommend that current drunk driving laws and their enforcement be evaluated to identify gaps and loopholes and develop model state legislation. Such evaluation should include consideration of liability on the part of purveyors of alcohol for injuries caused by drunk drivers. Similarly, liability for other alcohol-related injuries such as fires and shootings should be explored.

Home injuries are a serious risk to young children and to the elderly. Falls, fires, and drownings at home cause about 20,000 deaths each year. Injury control programs should be developed that focus on the home and that tie together in a cost-effective manner the diverse intervention strategies needed to deal with the many sources of injuries in the home. High priority should be given to building codes that require smoke detectors in all dwellings, as well as automatic fire extinguishing systems, hot water systems that cannot discharge water hotter than 120°F, childproof swimming enclosures, and designs that reduce falls.

Injuries from firearms kill 34,000 Americans every year. For ages 15–34, they are the second leading cause of death. For young adult blacks, they are the number one cause of death. The poor of all races bear a disproportionate share of the burden of firearm-related deaths and disability. The volatile issue of gun control has drawn attention away from the variety of approaches that might reduce firearm injuries. These range from reducing the importation of easily concealed handguns to designing guns so that they cannot be easily fired by young children.

Occupational injuries kill 13,000 workers each year and permanently disable many times that number. Certain groups of workers are at especially high risk of severe injury. Many job hazards have not been adequately addressed, including farms with fewer than 11 employees, who are not protected under the OSHA laws; pilots of light aircraft, for which occupant protection standards are more than 30 years out of date; and loggers, train operators, and firemen.

Although *Closing the Gap* chose to consider intentional and unintentional injuries separately for analytic purposes, the general injury prevention strategies in the following outline are applicable to both. This outline groups intervention strategies into categories to facilitate their consideration and discussion.

Regardless of the categories, it is worth noting the experience of experts in the fields of injury control, health education, and public health, who caution that strategies directed to the individual are less effective than those directed to groups, communities, or society as a whole. Interventions are most successful when they can be applied at the community level rather than at the individual level, when they concentrate on modifying environmental factors rather than altering human behavior, and when they require little or no individual effort.

Industry Efforts

1. Vehicle design
   a. Incorporate proven safety features into the design and manufacture of automobiles, including (but not limited to):
      (1) A single, centered rear brake light at eye level
      (2) A device that limits an automobile's maximum speed to that commensurate with the vehicle's ability to protect occupants from fatal frontal crashes
      (3) Passive restraints, including air bags and automatic seat belts
      (4) Bumper height under 21 inches to reduce injuries to adults
      (5) Improved exhaust systems that prevent toxic gases from leaking into vehicles
      (6) Warning devices that detect high carbon monoxide concentrations and automatically turn off the engine
   b. Build or modify boats to ensure stability, adequate lighting, and availability of flotation devices
   c. Incorporate rollover protection design into tractors, powered industrial trucks, and construction equipment (e.g., fork lifts, skip loaders)
   d. Incorporate state-of-the-art design for small airplanes to reduce crash injuries
2. Design of other equipment and products
   a. Reduce maximum water heater temperatures

to less than 130°F (preferably less than 120°F)

b. Require the manufacture of cigarettes that extinguish within four minutes

c. Promote manufacture and use of matches that burn at a lower temperature, self-extinguish when dropped, and are difficult for children to light

d. Increase the use of flame retardants in household furnishings

e. Reduce or eliminate the manufacture or sale of hazardous chemicals (e.g., change chemical formulation, as was done in leaded paints)

f. Limit the amount of dangerous drug or product per package (e.g., number of baby aspirin per bottle to less than a fatal dose; single-dose units of dangerous household products)

g. Encourage increased corporate responsibility for designing safe products for children

h. Encourage increased corporate responsibility for providing safe food products for children; label foods that are hazardous for young children

i. Place air holes in garment bags

j. Design guns to reduce the incidence of inadvertent discharge; make it difficult for a child or inebriated individual to fire a gun

3. Worker safety

a. Improve ventilation in high-risk areas to prevent the build-up of dangerous gases

b. Eliminate wage incentives that lead to increased risk-taking behaviors

c. Increase the use of robots for dangerous jobs

d. Limit noise levels so they cannot obscure sounds from warning devices

e. Design worksite layouts to increase the operator's visibility of hazardous portions of machinery

f. Provide and require the use of protective clothing and equipment

g. Provide lifelines for workers near bodies of water

h. Protect workers not currently covered by OSHA

i. Identify workers and injury risks that are not being addressed adequately

Environmental Design Strategies

1. Roadways: Incorporate modern roadway design and safety features in the development of new roads and remove hazards from existing roads

a. Remove roadside structures or use only those that decrease crash forces

b. Increase the duration of the yellow phase of traffic light sequence

c. Separate pedestrians from vehicles by physical barriers

2. Home and community

a. Promote the use of increased illumination, handrails, childproof barriers, walkways, window guards, and nonskid surfaces on stairs and tubs; promote the rapid removal of ice and snow from sidewalks; promote sand playground surfaces

b. Install smoke detectors and sprinklers and automatic fire extinguisher equipment, especially in high-risk buildings. Develop and implement standards for safe swimming pool use and design, including:

(1) High fences with self-latching childproof gates

(2) Ready availability of rescue and resuscitation equipment

(3) Adequate lighting within and around pools

(4) Slip-resistant surfaces around pools

c. Post signs identifying depth, undertow, or slippery bank where warranted

d. If guns must be kept in the home, keep all guns and ammunition locked and inaccessible to children

e. Support the reauthorization of Consumer Product Safety Commission and increase its funding

Education

1. General public

a. Broaden the availability and use of cardiopulmonary resuscitation (CPR) training

b. Teach and publicize the proper treatment for burns and common injuries

c. Communicate the nature of imminent hazards with minimal confusion and a minimum of false alarms

d. Combine educational efforts with other strategies, including community organization and involvement

e. Accurately portray injury risks in the media and provide role models for injury prevention

f. Increase knowledge of injury control in the community and as part of high school and college science curricula; teach injury prevention and control in public health, medical, and law schools

2. Targeted groups and individuals

a. Instruct high-risk groups of their increased risks (e.g., advise epileptics to shower rather than bathe to prevent drowning; advise parents of the potential of children choking from common foods)

b. Teach the Heimlich maneuver to parents, child care providers, and restaurant workers

c. Provide trial lawyers with the epidemiologic data on which to base litigation against automakers who fail to provide the most effective methods of reducing motor vehicle injuries and death; apply this strategy for other industries or manufacturers

Health Intervention Strategies

1. Health professionals
   a. Encourage health professionals to discourage the misuse and abuse of alcohol
   b. Restrict antidepressant prescriptions
2. Health care system
   a. Implement and expand alcohol rehabilitation programs; widen their availability
   b. Support poison control centers
   c. Increase the availability of emergency medical services and preplanned protocols for emergency situations

Economic Measures to Reduce Injuries

1. Public programs
   a. Fund and provide safe, convenient public transportation
   b. Help low-income persons pay winter heating costs
   c. Provide air-conditioned shelters for individuals at risk for heat-related morbidity or mortality, and provide transportation to these shelters
2. Incentives and disincentives
   a. Encourage insurance companies to cancel liability coverage for manufacturers of faulty or dangerous goods
   b. Provide tax incentives for implementation of new safety designs
   c. Base the tax on wine, beer, and liquor on alcohol content
   d. Increase the cost of alcoholic beverages and index the price to inflation

Restrictive Policies and Their Enforcement

1. Vehicle use
   a. Promote seat belt laws
   b. Enforce motorcycle headlight laws
   c. Enforce child restraint laws
   d. Require helmet use for motorcyclists, moped drivers, bicyclists, and horseback riders
   e. Raise the minimum driving age
   f. Reduce the exposure of teenage drivers to high-risk situations through curfews, etc.
   g. Strictly enforce speed limit laws and lower the speed limit in high-risk areas
   h. Require a physical exam for the elderly before issuing driver's licenses
   i. Remove or separate roadside hazards (unyielding posts, ditches that cause rollover, etc.)
   j. Evaluate current drunk driving laws and their enforcement, and develop model laws
2. Alcohol use
   a. Raise alcohol purchase age to 21
   b. Restrict advertising that depicts alcohol as socially desirable and harmless
   c. Restrict the sale and consumption of alcoholic beverages in boating, pool, harbor, marina, and beach areas; impose penalties for operating a boat while intoxicated
   d. Prohibit the sale of beer and wine at convenience stores, gas stations, and fast food outlets
   e. Reduce driving under the influence of alcohol through identification and elimination of loopholes in laws and enforcement
   f. Encourage and enforce provider liability for damages resulting from serving alcohol to a driver who subsequently sustains or causes injury or death while intoxicated
3. Building design and upkeep
   a. Stringently enforce heat and electrical standards for old and new homes
   b. Enforce building codes for fire doors, fire walls, clearly marked exits, fire extinguishers, and sprinkler systems
4. Firearms
   a. Reduce the availability of guns, especially easily concealed handguns
   b. Reduce the availability of ammunition and make it less lethal
   c. Require hunters to wear helmets and bulletproof vests

PREVENTIVE HEALTH CARE

Chairperson: Lester Breslow, M.D., M.P.H.
Rapporteur: William Herman, M.D.

The American people are increasingly aware of the need for health maintenance, particularly through prevention. The prevalence of cigarette smoking is declining, cholesterol levels are lower, high blood pressure is better controlled—trends that result in overall improved health. For example, heart disease is decreasing at the rate of 2.5 percent a year, and, except for lung cancer, the total mortality from cancer is declining. Life expectancy is increasing. The role of health professionals is to help accelerate and magnify these favorable trends.

The ultimate decisions affecting prevention are often personal, made by individuals or families. But these choices are not made in a vacuum—they must be considered in the social context in which they take place. These decisions should encompass what we ordinarily call medical care, as well as the whole array of personal health practices.

We believe that prevention should include not only the avoidance of disease where possible (primary prevention) but also the detection of pathologic processes early enough so that corrective action can be taken (secondary prevention). In addition, surveillance is an essential component of prevention, because it provides information on changing trends in disease incidence so that appropriate responses can be initiated. Finally, prevention requires action through the entire social system—not just the health care field but the educational system, industry, and local government.

We propose several strategies to reach our goal of preventive health care for all persons. We seek a consensus on standards for personal and environmental health services and for education directed toward health maintenance and disease prevention. For each period in life, it is possible to define specific sets of services appropriate for health promotion. We believe that people should be involved in deciding what they need. Objectives regarding bodily, behavioral, and environmental risk factors for health should be established and periodically revised.

We should extend present preventive efforts (e.g., immunization programs and fluoridation) to the entire physical environment, including the workplace. Present efforts to define health considerations should also extend to broadcasting and other mass media.

Adequate public and private funding for effective preventive health services is needed, with particular attention to universal coverage for specified services. We must also develop and implement prevention-oriented school health services with special attention to food services and physical education. It seems inconsistent to teach youngsters about nutrition in the classroom and then send them to a cafeteria where various types of junk foods are offered.

Let us seek new incentives for health professionals to provide preventive services and offer financial incentives to individuals and groups for undertaking preventive activities, for example, through insurance incentives.

The following outline provides a basis for discussion of possible strategies to improve preventive health care.

Availability, Accessibility, and Utilization of Preventive Health Services

1. Availability and access to care
    a. Ensure the adequate provision of public funds for health services known to be cost beneficial (e.g., immunizations, fluoridation); provide entitlement funding for these services
    b. Develop new approaches to the funding of preventive health services

(1) Develop and incorporate into third-party packages the preventive services that meet people's needs
(2) Encourage organization and funding of preventive services through industry (e.g., employer-sponsored programs and labor–management-negotiated programs)
(3) Offer financial incentives to individuals and groups for undertaking preventive activities
(4) Develop alternate methods of covering individuals for preventive services
    c. Increase and improve the range of preventive health services available (e.g., preventive dental care; screening and early detection of diabetes, cancer, and hypertension; care for patients with arthritis or back pain; care for the diabetic patient)
    d. Improve the distribution of providers of preventive health services
    e. Provide preventive services during hours convenient to the public
    f. Provide incentives that reward health professionals for utilizing appropriate preventive health services
    g. Provide transportation for those requiring assistance
2. Utilization
    a. Provide reimbursement by health insurance plans for essential preventive health services (e.g., screening and early detection programs, preventive dental care, calcium supplements to prevent osteoporosis)
    b. Educate the public on the benefits of preventive health services
    c. Promote awareness in the community of available preventive health services
    d. Encourage greater public utilization of preventive services
    e. Encourage community sponsorship of preventive health activities
    f. Increase utilization of services by individuals at high risk for preventable health problems by linking social support programs to preventive health services
    g. Support health departments, both legislatively and financially, in training of personnel and redirection of services as a key resource for prevention
    h. Explore new ways of providing preventive services (e.g., utilizing new as well as traditional professionals)

Improving the Quality of Preventive Health Services

1. Develop standardized recommendations for preventive health services

2. Professional education

a. Ensure that medical and other health schools educate health professionals to deliver comprehensive preventive services that reflect known interventions for preventable morbidity and mortality (e.g., incorporate essential information into medical school curricula)

b. Stress the health consequences of lifestyle and behavioral factors known to be associated with preventable morbidity and mortality in the education of health professionals

c. Encourage health professionals to utilize available, standardized recommendations for preventive health care

Preventive Health Programs

1. Primary and secondary prevention

a. Expand and maintain programs requisite to the delivery of quality preventive health services (e.g., immunization, fluoridation, diabetes control programs)

b. Ensure the provision of adequate public funds for programs known to be cost beneficial (e.g., immunization, fluoridation)

c. Develop and implement disincentives for unhealthful decisions in addition to incentives for healthful ones

2. Surveillance

a. Expand and maintain surveillance activities to identify and evaluate preventable health programs (e.g., hospital-acquired infections, tuberculosis, sexually transmitted diseases)

b. Expand current surveillance activities to ensure the ability to identify new and unusual problems of public health significance

ALCOHOL MISUSE

Chairperson: Frederick C. Robbins, M.D.
Rapporteur: Patricia Ramia

Alcohol accounts for as many deaths each year as did the entire Vietnam War. Half of these deaths are the result of alcohol-related accidents, particularly automobile accidents. Many of these deaths are among youth, awarding alcohol the number two spot in the ranking of risk factors leading to the loss of productive years of life.

The health consequences of alcohol misuse and abuse may also include intentional or unintentional injury to self, family, friends, or others. The morbidity and mortality resulting from injury in motor vehicle accidents, fires, drownings, falls, and vio-

lence are excessive. Other health consequences resulting from alcohol misuse or abuse include cancer, pregnancy-related disorders, diseases of the digestive system, and heart disease. Even when these health consequences are not fatal, serious, permanent disability associated with alcohol misuse can significantly reduce the quality of life for the affected individual.

Five key assumptions guided us in our examination of the use and abuse of alcohol. First, we have to recognize that our society accepts the moderate consumption of alcohol in low-risk populations. Unlike tobacco use, which is detrimental in any amount, some use of alcohol is acceptable in our culture and almost every culture. Second, any consumption in high-risk groups should be discouraged. Third, the option of not drinking should be socially acceptable. Fourth, heavy use is to be discouraged in all situations. And last, safety and health protection measures that apply across our entire population should be a high priority.

Our recommendations to decrease the abuse of alcohol centered on three broad goals: alter the individual and public perception of alcohol use, align public policy with health priorities, and provide appropriate prevention and treatment measures. It is important to note that in order to reduce alcohol-related death and disease, we must work closely with two high-risk populations: young people who drink to excess and account for many vehicle crashes, and pathologic drinkers who are dependent or addicted.

In the past, education of the individual has been seen as necessary and sufficient to deal with alcohol problems. We know that it is necessary but not at all sufficient.

There are actually three educational approaches to be considered. The first approach, aimed at the individual, teaches that alcoholism is a disease and that alcohol is a major drug: alcholism is treatable, and it is socially acceptable for a person to seek treatment. The second message is that alcohol problems are linked to other social problems such as unemployment, economic conditions, and consumer product safety issues. Alcoholism must therefore be considered in its social context. The third approach needs to focus on educating special populations about alcohol abuse: those people who make decisions that affect the lives of others, such as family members, state and local politicians, and appointed officials.

Our specific recommendations for developing a public policy to discourage alcohol consumption include raising the price of alcohol through tax policy, especially by increasing the federal excise tax on beer and wine. At present, alcoholic beverages are priced competitively with soft drinks. This makes the symbolic statement that alcohol is a legitimate alternative in any situation where soft drinks are consumed.

We also recommend removing the tax deductions for alcohol as a business expense. Corporations now purchase 12 percent of all alcohol in the United States, which amounts to a tax write-off of $5.6 billion through expense accounts, for gifts, and at conventions. In addition, the alcohol industry legally deducts advertising costs totaling about $1.5 billion a year.

We strongly encourage the development of server intervention programs. This includes not only the Dram Shop Third Party Liability laws, which place the responsibility and liability on the server for providing alcohol to an intoxicated person, but also the proper education of servers and improving the environment in which alcohol is served. We need to provide training for servers. They are handling a dangerous drug, sometimes serving it to very young people or those who may have been using other medications. Servers need much more information about dispensing this drug. Bars should be designed to create an environment conducive to lower levels of consumption and safer kinds of drinking behavior.

People from the retail industry, the alcoholic beverage industry, and community representatives should be brought together to discuss ways that server intervention and other approaches to the more sensible use of alcohol can be promoted. A similar approach could be used with representatives of the media to encourage the proper portrayal of alcohol use and abuse, especially in the mass media.

The following outline categorizes strategies to reduce the problem of alcohol misuse to a framework that allows meaningful discussion. The categories themselves are provided only to help organize ideas and discussion.

Education and Information

1. Mass media efforts
   a. Increase knowledge of the risks and hazards of alcohol misuse and abuse through public service messages, program content, and advertising
   b. Alter public attitudes and awareness of problems associated with alcohol use
   c. Provide incentives for nondrinkers (especially youth) not to start
   d. Stimulate public participation in programs to reduce the prevalence of alcohol misuse

2. National health education efforts
   a. Promote educational activities in primary and secondary schools
   b. Promote educational activities in the workplace and the community
   c. Institute educational programs that help to develop coping skills to resist peer pressure using community resources (e.g., schools, churches, community organizations)
3. Server education: Require adequate server education by licensing boards
4. Societal norms
   a. Establish acceptable social definitions of alcohol use and misuse
   b. Increase the social unacceptability of alcohol misuse

Economic Incentives and Disincentives

1. Taxation
   a. Equalize the taxation on beer, wine, and distilled spirits
   b. Increase taxes on all alcoholic beverages
   c. Remove any tax advantages associated with entertaining with alcohol

Restrictive Policies on the Marketing, Promotion, and Use of Alcohol

1. Restrict the marketing of alcoholic beverages
   a. Restrict the hours of sale and serving of alcoholic beverages
   b. Increase the legal age limit for puchasing alcoholic beverages
2. Restrict the promotion of alcoholic beverages
   a. Limit the advertising of alcoholic beverages
   b. Limit the extent and manner in which alcohol may be portrayed by the media, the entertainment industry, and in the sponsorship of public events
   c. If advertising is to continue, require compensatory time and space for health education messages regarding the risks associated with alcohol
   d. Restrict the promotion of alcohol consumption by establishments that serve alcoholic beverages (e.g., happy hours, consumption contests)
3. Institute policies requiring the labeling of alcoholic beverages to include alcohol content, ingredients, and a warning regarding the hazards associated with alcohol misuse
4. Institute policies that place responsibility on the server or provider for providing alcohol to individuals who subsequently sustain or cause injury or death as a result of intoxication
5. Increase and consistently enforce existing laws and penalties for violations incurred while the offender is intoxicated, especially drunk driving laws

Integrate Intervention Activities into Existing Social Systems

1. Health care system
   a. Provide counseling or aid for alcohol abusers or, if more appropriate, referral to persons or programs offering such aid
   b. In the education of health professionals, stress the health hazards of alcohol misuse
      (1) Provide complete information regarding the health consequences of alcohol misuse and methods for treating this problem
      (2) Challenge health professionals to be role models
   c. Make health professionals aware that they are at particular risk for misusing alcohol, and educate them regarding alternative coping skills and behaviors
2. Workplace
   a. Make educational programs available to all employees
   b. If possible, provide financial support for treatment programs
3. Voluntary agencies
   a. Coordinate education efforts on the health hazards of alcohol misuse and abuse
   b. Coordinate a professional media campaign to discourage alcohol misuse
   c. Coordinate counseling and treatment programs at appropriate sites
   d. Act as a referral network for professionals and the public regarding counseling and treatment programs, and establish financial incentives for nondrinkers.
4. Insurance: Encourage insurance companies to lower premiums for nondrinkers

VIOLENCE, DEPRESSION, AND SUBSTANCE ABUSE

Chairperson: Thomas E. Bryant, M.D., J.D.
Rapporteur: Nancy Fajman, M.P.H.

The impact of violence, depression, and substance abuse on our society is staggering. Not only are these problems important causes of death, they are also major causes of years of life lost prematurely. The result is high morbidity, loss of productivity, and billions of dollars spent on treatment. The involvement of young people and minority groups in these disorders has important social implications beyond the measures of morbidity or mortality. These disorders result in lost productivity and lowered quality of life—important elements that cannot easily be demonstrated with statistics.

The following intervention strategies have been categorized into broad classes to facilitate discussion. These classes consider both general intervention strategies applicable to all three problems and specific strategies applying to only a single problem.

Depression. We must first reduce the stigma associated with depression. Given the nature of depression, one of the variables that seems most amenable to change is the public's perception of this disorder. People need to realize that depression is a treatable and understandable disease, and one for which they should not be ashamed to seek treatment.

We need to increase the recognition and treatment of depression by our primary care physicians. This can be accomplished in part by an active program in medical school curricula and continuing education. Because most people with severe depression go to their family doctor rather than to a psychiatrist or a psychologist, family doctors and their nurses need training to better identify and treat this problem.

We also need to present a positive concept of mental health as a desirable quality of life and promote meaningful social roles in the community for persons who are not able to work.

Violence. We must limit the availability of lethal agents, including medication and firearms. Both suicides and domestic violence increase as the means of destruction proliferate. We also believe it is important to research the epidemiology of firearm injuries, an almost completely neglected area.

Educational efforts to criminalize family or domestic violence should be undertaken. In the past, family violence has been somewhat ignored by the courts, but this is changing. We would like to encourage this new realization, and we believe a number of positive results will follow if we can criminalize family violence.

An important recommendation is that we undertake efforts to empower women. For example, adequate safety and income opportunities are needed by women who are victims of family violence. In addition, the availability of shelters for battered women and their children should be expanded.

Substance abuse. Our primary recommendation is to increase the percentage of drug users who go into drug abuse rehabilitation programs. Efforts should be made to identify users early in their drug careers with the expectation that intervention efforts are more effective at that stage.

We recommend increased funding for youth programs, such as recreational programs that provide alternative activities for young people. We also feel that, because of the high incidence of bacterial and viral infections, we should decriminalize the possession and purchase of paraphernalia associated with illicit drug use (syringes and needles).

On the advice of social scientists who have studied these problems, we have chosen interventions that act on the community level rather than the individual level. These interventions are aimed at modifying environmental factors rather than changing human behavior. The following outline presents our specific suggestions.

Education and Information

1. General public
   a. Increase education regarding family life, family planning, and child rearing
   b. Promote education on the importance of parent–child bonding and family stability
   c. Educate parents and children to identify and acknowledge violent behaviors and impulses (e.g., suicide, domestic violence)
   d. Teach appropriate coping and conflict resolution skills
   e. Enhance public education on the causes, manifestations, and treatment of violent behavior and impulses, depression, and substance abuse
   f. Integrate psychological education, including stress management, into the public school curriculum
   g. Develop and promote a broad-based public education campaign to reduce the stigma associated with depression and other mental disorders
   h. Decrease media portrayal and acceptance of violence as a regular and reasonable element of life
   i. Restrict programming that includes violent behavior to limit the exposure for youth
2. Professionals
   a. Improve recognition of the victims of violence, depression, and substance abuse by health care professionals, teachers, and clergy
   b. Improve health care professionals' management and treatment of victims of violence, persons with depression, and substance abusers

Restrictive Policies and Societal Factors

1. Handguns
   a. Limit the availability of handguns and small arms ammunition
      (1) Sell handguns only to groups requiring their use (e.g., military, police)
      (2) Require difficult and expensive registration or licensing of firearms
      (3) Sell ammunition only during hunting season or at approved target practice sites; increase the price of ammunition significantly
      (4) Decrease the production, manufacture, and importation of firearms and ammunition
   b. Implement strategies to reduce the injury potential of handguns and small arms ammunition
      (1) Place safety guards on guns that require several steps to remove, making removal beyond the ability of children and intoxicated adults
      (2) Develop (and require the use of) ammunition that is less likely to penetrate the skin and requires less velocity to fire
      (3) At the least, require the use of only fully jacketed bullets (as required by the Geneva Convention and used by the military)
      (4) For general use, sell only guns that require reloading
      (5) Reduce the muzzle velocity of guns provided for general use
2. Social changes
   a. Decrease the cultural acceptance of violence
   b. Define high-risk settings and occupations for violence, depression, and substance abuse, and determine appropriate interventions
   c. Discourage the acceptance and portrayal of males as overly dominant and physically aggressive in societal roles

Economic Factors

1. General: Increase funding for youth recreation programs
2. Violence: Train high-risk adolescents in job-related skills and make jobs available to them
3. Depression
   a. Improve insurance coverage for psychological disorders
   b. Fund efforts to promote public education on, research into, and treatment of depression
4. Substance abuse: Improve insurance coverage and expand funding for employee assistance programs

Health and Social Services

1. General
   a. Develop outreach and support organizations for groups at high risk for depression, suicide, and drug abuse (e.g., the unemployed, recently bereaved, divorced, chronically ill, children of the mentally ill, children of alcoholics)
   b. Reduce consumption of alcohol and other drugs
2. Violence
   a. Develop and strengthen existing programs for the detection and treatment of child abuse
   b. Expand the number of shelters and their scope of services for battered women

c. Interact with police departments and schools to record, intervene in, and help prevent violent incidents

3. Depression: Improve screening and intervention efforts in primary medical care settings to promote prevention of depression and recognition of depressed and otherwise emotionally disturbed individuals

4. Substance abuse

a. Identify users early in their drug-using careers

b. Improve access to and increase utilization of substance abuse treatment programs

Criminal Justice System

1. Violence

a. Have police, courts, and laws treat family violence as criminal behavior

b. Train police and citizen intervention teams

c. Increase clearance rates for cases of murders and robberies

d. Improve linkages between police and social services in response to violence

e. Initiate informal citizen surveillance and silent witness programs

f. Educate prosecutors, judges, and juries about woman battering and child abuse

g. Facilitate access of victims to legal services

h. Initiate victim and witness assistance programs

i. Increase and consistently enforce penalties for the use of handguns in the commission of crimes

j. Create alternative assistance for perpetrators within the context of criminalizing the behavior

2. Substance abuse

a. Decriminalize the possession of drug-related paraphernalia

b. Allow over-the-counter sale of needles and syringes without prescription to prevent the spread of infectious disease

UNINTENDED PREGNANCY

Chairpersons: Luella M. Klein, M.D., and Martin Smith, M.D.

Unintended pregnancy is a national problem that requires national attention. In 1980, of the 6 million pregnancies in the United States, 3.3 million were either unwanted or mistimed (occurring before the woman wanted to have a child). Of these 3.3 million unintended pregnancies, 1.5 million were terminated by legal abortion.

During any given year, 36 million of the 55 million women of reproductive age in the United States wish to prevent pregnancy. We need to understand that women spend most of their reproductive lives preventing pregnancy.

Both as health care providers and as part of the public, we must be mindful of teenagers. More than 1 million pregnancies occur among teenagers each year, 80 percent unintended. Data show that a woman who has a child before she is 18 has only a 50 percent chance of completing high school. Without at least a high school education, she has fewer opportunities to get a productive job and to provide for herself and her children. She is usually unwed and often faces a future of public support, perhaps subjecting herself and her children to poverty for the rest of their lives. About half the women in families receiving Aid to Families with Dependent Children (AFDC) have given birth as teenagers.

We can reduce unintended pregnancy. Social scientists who study population changes recognize four major ways of preventing childbearing: (1) postponing marriage, cohabitation, or age of first sexual intercourse; (2) contraception, including barriers, withdrawal, intrauterine devices, oral contraceptives, injections, and sterilization; (3) induce abortion; (4) frequent and prolonged breast feeding to extend the interval between pregnancies.

National and international forums have identified four key ethical rationales for national policies and programs supporting family planning. Consistent with basic American traditions is the right of individuals and couples to choose for themselves the number and timing of the children they have. The second is the health advantage to the mother, the infant, and the family that results from limiting family size and spacing children. The third principle is the foundation of public health in the United States, which promotes the reduction of differences in health problems between the affluent and the poor. The fourth principle is the intrinsic value of improving social and economic opportunities, which are facilitated by having smaller families and by delaying the age of childbearing beyond teenage years.

The promotion of sexual behavior along with the lack of any sense of responsibility about the consequences of sexual activity is a major element encouraging unintended pregnancies. We must alter the media presentation of sexual issues. In this country, everything is sold with sex, and every night television unveils instant intimacy with no discussion of the results. Television, radio, and the printed media seem to have almost a conspiracy of silence about responsible sex and pregnancy prevention. More important than simply advertising contraceptives would be the presentation and discussion of pregnancy prevention and sexual responsibility—topics avoided on television. It is also important that the media show the male partner having more responsibility and taking an active role in family planning.

Another obstacle to reducing unintended pregnancies is ignorance. We must break down myths that have prevailed in our society for decades, including the myth that contraception is more dangerous than pregnancy. In fact, oral contraceptives and intrauterine devices are safer (i.e., cause fewer deaths) than using no contraception, except in older smokers on the pill. We need to put these risks into perspective. More than 3 million women in the United States do not use effective contraception because of fear of complications—not complications themselves, but *fear* of complications. Moreover, many physicians do not know the mortality rate of various contraceptive methods or the mortality rate of pregnancy.

Life education, reproductive health information, and sex information should be available in schools, and information on these subjects should be presented to parents, teachers, counselors, and local PTAs.

It is important for us to enunciate a reproductive health policy with the goal that all pregnancies be intended and cared for. Such a policy needs emphasis throughout society, especially among health care providers. The fact that unintended pregnancy is prevalent in our society and is preventable should be a subject for discussion within every professional health care association.

One of the ways to decrease the risk of unintended pregnancy is to increase self-esteem among those with less education or lower socioeconomic status. We have found that if a woman feels she has few opportunities, that she cannot accomplish something in life or attain higher income and status, she is likely to see little use in preventing pregnancy. Therefore, we need to improve the educational level of women and provide greater access to jobs if we wish to make women feel responsible for themselves and choose contraception or postpone sexual involvement.

Some of us in the group were adamant that women should understand that control of their own lives and reproduction is now within their reach. We should not only maintain but improve access to contraceptive services and coordination with other health services. We support voluntary, confidential contraceptive services for all sexually active persons of all ages.

In this era of decreased funding for social programs, it is not popular to recommend more money for present programs and projects. However, we should examine these numbers closely: the cost of one unintended pregnancy to a teenager for her support, medical care, AFDC, housing, etc., is $18,000, while the cost of comprehensive family planning services is $63.

The goal of reproductive health is that all pregnancies in the country are intended and cared for so that women, men, and their families experience minimum mortality and morbidity.

The following is an outline of selected intervention strategies that should be considered in ameliorating the problem of unintended pregnancy in the United States.

Social Issues

1. Enunciate a reproductive health policy to reduce unintended pregnancies
    a. Professional associations should make reduction of unintended pregnancies a goal
    b. Family planning information should be presented
    c. State education departments should provide information about family planning
2. Decrease risk of unintended pregnancy
    a. Provide jobs for both men and women
    b. Increase self-esteem among men and women
3. Alter media presentation of sexual issues to include the consequences of sexual activity and responsibility for sexual behavior
4. Emphasize the role and responsibility of the male partner
5. Develop minority support for prevention of unintended pregnancy
6. Increase the educational level of women

Information and Education

1. Increase public awareness of unintended pregnancy as a high national priority
2. Use prototype of successful teen programs
    a. Encourage postponement of intercourse for both men and women
    b. Use positive peer influence
3. Stimulate the development of community-based initiatives
4. Educate children, PTA, teachers, parents, and professionals (group-specific education)
5. Educate women in the understanding that they control their lives and reproduction

Contraceptive Services

1. Increase access of all socioeconomic groups to contraceptive services
2. Coordinate contraceptive services with other

health services (i.e., screening, referrals, counseling) and offer screening and counseling for areas of concern surrounding contraceptives (i.e., sexuality, abstinence)

3. Support confidential contraceptive services for all sexually active persons of all ages

4. Provide alternatives for dealing with unintended pregnancy

5. Prevent the recurrence of unintended pregnancy in women who have already had one unintended pregnancy (i.e., target high-risk groups)

Specific Interventions

1. High-priority interventions

   a. Evaluate the efficacy of family planning programs and develop proposals to meet 1990 objectives for the nation

   b. Convene a meeting of media executives, writers, producers, sponsors, actors, etc., to promote responsible sexual portrayals in media

   c. Convene meetings of all interested groups such as Right to Life, Pro Choice, the American College of Obstetricians and Gynecologists, the American Academy of Pediatrics, and others to discuss areas of agreement

   d. Mobilize minority support for family planning programs

2. Other interventions

   a. Increase funding for existing probjects

   b. Establish a pilot project to determine the effectiveness of specific interventions

   c. Encourage the alliance of ACOG, AAP, and other interested organizations for leadership

   d. Encourage and provide better teacher and professional education

Afterword

William H. Foege, M.D., and Robert W. Amler, M.D.

Much has happened in the health field since November 1984, when "Closing the Gap" was held. For example, AIDS has emerged as our most rapidly growing health problem; and although a definitive treatment or cure for AIDS is not yet in sight, effective means of preventing it are already known.[1] Attention also has increasingly been focused on other problems, such as substance abuse, homeless people, and the case for healthier work sites, especially the smoke-free work environment. On the technology front, impressive gains continue to raise new questions in medical ethics and access to health care, such as surrogate motherhood and the selection of candidates for organ replacement. Moreover, innovative proposals are now under consideration to improve the quality of life by assuring catastrophic health care for all elderly Americans.

It is interesting, in retrospect, to note how successful the Carter Center consultants were in identifying many of the opportunities for prevention now being recognized by a growing number of leaders in business, education, and other fields, as well as in health. Government health agencies are reexamining their capacity to prevent premature death and unnecessary illness. Many professional and voluntary organizations are opposing misleading advertising and have intensified their own health promotion efforts. Television and radio stations no longer advertise smokeless tobacco products but are preparing to advertise condoms for the prevention of AIDS, other sexually transmitted diseases, and unintended pregnancy. By 1990 most automobile manufacturers are planning to equip their cars with air bags.[2] Health educators have documented measurable and substantial health benefits of school health education,[3] and there is additional evidence that students are supporting their efforts.[4]

Much of this recent surge in prevention activity is clearly not a result of "Closing the Gap" but closely parallels it in design and focus. For example, a U.S. Preventive Services Task Force has been formed to establish a rational approach to prevention by examining and categorizing the evidence for major preventive maneuvers.[5] The National Academy of Sciences has proposed a national agenda for injury research and control that has led to collaborative action between the Departments of Transportation and Health and Human Services.[6] The Indian Health Services has conducted a cross-sectional review of major health problems and precursors affecting Indian people, *Bridging the Gap.*[7,8] Perhaps of greatest interest has been the appearance of "prevention centers"—local consortia formed cooperatively with private and public resources—to design and implement disease prevention activities tailored to the needs of local populations.[9,10]

Since November 1984, the Carter Center has actively supported derivative activities in health promotion, global health, personal health risk appraisal, and conflict resolution. The first effort in health promotion was a one-hour television program on behavioral risk factors produced by the Georgia Public Television Network. Entitled *Kids Just Wanna Have Fun,* the program was targeted for school children and featured Bill Cosby and Jimmy Carter. In addition, a prevention guide for health officials is being developed with the American Public Health Association and the Centers for Disease Control. Discussions are also being held on how to best use health materials in educational efforts by schools and churches.

Global health activities began with a consultation on health problems in developing countries, "Risks Old and New," in April 1986. The consultants included many ministers of health and chief technical experts from developing countries. They examined the persistence of old risks like malnutrition, infection, and population pressures in developing countries, as well as the emergence of new risks like tobacco and alcohol products, injuries (whether intention or unintentional), and environmental and occupational hazards. Carter Center health activities are now under way or planned in Bangladesh, Pakistan, and Ghana. Related efforts are also underway to promote agricultural innovations in de-

From the Carter Center of Emory University (Foege) and the Centers for Disease Control (Amler), Atlanta.

Address reprint requests to Dr. Amler, Centers for Disease Control, Atlanta, GA 30333.

veloping countries, in connection with Global 2000 and the "Green Revolution."

To promote personal risk reduction, the Carter Center will soon complete a fully documented and updated Health Risk Appraisal (HRA) computer program for the public domain in collaboration with the Centers for Disease Control and 25 other health organizations. The computer program has been designed to be flexible enough to accommodate improvements in risk factor data and knowledge of risk reduction as the technology of prevention matures. A highly generalized, modular architecture was selected to ensure that the software could readily be adapted to a variety of uses and settings. The new Health Risk Appraisal is scheduled for release in September 1987.[11]

A unique outcome of "Closing the Gap" was a conflict resolution symposium on tobacco held in a Southern resort camp in September 1985. (The subject was suggested by an earlier conference held in Raleigh by the North Carolina Health Council.) Mr. Carter invited leading health officials and professionals, a U.S. Congressman, a U.S. Senate aide, tobacco farmers, auctioneers, state agriculture officials, and industry representatives. Under the guidance of professional mediators, the guests negotiated agreement in several important areas. These negotiations later were credited with stimulating action by the Congress (The Smokeless Tobacco Comprehensive Health Education Act of 1986) to ban television and radio advertising of smokeless tobacco and require warning labels on containers of these products.

Without a method to determine each cause and effect, it is nonetheless encouraging to note how far prevention has advanced since November 1984. Perhaps of greatest significance is the growing cooperative spirit between organizations and agencies, uniting people of diverse backgrounds and talents to act on generic precursors of preventable illness. Concerted action should reap substantial rewards as the gap is closed.

REFERENCES

1. Centers for Disease Control. Update: acquired immunodeficiency syndrome—United States. Morbid Mortal Weekly Rep 1986;35:757–60, 765–6.

2. Brown W. Airbag industry explodes as 18-year dispute fizzles. Washington Post 1987 Apr 12:H2.

3. Christenson GM, Gold RS, Katz M, Kreuter MW (eds). Results of the school health education evaluation. J School Health 1985;55:295–355.

4. Centers for Disease Control. Project graduation—Maine. Morbid Mortal Weekly Rep 1985;34:233–5.

5. Office of Disease Prevention and Health Promotion. ODPHP: A decade of progress. Washington, D.C.: Department of Health and Human Services, 1986.

6. Committee on Trauma Research. Injury in America: a continuing public health problem. Washington, D.C.: National Academy Press, 1985

7. Rhoades ER, Hammond J, Welty TK, Handler AO, Amler RW. The Indian burden of illness and future health interventions. Public Health Rep 1987;102:361–8.

8. Indian Health Service. Bridging the gap: report of the task force on parity of Indian health services. Washington, D.C.: Department of Health and Human Services, 1986.

9. Anonymous. The Henry J. Kaiser Family Foundation Annual Report 1985. Menlo Park, California: The Henry J. Kaiser Family Foundation, 1986.

10. Anonymous. Update CDC: Prevention center grants. Perspectives 1987;1:43–4, 50–2.

11. Centers for Disease Control. Health risk appraisal—new tool for chronic disease prevention. Chronic disease notes and reports. MMWR 1987;36.

12. Carter J, Carter R. Everything to gain: making the most of the rest of your life. New York: Random House, 1987.

Appendix: Closing the Gap

William H. Foege, M.D., Robert W. Amler, M.D.,
Craig C. White, M.D.

A national consultation on health policy was held at The Carter Center of Emory University, Atlanta, November 26 through 28, 1984.[1] National leaders from private, public, voluntary, and academic institutions met with specialists from many health fields to recommend and develop priorities for interventions directed at unnecessary morbidity and mortality in the United States. The consultation was the second in a three-part, five-year health project of research, planning, and implementation known as "Closing the Gap," and was cochaired by former President Jimmy Carter and Edward N. Brandt, Jr, MD, Assistant Secretary for Health. Contributions appear in this issue from President Carter[2] and Dr Brandt.[3]

Rather than seek technologic breakthroughs, the project seeks to focus national health policy on the "gap" represented by health problems that are unnecessary in light of knowledge that already is at hand. Consultants from various medical specialties conducted extensive investigations of the burden imposed by cancer, heart disease, diabetes, and 11 other priority health problems. They quantified preventable morbidity and premature mortality associated with specific risk factors or available interventions. Epidemiologists at the Centers for Disease Control, Atlanta, conducted a cross-sectional study to determine generic risk factors and generic problems with the greatest disease burden.

This report summarizes major findings and recommendations of the consultation. A detailed symposium will be published soon.

METHODS

A total of 14-high priority health problems was selected for study from an expanded list of health problems that included the *International Classification of Diseases, Ninth Revision,* and dental diseases. Se-

lection was based on five major selection criteria: (1) point prevalence and secular trends; (2) severity in terms of health impact and cost; (3) sensitivity to intervention using current scientific or operational knowledge; (4) feasibility of such intervention; and (5) generic applicability of such intervention to other health problems.

A study group of specialists led by a Carter Center consultant for each of the 14 health problems conducted an in-depth investigation to (1) report the impact of the health problem, (2) determine the preventable component of that impact, and (3) identify attributable risk factors and feasible interventions. The groups compiled existing data from a variety of sources, ranging from clinical case reports to vital and health statistics of state and local health departments and the National Center for Health Statistics. Additional comment was obtained from Carter Center project officers and a scientific review panel composed of epidemiologists from Emory University, the National Center for Health Statistics, and the Centers for Disease Control.

A cross-sectional analysis of the 14 position papers was conducted to determine the factors most responsible for the "gap" on the basis of their contribution to excessive morbidity and premature mortality. Where risk factors overlapped, a "cascade" priority system was used to assign attributable proportions of morbidity and mortality. This model was used with the recognition that it tends to underestimate the impact of factors that are lower in the cascade because it assigns a single underlying cause for each death or event. Although the analysis was driven primarily by mortality data, morbidity was thought to be roughly parallel in most instances. Exceptions to this were arthritis, dental disease, depression, and violence; the relative importance of these conditions was substantial when morbidity measures were applied.

Generic risk factors were assigned priority based on the extent to which the "gap" could be closed if such factors were eliminated. Certain quality-of-life issues (eg, depression) were considered as well as mortality and hospitalization. This procedure iden-

From the Centers for Disease Control.

Originally published in the *Journal of the American Medical Association,* 1985;254:1355–8. Reprinted by permission.

Address requests for reprints of the original article to Dr. Amler, The Carter Center of Emory University, Atlanta, GA 30322.

Table 1. Studied health problems and associated generic risk factors

Principal investigator	Health problem	Generic risk factors
John V. Bennett, MD	Infectious diseases	Lack of preventive services (tobacco, alcohol)[a]
Alfred W. Brann, Jr, MD	Infant mortality	Unintended pregnancy, tobacco, alcohol, improper nutrition, lack of preventive services, socioeconomic level
Lawrence S. Farer, MD, MPH	Respiratory diseases	Tobacco, lack of preventive services (alcohol)[a]
Michael E. Fritz, DDS, PhD	Dental diseases	Lack of preventive services
Paul J. Goldstein, PhD	Drug abuse	Lack of preventive/social services, socioeconomic level
Richard S. Johannes, MD	Digestive diseases	Lack of preventive services, alcohol, tobacco
Frederick C. McDuffie, MD	Arthritis	Lack of preventive services
Mark L. Rosenberg, MD, MPP	Homicide/suicide	Handguns, alcohol, lack of preventive/social services, socioeconomic level
Richard Rothenberg, MD, MPH	Cancer	Tobacco, alcohol, improper nutrition, lack of preventive services
Gordon S. Smith, MB Chb, MPH	Unintentional injuries	Injury risks, alcohol, tobacco, socioeconomic level
Alan Stoudemire, MD	Alcoholism	Alcohol, lack of preventive services
	Depression	Lack of preventive services
Steven M. Teutsch, MD, MPH	Diabetes	Lack of preventive services, improper nutrition, tobacco
Dennis D. Tolsma, MPH	Cardiovascular diseases	Tobacco, high blood pressure, improper nutrition, lack of exercise

[a] Problems listed in parentheses were too difficult to quantify.

tified four "highest priority" generic risk factors (tobacco, alcohol, injury risks, and unintended pregnancy) and two generic problems (mental health problems and delivery of prevention services).

At the November consultation, a working group was assigned to each of the six generic risk factors and problems. Each group considered strategies and methods required to implement effective interventions and recommended a set of objectives for the nation. In addition, future program activities were highlighted for The Carter Center.

RESULTS

The 14 health problems studied by The Carter Center consultants (Table 1) accounted for approximately 70% of hospitalization days, 85% of direct personal health care expenditures, 80% of deaths, and 90% of potential years of life lost before age 65 years in the United States in 1980. Roughly two thirds of reported mortality was due to potentially preventable causes—1.2 million deaths (65%) and 8.4 million years lost before age 65 years (63%). These totals are so large that short-term variations in disease occurrence or changes in the analytic model used have little impact on the distributions described below.

Tobacco was identified as the leading generic risk factor associated with mortality, according to either measure (Figure 1). Other principal risk factors associated with unnecessary deaths were high blood pressure, improper nutrition, and lack of screening. Other principal risk factors associated with unnecessary years lost before age 65 years were alcohol, injury risks, and lack of prevention services. Some of the salient findings and recommendations of the consultants are highlighted below.

Tobacco

Tobacco is the leading single cause of premature death in the U.S. population, causing over 1,000 unnecessary deaths every day.[4,5] Most of these deaths occur as cardiovascular events (heart attacks, strokes, and complications of diabetes); cancer; and chronic lung disease. Tobacco causes more deaths by circulatory diseases than by cancer, though the toll from cancer is substantial. Tobacco is the leading carcinogen of man and accounts for the alarming rise of lung cancer in women.[6] Moreover, tobacco causes almost all chronic lung disease. Two additional tobacco-induced health problems, infant mortality and deaths due to house fires, account for a substantial number of premature deaths. Tobacco also causes considerable morbidity from peptic ulcer disease and vascular disease, which often necessitate surgery or amputation of a limb.

Major recommendations of the working group. (1) Make nonsmoking the social norm and reduce all opportunities for consumption of tobacco. (2) Compensate victims of diseases caused by tobacco. (3) Explore the moral dilemma posed by the continued production of tobacco for profit. (4) Neutralize misleading advertising and increase public knowledge about the risks.

Injuries

Injuries are the leading cause of death for at least half of the American life span (ages 1 to 44 years).[4,7,8] One third of these deaths are related to use of motor vehicles, making the motor vehicle the most deadly nonnuclear machine in this century.[8] Because injury mortality occurs disproportionately

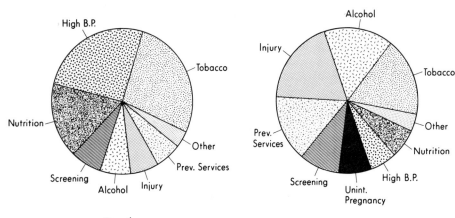

Figure 1. Graphic representation of causes of unnecessary mortality.

Deaths

Years of Life Lost Before Age 65

among the young, it is also a leading cause of premature death. Many of the nonfatal injuries result in serious and premanent disability. Unintentional injuries are a major concern for every facet of society.

Major recommendations for the working group. (1) Promote safer design and use of vehicles and homes (eg, airbags, seat belt laws, home and product safety). (2) Reduce exposure of teenagers to high-risk driving situations. (3) Improve accuracy of media portrayal of injury risks. (4) Increase knowledge of risks and prevention among teenagers and the general public.

Alcohol

Alcohol is the second leading cause of premature death, accounting for about 1.5 million potential years of life lost before age 65 years.[4,9] Roughly one third of this loss is due to motor vehicle fatalities and one third to other unintentional injuries (eg, falls, fires, drownings).[7-10] The remaining third includes alcohol-related violence, cirrhosis, and cancer of the mouth, larynx, and esophagus. In addition, serious, permanent disability resulting from alcohol misuse may substantially reduce the quality of life for the individual, the family, and society.

Major recommendations of the working group. (1) Modify government policy toward taxation, advertising, and merchandising. (2) Disseminate action strategies for local comunities. (3) Increase knowledge of risks and prevention among teenagers and the general public.

Preventive Care

Preventive care is of major importance in reducing the burden of unnecessary illness and premature death due to such diverse health problems as infectious diseases, dental disease, and cancer. It also contributes to the control of disease and health

problems (eg, diabetes, arthritis, infant mortality). Prevention may be primary in that the disease itself is entirely prevented (eg, immunization, fluoridation), or secondary in that the disease, though no prevented, is detected early enough to prevent or modify serious health consequences (eg, diabetes, sexually transmitted diseases, cancer of the cervix). In addition, disease surveillance is an essential component of prevention in that it elucidates changing trends in disease occurrence so that appropriate responses may be implemented (eg, acquired immunodeficiency syndrome, hospital-acquired infections).

Major recommendations of the working group. (1) Develop standard protocols for personal and environmental health services and health promotion. (2) Achieve adequate, appropriate public and private funding for effective prevention services. (3) Explore new opportunities for prevention. (4) Increase knowledge of healthful practices among health professionals and the general public.

Unintended Pregnancy

Unintended pregnancy, including all unwanted and mistimed pregnancies, accounts for 55% of all pregnancies in the United States.[11] The consequences are particularly serious for teenagers. Parenthood before age 18 years reduces high school completion rates by 50% for women and by 25% for men, and reduces income by 80% for families headed by teenaged mothers.[12] In 1975, families of teenaged mothers received roughly half of the $9.4 billion in payments for Aid to Families with Dependent Children.[12]

Major recommendations of the working group. (1) Enunciate a reproductive health policy to reduce the incidence of unintended pregnancy. (2) Increase access to preventive services. (3) Improve accuracy of media portrayal of sex and its consequences. (4) Increase knowledge of the hazards of unintended

Table 2. The Carter Center health policy program goals

1. Establish a program using health fellows to evaluate, structure, and support domestic and foreign health policies.

2. Promote nonsmoking and other healthful behaviors as the social norm, in concert with media, academic centers, government, and health institutions.

3. Conduct seminars in conflict resolution to discover areas of agreement on health-related topics between groups that are customarily opposed to one another. Include tobacco and firearms as topics.

4. Disseminate the data and findings to four essential groups:
   Clinicians: Incorporate preventive medicine in daily practice.
   Educators: Implement established effective health education curricula in primary and secondary schools.
   Clergy: Explore the ethical relationships of society, community, industry, and health of the individual.
   Public: Recognize significant health-related decisions and behaviors, and make informed choices.

pable to facilitating changes in health policy and practice. This consultation defined the current burden of health problems that are unnecessary in light of knowledge that is already at hand. This "gap" is substantial in medical, economic, and human terms. It involves more than half of all deaths and major illnesses in this country and consumes resources that otherwise could be devoted to problems for which reliable preventive strategies are not yet known.

To help close the gap, each of the six working groups developed a strategy of detailed national interventions well beyond the scope of this brief report. These strategies, if implemented, would involve joint efforts by the private sector as well as government agencies; they would draw on the skills and resources of academic institutions and volunteer and professional organizations. The working groups highlighted four future program activities uniquely suited to The Carter Center (Table 2). Most of these activities are already under way.

pregnancy and available interventions among teenagers and the general public.

Mental Health Problems

Mental health problems, especially depression, violence, and substance abuse, are important causes of premature death. Nevertheless, the impact of these problems is difficult to gauge from mortality data alone. The combined morbidity and cost are at least equally burdensome. Moreover, the predilection of these diseases for the young and for minority groups has social implications that extend beyond the limitations of these data.

Major recommendations of the working group. *Depression:* (1) Improve recognition and treatment by primary care physicians. (2) Increase public knowledge. *Violence:* (1) Limit availability and use of potentially lethal agents. (2) Criminalize family violence and empower victims. (3) Increase the number of battered women's shelters. *Substance abuse:* (1) Improve and expand treatment centers and alternative activities for young people. (2) Identify users and intervene early. (3) Decriminalize possession of syringes and needles (to reduce infectious sequelae).

SUMMARY

The Carter Center offers a unique opportunity to bring together those individuals and groups ca-

REFERENCES

1. Tokarz W. Carter message to MDs: stress risk reduction to prevent major disease. Am Med News, Dec 28, 1984, pp 1,3,17–20.

2. Carter J. Closing the gap: The burden of unnecessary illness. JAMA 1985;254:1359–1360.

3. Brandt EN Jr. Why the Carter Center? JAMA 1985;254:1360.

4. Healthy people: the surgeon general's report on health promotion and disease prevention. Public Health Service, 1979.

5. Smoking and health: A report of the surgeon general. Public Health Service, 1979.

6. The health consequences of smoking—cancer: a report of the surgeon general. Public Health Service, 1982.

7. Baker SP, O'Neill B, Karpf RS. The injury fact book. Lexington, Massachusetts: Lexington Books, 1984.

8. National Research Council-Institute of Medicine Committee on Trauma Research: Injury in America: a continuing public health problem. Washington, DC: National Academy Press, 1985.

9. Surveillance and assessment of alcohol-related mortality, United States, 1980. *MMWR* 1985;34:161–3.

10. Alcohol and fatal injuries, Fulton County, Georgia, 1982. MMWR 1983;32:573–6.

11. Ory HW, Forrest VD. Making choices, evaluating the health risks and benefits of birth control methods. New York: Alan Guttmacher Institute, 1983.

12. Moore KA, Burt MR. Private crisis, public cost, policy perspectives on teenage childbearing. Washington, DC: Urban Institute Press, 1982

SUBJECT INDEX